Palgrave Studies in Literature, Science and Medicine

Palgrave Studies in Literature, Science and Medicine is an exciting new series that focuses on one of the most vibrant and interdisciplinary areas in literary studies: the intersection of literature, science and medicine. Comprised of academic monographs, essay collections, and Palgrave Pivot books, the series will emphasize a historical approach to its subjects, in conjunction with a range of other theoretical approaches. The series will cover all aspects of this rich and varied field and is open to new and emerging topics as well as established ones.

More information about this series at
http://www.palgrave.com/gp/series/14613

Emily Russell

Transplant Fictions

A Cultural Study of Organ Exchange

palgrave
macmillan

Emily Russell
Rollins College
Winter Park, FL, USA

Palgrave Studies in Literature, Science and Medicine
ISBN 978-3-030-12134-1 ISBN 978-3-030-12135-8 (eBook)
https://doi.org/10.1007/978-3-030-12135-8

Library of Congress Control Number: 2019932923

Cover credit: Victor Habbick Visions/Science Photo Library, Getty Images

This Palgrave Macmillan imprint is published by the registered company Springer Nature Switzerland AG
The registered company address is: Gewerbestrasse 11, 6330 Cham, Switzerland

Acknowledgements

This book could not have been completed without the support of a generous network of colleagues, students, and family. Jana Mathews is a tireless and enthusiastic collaborator. Her partnership enriches all aspects of my professional life and I owe her a tremendous debt of gratitude. As my thinking and research have evolved throughout this project, my students have inspired and challenged me. I am appreciative for the scores of Rollins undergraduate students who have been willing to take a chance on courses titled "Gruesome Anatomy" or "Body Snatchers: Literature and Medicine" and to the Department of English for their openness and encouragement. Finally, I want to thank my family, Phil, Will, and Ben Fibiger, and my parents, Bill and Kathy Russell.

Contents

CHAPTER 1

Introduction

The story of medical progress in the twentieth century nearly always places organ transplantation as the height of achievement. In the first round of breakthroughs, surgeons had to develop techniques to make impossibly tiny sutures in challenging, slippery conditions under a terrible time constraint. Once these first surgical techniques were mastered, a second round of challenges emerged: How to keep transplant recipients alive when their bodies constantly fought off the invading new organ. Even as the news media trumpeted the successful surgeries of the mid-century—a kidney transplant between the Herrick twins in 1954 or the "Miracle at Cape Town" heart transplant in 1967—doctors and patients struggled against the persistent problem of immune rejection. In the 1980s, a "miracle drug," cyclosporine, allowed doctors to manage the problems of rejection and prompted a third round of breakthroughs. Today, organ exchange has become a celebrated, even commonplace surgery, with tens of thousands of operations taking place in the USA each year.

In this story of setbacks and breakthroughs, however, it is easy to lose some of the truly radical nature of organ exchange. We celebrate the surgery as medical miracle, but there are other, darker stories that could be told of transplantation. After all, the bare realities of the surgery are the plot points of familiar horror narratives. Take a moment to truly consider this fact: We take organs from dead bodies and place them in the living. This practice flies in the face of many of our most enduring

E. Russell, *Transplant Fictions*,
Palgrave Studies in Literature, Science and Medicine,
https://doi.org/10.1007/978-3-030-12135-8_1

concepts, most particularly the strict separation between the dead and the living and between the self and others. Organ transplantation violates the most fundamental categories by which we understand health, identity, illness, and death. But how did we overcome these taboos? How did transplantation transform from something to be feared to something we celebrate? Although medical historians have told the story of transplantation as outlined above—the story of technical challenges and triumphs—*Transplant Fictions* tells the cultural story of how transplantation became not just medically, but conceptually possible.

The cultural study of organ exchange begins with a medical miracle in the most basic sense. Cosmas and Damian were twin brothers, practicing doctors, and outlaw Christians living in Syria in the second half of the third century. After the twins refused to make sacrifices to the gods, the Roman authority in Syria ordered their execution. They were tortured, burned, crucified, stoned, and shot with arrows before a beheading finally accomplished their martyrdom. Like donated cadaver organs, however, the lives of these saints do not end with their death. Centuries later, they are credited with the "miracle of the black leg," typically cited as the first documented case of imagined surgical transplantation.

Versions of this story proliferate between 1200 and 1400, but the most popular is recounted in the medieval bestseller, *The Golden Legend*. According to the tale, a Christian living in Rome sought relief from the martyred saints because his leg was being consumed by a cancer, or what we would likely call gangrene. One night, as he slept in a local church dedicated to Cosmas and Damian, they appeared to him in a dream. Carrying with them the salves and instruments of their surgical trade, one said to the other, "Where can we get flesh to fill in where we cut away the rotten leg?"[1] The other replied, "Just today an Ethiopian was buried in the cemetery of Saint Peter in Chains. Go and take his leg, and we'll put it in place of the bad one." He traveled to the nearby cemetery and returned with the "Moor's" leg. They cut off the leg of the sick man and attached the cadaver leg in its place. Then, they returned to the cemetery and attached the gangrenous leg to the body of the dead Ethiopian. Transplant accomplished, "the man woke up, felt no pain, put his hand to his leg, and detected no lesion. He held a candle to the leg and could see nothing wrong with it, and began to wonder whether he was himself or somebody else."[2] He leapt overjoyed from his bed and ran out to tell the tale of his miraculous dream and cure. Finally, the community rushed to the Ethiopian's tomb where they found his leg indeed cut off and the sick man's laid in its place. A miracle of transplantation had occurred.

Even though written centuries ago, this first story of organ exchange reveals the many conceptual crossings required to even imagine transplantation. The doctor-saints are able to overcome differences of living and dead, diseased and healthy, Christian and Moor, European and Ethiopian—categories that constitute many of our most enduring ideas of life and social organization. Despite an initial moment of deep insecurity, of wondering whether he is himself or somebody else, the cured patient and his community embrace the operation and celebrate the doctors for their miraculous achievement. By breaking down the steps of this evolution, my cultural study of transplantation chronicles the conceptual sleights of hand through which organ exchange becomes the crowning achievement of twentieth-century medicine. Quiet ruptures in our understanding of medical authority, funerals, and death have paved the way for a widespread embrace of a procedure as radical as organ transplantation. But it did not have to be this way.

Transplant Fictions brings together a diverse set of cultural representations to understand how organ exchange became possible. By "possible" I do not mean the history of vein suturing, tissue typing, and immune suppression that has made this once-radical surgery now relatively routine. I mean: What concepts have emerged that allow us to overcome the profound ideological violations represented by transplantation? What changing notions of identity, death, medicine, and the social body have paved the way from imagination to experimentation to clinical practice?

These questions are embedded in the earliest seeds of our imagining. Even a millennium ago, we understood transplantation as a miracle with the power to remake fundamental categories. As the founding text in the genre, the miracle of the Black Leg deserves a closer reading. Perhaps the most resonant moment in the legend comes at the patient's awakening to a new understanding of his embodied self. The seventeenth century *Acta Sanctorum* offers a slight elaboration of this scene: "Waking up, when he felt himself without pain, he placed his hand on his leg, and found no lesion. Putting a candle then nearby, when he saw nothing wrong in the leg, he thought that he was himself not who he was, but that he was rather someone else."[3] There are two phases of "discovery" here. First, the sufferer becomes aware of multiple absences: the lack of pain and the lack of lesions. Then, under the light of a candle, he visually confirms the health of the leg, but in so doing experiences a radical revision of self: "he thought that he was himself not who he was, but that he was rather someone else." This troubling of individual identity is not simply the product of medieval superstition. Interviews with contemporary transplant recipients both before and after surgery reveal anxieties about sense of self. Commonly reported post-surgical changes include changes to personality and taste, often attributed to taking on aspects of the donor. Vegetarians become meat lovers, and punk rockers develop a love for classical music. Even in the least sentimental accounts, the relatively immediate transformation from end-stage organ failure to relative health marks a radical change. In these reports, patients describe a profound sense of alienation from their pre-surgical self, often in terms that emphasize the play of opposites.[4]

In addition to asking what it means for the ill patient to incorporate the flesh of another body, the legend of the Black Leg attends to the body of the donor as well. In most retellings, the miracle is a true exchange, where Cosmas and Damian return the gangrenous flesh to the entombed corpse. As Leonard Barkan, a scholar of Early Modern culture, reminds us, the symmetry of this exchange reflects two fundamental concerns of the period: A belief in the completeness of the physical body and the doctrine of the original body needed at the second coming of Christ. In the latter formulation, each individual's perfected body will rise to heaven at the resurrection. While this attention to the afterlife of the exchanged limbs may seem rigid or oddly specific, anxieties about the religious future of the body are not merely the province of the medieval era. In fact, the online frequently asked questions (FAQ) sections for many organ procurement organizations take such religious anxieties seriously, understanding the importance of such concerns for many prospective donors and their families. Today, every major world religion endorses transplantation, but it is important to place this endorsement in the context of centuries of understanding the corpse as sacred and inviolable. The early chapters of this book more closely explore the sea change necessary to move from reverence and clerical authority over the corpse to acceptance of near total medical authority over death and the body.

In the Cosmas and Damian story, transplanting the gangrenous leg onto the Ethiopian corpse also signifies a commitment to the principle of somatic wholeness. This notion is less doctrinally specific and, perhaps for that reason, more widespread and enduring. In modern Western conceptions, the body is understood as a sovereign self: closed, contained, unified, and under rational control. In restoring diseased flesh to a cadaver, Cosmas and Damian reflect an understanding of physical integrity rooted in wholeness. The same online FAQ sections are careful to assure families that open casket funerals are possible after donation. While failing organs are obviously not swapped back to donor cadavers, procurement and funeral personnel are careful to mask the intrusions caused by organ retrieval surgery. It is the symmetrical exchange of diseased and healthy flesh in this first imagined transplantation that reveals our deep-seated attachment to bodily integrity. After all, why transplant the diseased flesh to the corpse unless guided by a strong ideological preference for wholeness? The very conceptual categories of somatic wholeness and inviolability that are challenged by the achievement of transplantation are first emphasized in this earliest imagining. In particular, removing part of one body and locating it inside another raises important questions about the nature of identity. Where does the self reside and what level of incursion or addition will change that sense of self? What does it mean to wake up (e.g., from surgical anesthesia) and be restored to health? Is the patient "himself or somebody else"?

After its late medieval inception, the legend of the Black Leg finds popular expression once more in Renaissance painting. The visual appeal of the story is evident as visual artists take advantage of the striking contrast between the white skin of the Christian sufferer and the black skin of the Ethiopian donor. Although many artists play with the scale and shape of the mismatched legs, thus emphasizing the fundamental difference between the donor and recipient, others take a different approach. As Leonard Barkan notes in his analysis of artwork depicting the miracle, these artists use strategies of mirroring and symmetry, placing the donor and recipient "in that curious territory where opposites are identical" (240). Barkan is also careful to caution us away from reading the racial origin of the Ethiopian gladiator through an overdetermining lens of race in the West. But even without the intervening history of chattel slavery and Civil Rights struggles, we can understand the terms "Ethiopian" and "Moor" as signs of social difference. In this convergence of self and unfamiliar other, it is important to see that difference is both emphasized and overcome in organ exchange.

The emergence in the early 1980s of cyclosporine accomplishes a modern path to overcoming difference in the world of transplantation. Hailed as a "miracle drug" (one that further enables the "miracle" surgery), cyclosporine allows doctors to conquer the immune rejection that sunk the outcomes of so many early transplantations. For example, in his testimony during the congressional proceedings for the National Organ Transplant Act, Al Gore told his colleagues, "then with the discovery of the new miracle drug, cyclosporin, the problems of rejection were almost completely solved."[5] Such optimism is bound up in the rhetoric of "miracles" and encapsulates the extent to which contemporary society has embraced medical technology as both the height of technological achievement and beyond lay understanding. Decades after the first successful transplantation between identical twins in 1954, doctors in the 1980s could now achieve good outcomes for organ exchange between strangers removed by our most fundamental categories of difference. Tissue typing and the process of matching look for some similarities to achieve better outcomes, but the realities of transplant technology allow for surgeons to operate in the "curious territory" Barkan describes, where "opposites" can be literally incorporated.

A Modern Miracle

Nearly one thousand years after Christians imagined the miracle of transplantation, Dr. Christiaan Barnard achieved "The Miracle at Cape Town" with the first successful heart transplant surgery. On December 3, 1967, Barnard and his team conducted a nine-hour operation at Groote Schuur hospital in Cape Town, South Africa. Their patient, Louis Washansky was a 54-year-old grocer; his donor was Denise Darvall, a 25-year old who was struck by a car while out on errands with her parents. In describing his landmark surgery for the *South African Medical Journal*, Barnard turns to poetic expression in his introduction:

> The dream of the ancients from time immemorial has been the junction of portions of different individuals, not only to counteract disease but also to combine the potentials of different species. This desire inspired the birth of many mythical creatures which were purported to have capabilities normally beyond the power of a single species. The modern world has inherited these dreams in the form of the sphinx, the mermaid and the chimerical forms of many heraldic beasts. Modern scientists have a more realistic approach and explored the possibility of treating certain diseases affecting specific organs by replacement of these organs with grafts.[6]

Even when addressing a specialist audience, Barnard recognizes that dreams, desires, and myths connect to the "more realistic approach" used by surgeons. The path to surgical execution has been laid by this "dream of the ancients" and, for a lay audience, is understood as no less miraculous.

Even the phrase "medical miracle" contains within it an oxymoron. In our example from the middle ages, Cosmas and Damian do not simply achieve a miraculous cure through prayer and faith. They are figured specifically *as* medical practitioners, bringing their salves and instruments and anointing the diseased leg before placing it in the tomb. Once twentieth-century surgeons achieved the imagined feat, sources ranging from international news coverage to political officials consistently describe the operation as a "miracle." In a typical example of popular celebration and optimism, Henry Waxman tells his colleagues in the US Congress, "Today, the transplantation of human organs represents nothing short of a scientific miracle. It promises to revolutionize medical practice and human existence."[7] Pioneering surgeons like Christiaan Barnard, Thomas Starzl, Samuel Kountz, and Norman Shumway were heralded as messianic figures, a comparison Barnard may have encouraged through remarks like, "Adam was the donor, God the surgeon, and he made Eve out of Adam's rib."[8] The very quotidian use of "medical miracle," however, belies the term's strangeness, performing a kind of mystical hand wave over the truly radical nature of the practice it describes.[9] Transplanting an organ from a dead body to a living one; giving up one's kidney to help a dying loved one or even a stranger; receiving tissue from a pig, baboon, or grown from stem cells—each of these practices has long been imagined with both wonder and horror. The often-ignored internal contradiction in the phrase "medical miracle" signals that some of this sublime character has been retained in our contemporary approach to organ exchange. But the trouble with the sublime lies in its ineffability, in the way in which "medical miracle" becomes a catchall term that obscures many of our complicated ideas about the realities of transplantation.

When we look more closely, however, we can unravel the complicated strands through which we understand organ transplantation—both in concept and in practice. As a paramount instance: Nearly every piece written on transplantation follows the insistent drumbeat of scarcity. "Every ten minutes someone is added to the national transplant list," "Twenty-two patients die each day waiting for a transplant," "Just 54% of Americans are organ donors."[10] Recitation of figures like these becomes the rhetorical foundation upon which we build our understanding of organ exchange. As a consequence, the perceived gap between supply and demand has driven profound changes, including everything from ethical debates to the way we define death itself. In the latter case, a committee of academics at Harvard Medical School was driven to invent the now-familiar concept of "brain death" in 1968. Part of the express motivation of the committee was to produce a new supply of cadaver organ donors. And so they set about the task of identifying a new set of criteria for diagnosing death among a specific class of patients. The trope of scarcity similarly shapes both culture and policy. Horrifying fictional tales of exploitive medical syndicates and mad doctors emerge from worries about insufficient supply. True-life and no less frightening stories of the illegal global organ trade are set in the conditions of two desperate populations: Organ sellers seeking a path out of poverty and recipients facing fatal illness and no readily available organs. In a final example, new categories of familial connection emerge as relatives seek to beat the low odds of cadaver donation through a live, directed donation.

These diverse fictions and realities are all rooted in the premise of scarcity, the concept from which most discussions of transplantation proceed. Medical anthropologist Lesley Sharp has reflected that nearly all professional gatherings of transplant professionals include airing of deep anxieties over scarcity. In these discussions, organs are often discussed as "scarce natural resources," placing human organs into seemingly incommensurate spheres like oil reserves, water disputes, and land use policies.[11] It is important to acknowledge, however, that while "scarcity" has dogged stories of transplantation since its earliest days, the meaning of that term has shifted. Although the number of donors has increased over time, changing policies around eligibility and improved overall outcomes have increased demand at a greater rate. Organ supply, then, is a constantly moving target and instead of closing, the gap is growing. Evocations of "scarcity," though, often fail to address this history and take the need to close the gap between supply and demand as a first principle.

In concert with discussions of the gap between organ supply and demand, we also find an important and oft-cited gap between expressions of enthusiasm for transplantation in concept, but lagging numbers of real donors when the question becomes more material. While surveys consistently document near-universal positive attitudes about transplantation (typically around 95%), donor rates among families of eligible patients or as expressed on voluntary declarations like driver's licenses are much lower. Our diverse cultural representations of transplantation can help explain why rates of donation so consistently lag behind expressed support. Lesley Fiedler, unsurprisingly for a literary scholar, also comes to this problem by way of culture. In an essay called "Why Organ Transplant Programs Do Not Succeed," published in 1996, Fiedler emphasizes the role of myth as the animating force behind our lingering resistance to donation in practice. Fiedler writes:

> This [gap] is not mere hypocrisy. Rather it results from a profound, though quite unsuspected, contradiction between the conscious acceptance and the unconscious repulsion many of us—perhaps, to some degree, all of us—feel when confronted with a presumably benign surgical procedure that challenges our most deep-seated, primal notions about life and death, the self and the other, body and spirit: a procedure, moreover, conducted without any of the consoling rituals traditionally accorded the cadavers of our loved ones.[12]

Fiedler goes on to consider "rejection" as an organizing metaphor for conceptual resistance to transplantation. Given the extent to which physiological organ rejection has been the dominant crisis in transplantation for decades, it is appropriate that several scholars have been inspired to use the term in this way. Joining Fiedler, both Susan Squier and Donald Joralemon explore different forms of cultural rejection of transplantation and the possibility of developing the "ideological equivalent to cyclosporine" as a way of suppressing the negative reaction.[13]

Examining cultural representations of organ exchange can explain this form of "rejection" by attaching clearer images and myths to that unconscious resistance. Cultural study of the kind conducted here can tell us why people do not donate; it can reveal the enduring scripts that give shape to the public's lingering resistance. Perhaps more significantly, though, *Transplant Fictions* engages in cultural study to answer an even more surprising question: What ideological fictions drive people to donate at all? If we agree that transplantation challenges many of our "most deep-seated, primal notions," shouldn't the more surprising statistic be the 95% rate of acceptance? What fictions had to be written that would support such a dramatic departure from these foundational concepts?

When compared to other boundary shaking medical questions—like abortion or euthanasia—organ exchange is remarkable not only as a technical feat, but in how very uncontroversial it has been.[14] *Transplant Fictions* studies the role of culture in producing the ideological pathways by which we arrived at this point of near-universal acceptance of a practice that we should find strange, if not horrifying. This attention to fiction marks a departure from much of the scholarly work on organ exchange. More typically, transplantation is examined through the lenses of medical anthropology, sociology, history, and ethics.[15] While ethnographic field work and medical historians bring to light the lived experience and evolution of contemporary transplant practice, I focus on the ways that stories told about transplantation express concepts that we may not openly examine, but which circulate in culture and shape our experiences nonetheless.

A cultural studies lens can open up scholarship on organ exchange in a few key ways. First, while historians, anthropologists, and ethicists may reference fiction in their work, literary scholarship makes fictional texts the central object of study. The archive for organ exchange then expands, now including everything from influential classics like Mary Shelley's *Frankenstein* to popular thrillers like Robin Cook's *Coma* or Jodi Picoult's sentimental tearjerker *My Sister's Keeper*. I pay close attention to both the silly and the serious out of a deep-rooted conviction that if we want to know how we came to such widespread acceptance of a radically experimental procedure, we need to examine the cultural expression that reflects our most commonly held notions about death, medical intervention, and transplantation itself. The material realities of health and the drive for cure or survival are powerful forces pushing advancements in experimental medicine. But these materials realities of the body are inextricable with our culturally bound understanding. Cultural study can demonstrate how foundational concepts like life and death change over time.

The second contribution of a cultural study lies in its method. In addition to texts traditionally bound by the heading of literature, a method of literary critique offers a new point of entry into diverse texts like newspaper articles, political speeches, judicial rulings, or first-person accounts by patients and clinicians. By highlighting the metaphors and language used by these speakers, we can reveal the underlying concepts that structure their thinking and, by extension, our own. By engaging with many of the profound ethical questions of organ exchange, cultural study does not narrowly advocate for the merits of one side in a debate, instead it takes a careful look at language to find the ideological premises that determine the very terms of the debate itself.

A method of close reading drawn from cultural study is particularly valuable in this case because the founding ideologies of organ exchange are so often expressed through metaphor. In addition to the rhetorical premise of scarcity, two metaphors—the "gift of life" and the concept of "spare parts"—recur time and time again. We know that the power of metaphors lies in their ability to carry forward much more complex concepts than those few words would seem to express. The phrase "gift of life," repeated in news headlines, T-shirts, posters, and in conversation is one such example. But how did this phrase come to be so common? What does it mean to our notions of death that we see an organ from a dead body as a gift of life to another dying individual? Questions like these animate *Transplant Fictions*, which looks to metaphor and representation to understand the conditions of conceptual possibility, social acceptance, and resistance of organ exchange.

Politics of the Heart

Cultural study, with its emphasis on secondary layers of meaning, also serves as an important antidote to a narrowly technical account of transplant history and practice. Early heart transplantation offers an evocative case study for this introduction because the surgeries so clearly spark discussion of the social, political, and cultural dimensions at play. Although the first kidney transplant surgeries were also met with fanfare, many have acknowledged that the heart holds a special role in our public consciousness. The stakes of heart transplant are higher in a material sense because there is no fallback to dialysis in the case of failure and because of the radical nature of the surgery itself, which includes stopping a beating (if failing) heart. But very early heart transplantation also generated more passionate interest because "the heart, an enduring object of mysticism, spirituality, and emotionalism, was a more prominent, newsworthy, and dramatic organ."[16] This assertion by Nicholas Tilney, M.D., former director of the Center for Transplantation Research at the Brigham and Women's Hospital, illustrates the ways that symbolism acts unevenly on the field of medicine. Technical advances may open new pathways of surgical possibility, but these pursuits are caught in a web of meaning that can both enable and restrict their adoption as clinical practice.

Surgeons depend not only upon technical advances like the discovery of cyclosporine or new techniques like heterotopic transplantation (in which the original organ is left in place alongside the transplanted heart). They also depend on ideological changes, like the change that imagined a diagnosis of brain death and allowed for heart bypass without charging surgeons with murder. And they need families to understand the donation of a loved one's organ as a gift of life and not the work of body snatchers coming to steal the sacred remains. These founding concepts that create the conditions of possibility for transplantation serve as the organizing structure for this book. Starting with the assertion that transplantation is a significant violator of fundamental boundaries, *Transplant Fictions* examines cultural production to reveal how we make sense of these violations and, in most cases, reduce them to the status of the unremarkable and commonplace.

Life and death. Self and other. Progress and hubris. Man and machine. Health and illness. Agency and commodity. Organ exchange holds each of these categories in tension. Christiaan Barnard's second successful heart transplant reveals the intricate strands of these concepts as a way of making meaning out of a boundary-crossing surgery. In the first exchange from Denise Darval to Louis Washansky, the donated heart crossed at least two important lines of social difference: gender and age. Little news coverage, however, was dedicated to what it would mean for a man to live with a woman's heart beating in his chest (although there was plenty of room for those questions in later fictions of organ exchange). In the second Barnard surgery, by contrast, the fraught political context of apartheid South Africa meant that much of the coverage emphasized the racial dynamics of the case. On January 2, 1968, just weeks after the first surgery, a white dentist named Philip Blaiberg received the heart of Clive Haupt, a 24-year-old man considered "Coloured" (or mixed race) under apartheid racial categorization.[17]

Most of the international comment centered on the tragic irony of this particular crossing of racial boundaries. An article in *The Guardian* titled "Brothers Under the Skin" asks, "If a White man can use a Coloured man's heart after death, can he sit on the same park bench with him while they are still living? Probably not."[18] In the USA, *Ebony* magazine editorialized, "If Dr. Blaiberg completely recovers and again walks the streets of Cape Town, a most ironic situation will ensue.... Haupt's heart will go literally to hundreds of places where Haupt, himself, could not go because his skin was a little darker than that of Blaiberg."[19] In response to this strain of coverage, the anti-apartheid leaning *Cape Times* wrote, "Some of the foreign comment on the second heart transplant suggests a greater general obsession with apartheid than even the South African Government habitually shows; and that is saying a lot."[20] Taken together, these comments illustrate the ways that transplant surgery cannot exist outside of the social and political contexts of the day. Two additional facts in the background of these cases demonstrate how unevenly social categories of difference play out in public response. First, Christiaan Barnard has revealed that days before the first landmark surgery he had another available donor for Washansky, but held back because the potential donor was nonwhite. For this historic "first," Barnard worried the political dimensions would swamp the story of medical accomplishment. Second, few outlets that focused on the racial contours in the later case discussed the fact that Denise Darvall had in fact donated two organs: the heart received by Louis Washansky and a kidney that was successfully transplanted into a 10-year-old "Coloured" boy. The story of a "Coloured heart" transplanted into a white man successfully supported two divergent ideological arguments: universal humanity, on the one hand, and a mechanistic view of the body on the other. Because Darvall's kidney donation lacked the racial ironies so evident in the Blaiberg case and lacked the symbolic weight attached to the heart, it fell from notice.

For some commenters, the Blaiberg/Haupt operation served as a metaphor for their hopeful vision of racial integration. One Australian newspaper wrote, "Out of a family's tragedy has come new hope for mankind in circumstances of high drama and great expectancy. As surgeons pioneer new frontiers they are reminding us that God's creatures are brothers and sisters under the skin and that, in the long run, racial barriers and unconquered disease may not be impregnable."[21] This concept of universal humanity, imagined as an essential sameness "under the skin" served as a powerful metaphor in the critique of racist policies. In this case, hope for social change is tied to medical advances and the dominating structure of a progress narrative. Dorothy Haupt, widowed after only three months of marriage, uses similar terms to describe the surgery: "I am glad that my husband's Coloured heart could save the life of a White man. I am also glad because it has changed the whole idea of 'apartheid. Now everyone can see that all of us—White, Black, or Brown—have the same heart."[22] The medical practice of tissue matching seemed to support this universal thesis; whereas differences among races were paramount in political contexts, "race differences were insignificant in tissue matching.... It was possible that a greater difference could exist between the tissues of two brothers of the same race than unrelated people from different races."[23] Organ exchange, then, could serve as a powerful new script, rewriting the racist fiction of essential difference rooted in the blood.

This idea of a universal sameness under the skin also underscores the principle of altruism that governs organ exchange around the world. From its earliest practice, organ exchange has been a gift economy, a concept expressed most concretely through metaphor: the "gift of life" that has become ubiquitous in donation campaigns. Medical anthropologist Nancy Scheper-Hughes asserts:

> Organ transplantation is the most intensely social of all medical practice. Its existence presupposes a unique trust between society and its physicians, and it is dependent upon the willingness of ordinary people to share their organs and tissues either with a mortally sick loved one or with an unknown "stranger," who was, nonetheless, a member of a larger ... social body ... of organ trading partners within a system of open-ended reciprocity.[24]

Cadaver organs donated by grieving families to anonymous strangers are by far the most common source of organs for transplant. A second source, directed gifts by loved ones, is also an expression of altruism, although through a more intimate relation. The National Organ Transplant Act of 1984 was established to support and protect both forms of altruism. As an immediate goal, it established a more efficient national system for the distribution of donated cadaver organs. The United Network for Organ Sharing (UNOS), which now directs cadaver donations across the country, grew from this provision. The "gift of life" metaphor encapsulates this complex system of donation, offering families and prospective donors an ideological anchor for their choice.

As transplant surgeon Thomas Starzl reminded the committee during the congressional proceedings, "There is only one set of donors for all the needed organs and the organs are a resource of the entire United States. This concept has to be built into the system."[25] Once donated, organs belong to the public and must be allocated according to an equitable and transparent system. But altruism as a foundational principle, one that was literally "built into the system," was not the only option.

The law also expressly outlawed the sale of human organs in the USA, a legal prohibition almost universally shared across the international community. Advertisements from a local doctor to serve as a broker for sold kidneys reminded early 1980s legislators that commodification was another competing principle. This model, though, was considered and roundly rejected by all of the expert witnesses before the committee. Organs would continue to be a precious gift, granted to the social body. Strangers divided by social and political categories of difference could be, for the purposes of transplantation, "brothers and sisters under the skin."

As the second dominant metaphor, texts covering organ exchange from across the spectrum of scholarship, fiction, media coverage, and policy debate deploy a "spare parts" analogy nearly as often as they evoke "the gift of life." Both metaphors play influential roles in directing the thinking of the public, as well as organ donors and recipients. In the spare parts analogy, a mechanistic view of the body assimilates many of the most radical elements of the surgery, reimagining it as a simple and straightforward procedure without troubling violations of boundary categories. Following Barnard's first successful heart surgery, the Vatican newspaper used this rhetoric to justify its support for the groundbreaking operation, writing, "the heart is a physiological organ and its function is purely mechanical." *Time* magazine echoed this sentiment with another typical assertion: "In fact, the heart is nothing more than a pump. There is no more soul or personality in a heart than in a slice of calf's liver."[26]

Some supporters of apartheid, however, used the spare parts analogy to accept the history-making operation without being forced to consider its challenge to their racist views. One right-wing South African politician places a local spin on the comments above in saying, "The heart is merely a blood-pumping machine and whether it comes from a White, Black or Coloured man—or a baboon or a giraffe for that matter—has no relevance to the issue of race relations in the political or ideological context. The question of colour is not at issue here."[27] Here, the baboon and giraffe are used as signals of absurdity, an attempt to wash out the relevance of the racial debate. But Barnard, like many other researchers then and now, *did* explore animals, specifically baboons, as sources for transplantation; and so the politician's exaggeration falls flat, recasting his essentialist and racist logic as the absurdity. Ugandan deputy foreign minister Vincent Rwamaro also expressed his fears of racial exploitation in terms of this analogy. Worried that blacks would serve as "spare parts for whites," the Haupt/Blaiberg transplant prompted Rwamaro to imagine a scenario in which a Black African would be "dragged from his house to a hospital and his heart pulled out to save a dying white man."[28] Although apartheid supporters would likely dismiss Rwamaro's concerns as hyperbolic, medical history is littered with examples of exploitation of vulnerable populations in the name of progress. Barnard's third transplantation, in which the heart of a Black African was placed into the body of a Colored man, was clouded by accusations from the donor's widow that she was not informed about the removal of her husband's organs.[29] In the USA, the 1972 case of *Tucker v Lower* became a bioethical landmark. In this case, a brain-dead black man in Richmond, VA was declared one of the "unclaimed dead" and his heart was transplanted to a white man without the permission of his family. The public circulation of these stories has real-life impacts. Both actual donation rates and public opinion polls consistently show lower rates of acceptance of transplantation among people of color in the USA. Fears that rules of consent will be violated or that doctors will not work as hard to save their lives are marked among people of color, and with good historical reason.[30] These exploitive practices are in part rooted in the dehumanizing logic of the spare parts analogy, a logic that will first target those already dehumanized by racist policies and ideologies.

In the spare parts analogy, repeated terms like "merely," "purely," and "just," reveal rhetorical attempts to diminish the ideological implications of the surgery. The widespread nature of the analogy suggests that such attempts to diminish are an important mechanism supporting broad acceptance of the practice. This is one of the ways in which such radical surgery becomes conceptually possible. Anxieties about dehumanization are not only common among those most subject to exploitation; the concept of humans as machines with interchangeable parts also raises red flags among policy makers and ethicists. The spare parts analogy emerges explicitly in discussion surrounding the National Organ Transplant Act (1984). As the founding piece of national legislation on transplantation, the proceedings for this bill in many ways reflected and entrenched how Americans talk about transplantation. In his remarks, Congressman Henry Waxman turned to metaphor to express his strong condemnation of organ sale: "Human organs should not be treated like fenders in an auto junkyard."[31] Using a similar metaphor, then-Congressman Al Gore told the *New York Times*, "We must not allow technology to dehumanize people so that we erode the distinction between things and people. People should not be regarded as things to be bought and sold like parts of an automobile. If this were allowed, it would seriously undermine the values of our society."[32]

Taken as a whole, this series of quotations shows how the same analogy can be used to animate very different ends. For the apartheid supporters, conceiving of the heart as "just a pump" makes space for the surgery without forcing a reconsideration of racist ideology. But the same metaphor of interchangeable parts in the context of US political dialogue serves as a vehicle to preserve notions of human dignity and social values. The striking flexibility of this metaphor demonstrates how cultural study can provide the tools to reveal layers of meaning in even the most commonplace phrases surrounding organ exchange. Such close reading serves as the major methodology employed throughout *Transplant Fictions*, as a series of highly diverse cultural texts become subject to examination that reveals the driving cultural assumptions that constitute our approach to transplantation.

* * *

This book falls into two major parts. The first explores changing approaches to death and dead bodies up to and including the invention of brain death in 1968. Beginning with the age of anatomy in Britain and the USA, the first three chapters explore how new ways of handling corpses—including dissection, embalming, death photography, artificial respiration, and lavish funerals—anticipate the structuring concepts that support organ exchange. The second half of the book identifies three genres—sentiment, horror, and romance—as the formal conventions by which we make sense of transplantation in practice. Once organ exchange moved from the realm of imagination to a relatively commonplace clinical practice, society has needed terms by which to channel both acceptance and resistance. These genres have provided those terms and created legible scripts to both open up the conceptual possibility of this radical medical innovation and to manage our lingering anxieties about it.

For all of our discussion of "the gift of life," *Transplant Fictions* starts by acknowledging that organ exchange involves multiple forms of death. Cadaver donors come to the operating table following a variety of scenarios, but the realities of artificial respiration and the emergence of "brain death" mean that the diagnosis of death has changed and often feels at odds with the breathing, heart-beating body to which loved ones say good-bye. A *Time* magazine article describing Barnard's first heart transplant anticipates many of the ethical issues surrounding donation and death:

> The real moral and ethical difficulty in heart transplants arises from medical uncertainty. Even when the heart has "stopped cold" and there is no more respiration, the condition is often reversible—as is proved countless times every day by first-aid squads and lifeguards as well as doctors. The surgeon wants the donor's heart as fresh as possible, before lack of oxygen causes deterioration or damage—that is, within minutes of death. This has raised the specter of surgeons' becoming not only corpse snatchers but, even worse, of encouraging people to become corpses. The question remains: Where should the line be drawn between those to be resuscitated and those not to be?[33]

The questions of what counts as an irreversible condition, whether doctors will work less hard to save the lives of potential donors, and what signs to read as true indicators of "death" have all converged in these discussions. For heart recipients, the surgery requires them to die on the table, their heart stopped intentionally by a surgeon who has vowed to "first, do no harm." And their new lease on life is predicated by the fact that someone had to die in order for them to live. These various deaths underscore the complexities of exchange. Chapters 2–4 offer a careful examination of the many evolving practices that have surrounded dead bodies and thus provide an important foundation from which to understand transplantation.

The reference to "corpse snatchers" in the *Time* article above evokes an important historical antecedent to transplant, one that I explore in closer detail in Chapter 2, "From Corpse to Cadaver." The rise of anatomy and surgical education in the eighteenth and nineteenth centuries created a new demand for corpses as objects of study. These practices created new logics for understanding death and dead bodies. In this scheme, cadavers and ill patients are understood as wholly under the control of doctors and medical technology. As Michel Foucault describes in *The Birth of the Clinic*, "Paradoxically, the presence of the corpse enables us to perceive it living—living with a life that is no longer that of either old sympathies or the combinative laws of complications, but one that has its own roles and its own laws."[34] There is much to take from Foucault's influential history of medicine, but it is perhaps this paradoxical notion of the "living corpse" that is most evocative in the case of organ exchange. What, after all, is the "gift of life," if not a once-dead organ that we can "perceive [as] living," a life with entirely new sympathies, and subject to new combinations, complications, and laws?

Along with a new sense of medical authority over death and the body came a new set of technologies for managing dying and its immediate aftermath. Chapter 3, "Making the Lifelike Corpse," explores the diverse ways in which death became something to be managed and (ideally) postponed inevitably. The medical principle that death should be avoided at all costs animated the pursuit of transplantation, especially in its earliest days when "success" was measured in days or months of life post-surgery. As a series of new technologies and rituals for managing the dying and dead came into public notice, organ donation emerged as an important alternative. Donation campaigns made values-based appeals, recasting transplantation not as the cutting edge of medical technology, but as the sentimental, generous, and even more *natural* way to manage dead bodies.

Chapter 4, "Mortal Signs: Transplantation and the Invention of Brain Death," uses a literary critical lens on political, legal, and news accounts of brain death to understand how a concept as profound as death could undergo a redefinition at the end of the twentieth century. In 1968, Harvard Medical School convened an ad hoc committee who identified a series of criteria for what they called "irreversible coma" and which became the law of the land under the term "brain death."[35] The Harvard Criteria defines death as a series of signs to be read in the patient and as something to be declared—a true performative utterance out of literary and linguistic theory. As such, a condition as seemingly fixed as death itself becomes located in the sphere of cultural construction and subject to literary analysis.

The second half of the book largely examines cultural representations that have emerged since the achievement of transplantation in the mid-twentieth century. If the first half explores somewhat distant concepts and practices as a winding path leading to the conceptual possibility of transplantation, the second half focuses much more directly on representations of organ exchange itself. Chapters 5–7 take up sentiment, horror, and romance as genres that structure our acceptance of and resistance to organ exchange. In a fascinating collision of the imaginative and the historical, we again find Dr. Christiaan Barnard, who turned to novel writing toward the end of his surgical career. In 1996, he published *The Donor*, a medical thriller that incorporates many of the generic elements discussed in the chapters to follow here.[36] The novel follows

Dr. Rodney Barnes, a brilliant celebrity transplant surgeon working at an imagined version of Barnard's own hospital in Cape Town, South Africa. At one level, the novel includes elements of sentimental romance as it follows Dr. Barnes's growing love for his transplant coordinator, Karen van der Waalt, and their early romance. The story turns to horror, however, when Karen gets into a fatal car crash and a manipulative, mad-scientist colleague takes advantage of Barnes's grief to embark on a bizarre set of medical experiments on the brain-dead cadaver. Just as his landmark heart surgery demonstrates many of the founding achievements and challenges of organ exchange, so does Barnard's fiction anticipate several of the most important concepts in our ideological grappling with the practice.

As is possible in the world of fiction, Karen is not only a transplant coordinator, she is also the widow of an organ donor and eventually becomes brain dead herself. While this conflation of circumstances is extraordinary, the descriptions of conversations with family and emotional responses to the donation decision ring true to life. When she is in the position of potential donor kin, Karen recoils from what she sees as the predatory practices of organ procurement: "The body was still warm and here [the surgeon] was hanging around more like a ghoul than a friend. He had just told her that she had lost her husband and, almost in the same breath, had asked her permission to invade his body, pluck out his organs, cause even more destruction to that wonderful being who had shared her life" (44). Despite laws requiring medical professionals to request donation from the families of brain-dead patients, many express discomfort with the conversation and compliance rates are unclear.[37] Doctors and nurses worry about being cast as the predatory corpse snatcher.

Eventually, however, Karen agrees to donate her brain-dead husband's organs and finds herself so moved by the experience that she seeks work with the transplant team. Now on the side of the "ghouls," Karen uses a very familiar script to convince family members of donation. In one example, she tells grieving parents, "We depend on the love and understanding of people such as yourselves. Mr and Mrs Jooste, I am asking you to give the hospital permission to use the organs from your son's body to help other people to live" (49). Thirty years earlier, in a 1967 *Life* magazine article describing the first successful heart transplant, Dr. Barnard represents his conversation with Denise Darvall's father in nearly identical terms: "There is no hope for [your daughter].

You can do us and humanity a great favor if you will let us transplant your daughter's heart."[38] Darvall reportedly replied, "If there's no hope for her, then try to save this man's life." The language of sentiment drives all of these statements, both fictional and true to life. Notice recurring references to love, understanding, your son, your daughter, hope, life, and humanity. In Chapter 5, "'The Gift of Life': Sentiment and the Family," I draw from media accounts as well as high- and low-brow sentimental fiction to demonstrate how the founding principle of altruism in organ exchange gets channeled through the generic conventions of sentiment.

The social dimensions of donation are emphasized in these speeches as well. "We depend." "Do us and humanity a great favor." Altruism expresses a sense of social responsibility, one that often imagines social ties through the sentimental metaphor of family. Relationships also emerge in donation decisions through the creation of a new social category: the donor family. As Karen reflects on her decision to become part of a "donor family," she thinks, "She never regretted her decision. It was as if part of [her dead husband] was still alive and advancing what he believed in as the goal of medicine: improvement of the quality of life" (47). Although it's most succinctly signaled in the phrase "gift of life," this belief in the continuation of life of a loved one through donation is a compelling motivator for donor families. An oblique expression of resistance to the dehumanizing elements of the spare parts analogy, donor families very commonly believe in the transfer of something of the donor to the recipient. In some cases, relationships emerge between the donor family and the recipient, often understood through metaphors of siblings or parents. Writing of these new forms of sociality, Lesley Sharp reminds us, "Whereas these relationships may seem strange and unsettling to the uninitiated, within the realm of organ transfer they are natural responses to an extraordinary form of death, to the medical ability to revive human life, and to the fact that organ transfer is about sharing hidden parts of oneself with a community of anonymous strangers."[39] Transplant scholars Renée Fox and Judith Swazey also take up the social dynamics of altruism, cautioning against the potential "tyranny of the gift" in both anonymous cadaver and directed living donation.[40] Although the complexities of these concepts are explored much more fully in Chapter 5, it is interesting to note that they exist in both early surgeries and in fictional representation decades later.

Of course, while imagining the essence of a loved one continuing in a new body can give comfort to donor families, it can also be a source of horror. Filmgoers and fiction readers in the twentieth story are familiar with a recurring trope in horror narratives in which someone receives a transplant only to discover that the violent characteristics of a criminal donor are transferred with the organ. New hands drive unwitting recipients to strangle or stab, transplanted corneas bring an inherited ability of tragic premonition.[41] In *The Donor*, Christiaan Barnard similarly employs this pulp fiction trope: In a medical experiment where the heart of a hanged murderer is transplanted into a baboon, the baboon "keeps scrabbling at its neck as if trying to remove something" (295), namely, the noose used to execute his donor. Later, the animal who has been nicknamed "The Killer" by his caretakers is used as a violent tool to dispatch a too-curious colleague.

In Chapter 6, "Murdering Hands and Mad Doctors: The Horrors of Organ Exchange," I explore more deeply how the concept of transmigration devolves from the sentimental context of donor families to an expression of enduring resistance toward the practice of transplantation. These recurring tropes serve as a powerful indication of anxiety about boundary violations, especially between self and other. A complementary trope in these horror narratives is the image of a mad or corrupt doctor, itself an expression of worry about the overwhelming power of medical authority. Again, *The Donor* provides us with prime examples of this figure: both in the form of Dr. Barnes, who violates ethical precepts in a drive for new procedures, and in the form of Dr. Kapinsky, the lab director under Barnes who (we come to learn) was literally raised under the tutelage of the Nazi physician Josef Mengele. An exchange between these two characters early in the novel emblematizes the paradoxically dehumanizing vision of radical medical experimentation in the name of progress and serving humanity. Barnes enthuses, "We'll have a living bank of human organs and tissue. There could be no objection to studies such as the effect of drugs and irradiation, and new surgical procedures could be attempted and performed on living humans" (107). Kapinsky worries, but what about the ethics committee? Barnes responds: "I don't see how they can object, as long as the relatives of the donors agree. After all, they're dead and we cannot harm them any further.... These patients will be nothing more than living corpses" (107). In this revealing oxymoron—"living corpses"—Barnard encapsulates a number of the troubling paradoxes that make horror such a compelling genre for narratives of organ exchange. Calling up material from Chapters 2–4, what does it mean for corpses to have a life after death? And how have we come to terms with a specialized category of death called "brain death? After all, why is it not just "death"? How should we feel about this dehumanizing use of human bodies in the service of medical progress? These questions, which manifest with different levels of specificity or intensity in a diverse array of practices surrounding death, come to a head in the case of transplantation.

Not only do horror films and novels serve as a recurring mode for investigating these boundary questions, but the tropes of this genre also structure real-life approaches to transplantation. Waking up after his heart transplant surgery, Louis Washansky famously said, "I'm a Frankenstein now. I've got somebody else's heart."[42] These touchstones of popular culture can serve people on the frontiers of medicine, individuals who suddenly fall entirely outside the realm of past human experience. For Washansky, Frankenstein's monster is the closest precedent for his unique experience and one of the few recognizable figures who can capture some of the wonder and terror of this new identity. Lawmakers facing similarly uncharted territory also draw on culture to animate their legislative agendas. During congressional hearings on the National Organ Transplant Act of 1984, Dr. Bernard Towers makes reference to the murderous Scottish body snatchers Burke and Hare along with Robin Cook's medical thriller *Coma* to argue against a practice of buying and selling organs. He tells the committee that the express aim of the Act is not "to prevent murder, although it may well do so in due course."[43] Compelling figures from film and literature serve as a reference point for crafting personal identity. Memorable plotlines become evidence in policy debates. These cultural forms both reveal the conceptual foundations of transplantation, but also become scripts that allow both individuals and the public to come to grips with profound changes in medical technology. Frankenstein is not an irrelevant fireside horror story; is it the articulation of important social anxieties about medical "progress" *and* a popular touchstone to make sense of the unknown for individuals living at the cutting edge of those changes.

Horror is also powerful as a genre in cadaver donation because it draws forth the often-denied reality that death and life are inexorably tied in this exchange. As one heart transplant social worker says of recipients: "They hardly ever deal initially with the fact that someone has to die. They know it, of course, but they don't want to have to think about it. This comes later, after the heart is in their body. But first and foremost, what they want to do is to live—and at just about any cost."[44] This powerful denial exists among both recipients and the public at large. As suggested above, the long-standing "gift of life" campaign works hard to recast the realities of donor death for all involved. But as bioethicist Stuart Youngner reminds us in his essay of the same title: "Some Must Die." Chapters 5 and 6 are in many ways paired; it is nearly impossible to think about the sentimental logic of support for organ donation in the USA without also acknowledging the lingering resistance that shows up in horror. Youngner finds a similar simultaneity: "Thus, for example, while the public service announcements and human interest stories extolling transplantation multiply, so too do the grisly cartoons, jokes, and tabloid horror stories about the same subject."[45] In the transplant era, we find a proliferation of cultural representations of the surgery, usually falling out according to these generic headings. On one day, the media will celebrate a bride being walked down the aisle by her dead father's heart recipient and then on the next day wring their hands about scientists creating monstrous human-pig hybrids. Such seemingly contradictory attitudes about the violations required in transplantation deserve closer examination—these expressions of contradiction serve as the major focus of this book.

Horror and sentiment serve as the structuring logics for legal, domestic organ exchange, but any discussion of transplantation ideology must also include the problems of commodification and the international black market. These twin phenomena motivate an extensive body of research in transplant studies, in many ways led by anthropologists Nancy Scheper-Hughes and Lawrence Cohen, both founding members of Organs Watch, a research group created in 1999 to track the international traffic in organs. In Chapter 7, "Kidneyville: Organ Exchange at the Margins," I study both real and fictional accounts of transnational organ exchange to discover a surprising third genre that structures our understanding of organ sale and transplant: romance. While the tragic stories of exploitation chronicled here seem at odds with romance in its most common sense, I identify how hope, transit, and the myth of a happy ending are often the unfulfilled motivators in these cases.

Again, Barnard's early heart transplants serve as emblematic examples of the ways that romantic transplant representation can sometimes be at odds with transplant realities. Post-surgery, a syndicated photograph swept through the world's press showing Philip Blaiberg splashing at the beach, showing off his successful recovery. An onlooker later described the much grimmer realities of the scene: “He was carried into the water, the entourage stepped back, cameras flashed, and he was hauled out before he disappeared helplessly under the waves.”[46] The volunteer system of donation on which legal organ exchange is predicated depends on popular understanding of transplant surgery as an unambiguous happy ending, of recipients enjoying days at the beach. Transplant professionals and recipients, however, are not the only ones invested in this rosy narrative. Organ sellers are similarly caught up in the act of kidney sale as a chance for mobility and hope: a path out of poverty, or a chance at immigration by “swapping [one’s] insides for a passport,” as in the case of the film *Dirty Pretty Things.* Romance, then, serves as a third genre by which we come to the practice of transplantation. The terms of hope, promise, and mobility can help explain how individuals across this exchange see their role in acts that are often rooted in desperation and require violation of both laws and the body itself.

Transplant Fictions starts from an oddity in contemporary culture: the near-universal acceptance of organ exchange. How did we come to celebrate a radical and experimental surgery—one that violates our most sacred categories of life and death, self and other—as a medical miracle? What pathways had to be laid in order to make transplant surgery not just technically, but conceptually possible? And, once we could achieve the surgery in fact, how did our celebration of the practice persist through decades of poor outcomes, of patients dying when up against the seemingly intractable problem of immune rejection? Finally, how does cultural representation express the sentimental logic that drives donation while also exorcising the lingering horror revealed in relatively low rates of donation? The stories we tell about transplantation range from the silly to the profound, sold in supermarket checkout aisles or spun from the imaginations of award-winning writers. But while these narratives are diverse in their quality and scope, they all serve as important new analytic ground by which to answer these animating questions. Transplant ideology is not only expressed in patient testimony or bioethical debates, it emerges through television medical dramas and sentimental tearjerkers, *People* magazine headlines and monster movies of the week. This is the ground upon which we reconcile the violations of transplantation and find new ways to occupy the liminal space of these boundary categories.

Notes

1. Jacobus de Voragine, *The Golden Legend: Readings on the Saints*, trans. William Granger Ryan (Princeton: Princeton University Press, 1993), 198.
2. Ibid.
3. Leonard Barkan, "Cosmas and Damian: Of Medicine, Miracles, and the Economies of the Body," in *Organ Transplantation: Meanings and Realities*, ed. Stuart J. Youngner, Renée C. Fox, and Laurence J. O'Connell (Madison, WI: University of Wisconsin Press, 1996), 244.
4. Studies of organ transplant, especially heart transplant, regularly document personality changes among recipients. See Renée C. Fox and Judith P. Swazey, *Spare Parts: Organ Replacement in American Society* (New York: Oxford University Press, 1992); Margaret Lock, *Twice Dead: Organ Transplants and the Reinvention of Death*, 1st ed. (University of California Press, 2001); Margareta Sanner, "Exchanging Spare Parts or Becoming a New Person?: People's Attitudes Toward Receiving and Donating Organs," *Social Science & Medicine* 52, no. 10 (May 2001): 1491–1499; Lesley A. Sharp, *Strange Harvest: Organ Transplants, Denatured Bodies, and the Transformed Self* (Berkeley: University of California Press, 2006); Margrit Shildrick, "Corporeal Cuts: Surgery and the Psycho-Social," *Body and Society* 14, no. 1 (March 2008): 31–46.
5. US Congress, "National Organ Transplant Act: Hearing before the Subcommittee on Heath of the Committee of Ways and Means, House of Representatives, Ninety-Eighth Congress, First Session, on H. R. 4080, July 29, October 17 and 30, 1983" (1984), 109.
6. Christiaan Barnard, "Human Cardiac Transplant: An Interim Report of a Successful Operation Performed at Groote Schuur Hospital, Cape Town," *South African Medical Journal* 41, no. 48 (December 1, 1967): 1271.
7. US Congress 1983 Rep. Henry Waxman. Gail Moloney and Iain Walker also note the ubiquity of the term "medical miracle" in early Australian newspaper coverage of the procedure. Gail Moloney and Iain Walker, "Messiahs, Pariahs, and Doctors: The Development of Social Representations of Organ Transplants," *Journal for the Theory of Social Behaviour* 30, no. 2 (2000): 210.
8. "Barnard Pays Visit to Jail on NY Isle," *Chicago Tribune* (December 10, 1968).
9. In his examination of the Cosmas and Damian legend for *Organ Transplantation: Meanings and Realities*, Leonard Barkan offers a similar point: "While we observe the life of this story then, we are in effect

deconstructing what is to us the exceedingly banal expression *medical miracle*; in other words, we are reminding ourselves how that expression might be in rhetorical terms an oxymoron or in cultural terms a lived contradiction or paradox" (227).

10. Figures asserted in June 2017 according to the Web sites for the Organ Procurement and Transplantation Network, a division of the US Department of Heath and Human Services, and Donate Life, Inc.
11. Lesley A. Sharp, *Transplant Imaginary: Mechanical Hearts, Animal Parts, and Moral Thinking in Highly Experimental Science* (Berkeley: University of California Press, 2014), 20.
12. Leslie Fiedler, "Why Organ Transplant Programs Do Not Succeed," in *Organ Transplantation: Meanings and Realities*, ed. Stuart J. Youngner, Renée C. Fox, and Laurence J. O'Connell (Madison, WI: University of Wisconsin Press, 1996), 58.
13. Donald Joralemon, "Organ Wars: The Battle for Body Parts," *Medical Anthropology Quarterly*, New Series, 9, no. 3 (September 1995): 336.
14. Margaret Lock's comparative anthropological work on brain death in North America and Japan reminds us that this lack of controversy was not a given. She also offers the important historical context that while there was an initial, worldwide flush of celebration following Barnard's initial transplantation, failures to achieve gains in survival rates for patients in subsequent years led medical groups to consider banning research on heart transplantation altogether. Lock, *Twice Dead*, 86.
15. Notable exceptions include article or chapter-length studies by literature scholars, Catherine Belling, "The Living Dead: Fiction, Horror, and Bioethics," *Perspectives in Biology and Medicine* 53, no. 3 (Summer 2010): 439–451; Pete Boss, "Vile Bodies and Bad Medicine," *Screen* 27, no. 1 (January 1, 1986): 14–25; Susan Squier, "Transplant Medicine and Transformative Narrative, or Is Science Fiction 'Rubbish'?," in *Biotechnological and Medical Themes in Science Fiction*, ed. Domna Pastourmatzi (Thessaloniki: University Studio Press, 2002), 87–110.
16. Nicholas L. Tilney, *Transplant: From Myth to Reality* (New Haven: Yale University Press, 2003), 176.
17. In apartheid South Africa, The Population Registration Act of 1950 created an obligatory system of ethnic categorization divided into four categories of "White," "Asiatic," "Colored," or "Black." For more on race relations and categorization in South Africa, see Ellen Hellmann and Henry Lever, eds., *Race Relations in South Africa 1929–1979* (New York: St. Martin's Press, 1979); Charles V. Hamilton et al., eds., *Beyond Racism: Race and Inequality in Brazil, South Africa, and the United States* (Boulder, CO: Lynne Rienner Publishers, 2001).

18. Quoted in Marais Malan, *Heart Transplant: The Story of Barnard and the "Ultimate in Cardiac Sugery"* (Johannesburg: Voortrekkerpers, 1968), 112.
19. "The Telltale Heart," *Ebony*, March 1968, 118.
20. Malan, *Heart Transplant*, 113.
21. Moloney and Walker, "Messiahs, Pariahs, and Doctors," 212.
22. Malan, *Heart Transplant*, 116.
23. Ibid., 115.
24. Nancy Scheper-Hughes, "Consuming Differences: Post-Human Ethics, Global (In)Justice and the Transplant Trade in Organs," in *A Death Retold: Jesica Santillan, the Bungled Transplant, and Paradoxes of Medical Citizenship*, ed. Keith Wailoo, Julie Livingston, and Peter Guarnaccia (Chapel Hill: University of North Carolina Press, 2006), 206.
25. US Congress, "National Organ Transplant," 228.
26. "Surgery: The Ultimate Operation," *Time*, December 15, 1967.
27. Quoted in Malan, *Heart Transplant*, 115.
28. Susan E. Lederer, *Flesh and Blood: Organ Transplantation and Blood Transfusion in Twentieth Century America* (Oxford: Oxford University Press, 2008), 174.
29. Tilney, *Transplant*, 185.
30. See Lederer, *Flesh and Blood*; Susan E. Morgan, Jenny K. Miller, and Lily A. Arasaratnam, "Similarities and Differences Between African Americans' and European Americans' Attitudes, Knowledge, and Willingness to Communicate About Organ Donation," *Journal of Applied Social Psychology* 33, no. 4 (April 1, 2003): 693–715.
31. US Congress, "National Organ Transplant," 285.
32. "Network Is Proposed for Organ Transplants," *New York Times*, October 6, 1983, Sec. A.
33. "The Ultimate Operation," *Time*, December 15, 1967.
34. Michel Foucault, *The Birth of the Clinic an Archaeology of Medical Perception* (New York: Pantheon Books, 1973), 149.
35. Henry K. Beecher, Raymond Adams, and Clifford Barger, "A Definition of Irreversible Coma: Report of the Ad Hoc Committee of the Harvard Medical School to Examine the Definition of Brain Death," *The Journal of the American Medical Association* 205, no. 6 (August 5, 1968): 337–340.
36. Christiaan Barnard, *The Donor* (London: Penguin Books, 1996).
37. See Youngner et al., "'Brain Death' and Organ Retrieval."
38. "The Gift of a Heart," *Life*, December 15, 1967.
39. Sharp, *Strange Harvest*, 32
40. Fox and Swazey, *Spare Parts*, 39–42.
41. See Maurice Renard, *Hands of Orlac*, trans. I. White, 1st edition (London: Souvenir Press Ltd., 1981); Charles Gardner Bowers, "The

Black Hand," *Amazing Stories* 5, no. 10 (January 1931): 909–911, 923; *The Eye*, directed by Moreau and Palud (2008, Lion's Gate).

42. "The Ultimate Operation," *Time*, December 15, 1967.
43. US Congress, "National Organ Transplant," 288.
44. Lee Gutkind, *Many Sleepless Nights: The World of Organ Transplantation* (Pittsburgh, PA: University of Pittsburgh Press, 1988), 184.
45. Youngner, "Some Must Die," 34.
46. Raymond Hoffenberg, "Christiaan Barnard: His First Transplants and Their Impact on Concepts of Death," *British Medical Journal* 323, no. 7327 (December 22, 2001): 1478.

CHAPTER 2

Corpse to Cadaver: From Body Snatching to *Body Worlds*

> It was a long and narrow room, with a lofty ceiling and snow-white floor.... Around the room, between the windows and along the walls, were placed some twenty oblong tables, each standing in the full glare of sunlight, which poured freely over the ghastly spectacles peculiar to the place. Bending over each table was a young man, whose long hair and characteristic look of frankness and restlessness combined, betrayed the Medical Student of the Quaker City.... [O]n each table, sweltering and festering in the sunlight, lay the remains of a woman and child and a man. Here was a grisly trunk, there an arm, there a leg, and yonder a solitary hand occupied the attention of the Student. Rare relics of the Temple which yesterday enshrined a Soul, born of the Living God!
>
> —George Lippard, *The Quaker City*

Behind most surgical innovations lies a disquieting string of failures, experiments, and transgressions. For transplantation in particular, the stakes of the surgery are so high and the boundary questions so profound that it pays to look back at the rise of surgery itself to understand how we have come to the contemporary embrace of this radical medical practice. During the eighteenth and nineteenth centuries in the USA and UK, dissection and anatomical science required massive changes in policy and attitudes toward death and dead bodies.

The above passage from George Lippard's 1845 bestseller *The Quaker City* reveals popular ambivalence about the medical use of corpses. On the one hand, the practice seems "ghastly," a violation of deeply held

E. Russell, *Transplant Fictions*,
Palgrave Studies in Literature, Science and Medicine,
https://doi.org/10.1007/978-3-030-12135-8_2

beliefs in the body as the temple of the soul. On the other, Lippard's chapter, called "The Dissecting Room," alludes to the increasingly common requirement of dissection as a valuable principle of surgical education and medical advancement. As the scene progresses, four or five hundred students fill the anatomy theater to attend a lecture on a possible new innovation in the treatment of disease (439). The role of sunlight in this passage perhaps best illustrates the ambivalence of the period. The figurative light of knowledge prevails in the sun-drenched space, but it is a glaring light that creates "sweltering and festering" human remains. Terms like "relic" and "yesterday enshrined a Soul" emphasize the liminal state of the corpse—the reference to the past suggests that they are no longer Christian subjects, but readers are reminded, "a Soul once shone from those eyes, a voice once spoke from those lips!" (437).[1]

Contrast this scene of ambivalence with another kind of surgical performance conducted over a century later. In February of 1976, Dr. Samuel Lee Kountz performed a live kidney transplant on *The Today Show*. In response, 20,000 people called NBC to offer their kidneys for donation. Such a full-throated endorsement of organ exchange marks how far popular opinion has shifted. In addition to technical achievements like protocols for re-implantation and the Belzer perfusion machine, Kountz understood the importance of popular attitudes toward advancing transplantation. In his quest to support increased donor registration, Kountz redeployed the public-facing strategies of the anatomy era. After all, what more mainstream audience exists than that of *The Today Show*? Surgical performance in this instance expresses a celebration of progress and an overriding belief in medical authority. But the life saved by Kountz's surgery required the death of another, a fact that is largely diminished in the embrace of medical progress. The fact that 20,000 people were inspired to direct their own organs to transplantation upon death means that much of the ambivalence toward the "ghastly spectacles" Lippard describes has been overcome.

It can be difficult to document long-standing attitudes about dead bodies, precisely because these attitudes are so deeply held as to seem natural and ahistorical. Few taboos are more deeply entrenched than those against the "improper" handling of corpses. We fear corpses as carriers of disease and reminders of our own fragility. We honor the dead with memorial services and imagine the grave as a secure place of endless repose. Centuries of ritual and culture in the West would suggest that corpses are objects that inspire fear or solemn mourning. While those cultural notions still predominate, transplantation requires a different understanding of the corpse, one in which death can be reimagined as a source of life. How, then, have we gotten to a place where instead of an object of disgust or reverence, a corpse can be embraced as a useful object? What have been the changing cultural, medical, and social conditions surrounding the corpse that ultimately make cadaver donation not only culturally acceptable, but celebrated?

This transition—in which transplantation is not just technically but also conceptually possible—is rooted in the change from "corpse" to "cadaver." The more specialized case of "cadaver," meaning a dead body used for scientific or medical purposes, signals the near-total authority assumed by medical technology over the failing human body. Of course, we still view such authority with resentment and skepticism, and medicine did not always occupy a primary interest in the life and death of individuals. In her book *Medicine as Culture*, Deborah Lupton reminds us that the near-total medical authority over both dying and the dead that we experience today is historically contingent: "In the 16th century and the first half of the 17th century in Europe, death was a largely non-medical ceremony. Both the Protestant and Catholic religions insisted that a member of the clergy should be in charge of the deathbed, rather than a medical practitioner, who left when it became clear that nothing more could be done."[2] As the Enlightenment values of reason and investigation took hold more deeply throughout the continent, medical authority was extended as an expression of those values.

Ultimately, the troubled rise of anatomy and dissection in the eighteenth century creates a path toward the practice of organ transplant in the twentieth century. As historian Ruth Richardson argues when describing the career of British surgeon and anatomist John Hunter, "The history of transplantation itself is rooted in the era of body snatching."[3] During this period, British surgeons like Hunter, Astley Cooper, and Robert Knox sought to drive medical knowledge forward by training themselves and their students with hands-on study and experimentation with the recently deceased. While this practice was not illegal, there were not enough political solutions that would supply fresh corpses to the increasing ranks of would-be doctors. To meet this demand, a new profession emerged: the resurrectionist, or body snatcher. Public outrage over the practice of body snatching was a catalyst for the passage of nineteenth-century Anatomy Acts in both the USA and Britain, giving more latitude to doctors and medical students by allowing them to procure unclaimed bodies, typically from prisons and workhouses. But this legal redress to the excesses of body snatching also met with public resistance. Historians, including Michael Sappol in the USA and Roy Porter in Britain, chronicle dozens of anatomy riots taking place on both continents.[4] Protestors saw dissection as an assault upon the dignity of the community and an example of government brutality toward the voiceless. These debates over problems with cadaver supply and demand offer an eerie anticipation of contemporary conversations about organ scarcity. In making some bodies the appropriate property of the anatomist's scalpel, Anatomy Acts elevated the public value of medical knowledge and took several steps toward the possibility of claiming corpses for diverse medical uses, including, a century later, organ transplant.

Two works of art from the seventeenth and eighteenth centuries demonstrate the enduring and complicated cultural relationship to the medical use of cadavers. Both works offer a glimpse into the public anatomy theater, spaces where medical students, and often the paying public, could observe an anatomy demonstration. In Rembrandt's *The Anatomy Lesson of Dr. Nicholaes Tulp* (1631), a cadre of seven physicians looks on with rapt attention as Dr. Tulp uses forceps to grasp the cadaver's exposed tendons.[5] In the image, the corpse is laid out naked on the table before the doctors, pelvis draped for modesty, and the skin of his left forearm and hand has been removed for the sake of the demonstration. The tone of the painting is somber and serious, with a strong play of light and shadow. The pale white flesh of the corpse stands out in strong contrast to the dark clothing of the onlookers, suggesting the body as a source of enlightenment. As a tribute to Dr. Tulp, the painting represents science and medical education as masters of the temporal and frail human body. Furthering this theme of enlightenment, the corpse's face is cast in the shadow of death, placing the body firmly as the object of scrutiny, not an active subject.

Another shadow lurking behind the painting is the historical context of the acquisition of cadavers for medical education. In Amsterdam in 1631, the Guild of Surgeons was allowed only one body for dissection per year and, as was consistent with other practices across Europe for several centuries, the body would have to be that of an executed criminal.[6] Thus, while the painting offers a demonstration of rising medical authority of the body, such dissections also served as a reminder of the similar authority of the state. For viewers of both the painting and the dissection itself, then, the event conveys a set of mixed messages about the social value of the corpse as a source of information but the lack of value of the criminal as individual. In this case, the demonstrative fascination of the onlookers and the orderly treatment of the corpse's physicality—laid out neatly, washed, only a small section of skin removed and just for the purposes of instruction—suggest the priority of medical knowledge over the interests of the individual body, if any can be said to remain. Writing of the practice of anatomy more broadly, Michael Sappol argues, "the *dissector*, the generator of meaning, was identified with *mind*, the dissected, those whose bodies were appropriated as the medium through which meanings were generated, were identified with the *body*" (2). Rembrandt's portrait of Dr. Tulp reinforces this scheme and serves as an important reinforcement of the importance of knowledge creation.

Such orderly treatment of the corpse, however, is only one mode in artists' depictions of the anatomy theater. Where Rembrandt wanted to convey respect for Tulp and medical education more broadly, English artist William Hogarth's satirical engravings of a century later are an effective skewering of the practice of dissection. In *The Four Stages of Cruelty* (1751), Hogarth tells the story of Tom Nero, a fictional villain who grows from a childhood habit of kicking dogs to adult life as a highwayman and murderer of his mistress. In the final plate, *The Reward of Cruelty*, Nero's hanged corpse is taken to a chaotic anatomy theater where he is dissected. One year later, the Murder Act of 1752 in Britain would require dissection or hanging the corpse by chains as a further punishment beyond execution for the crime of murder. The Murder Act was seen as a crime deterrent to a population that feared the anatomist's knife, but it also served the educational need among surgeons-in-training for an increased supply of cadavers. In Hogarth's image, Nero's heart has tumbled to the floor to be eaten by a dog, his eyes are being gouged out by a callous surgeon or preparator,[7] and another man wielding a knife has buried his own hand in the chest cavity to continue the extraction of organs. A motley collection of skulls and bones is boiling in a cauldron in the foreground, in preparation to join other skeletal specimens hanging about the room. The crowd in the room has grown from Rembrandt's attentive seven to more than two dozen, attending to the proceedings with varying degrees of interest.

Despite their apparent differences, in both works knowledge production emerges as an argument for the value of the practice of dissection. In *The Anatomy Lesson of Dr. Nicolaes Tulp*, a massive medical textbook dominates the right foreground of the painting. The text seems almost to be illuminated by the light reflected from the naked cadaver, suggesting a symbiotic relationship between textual study and hands-on demonstration. It would have been historically appropriate for the textbook to be Andreas Vesalius's 1543 *De Humani Corporis Fabrica*, the dominant text of anatomy instruction for centuries. In his painting, Rembrandt brings together the tropes of light, book, and body to make a case for medical authority. William Hogarth, too, structures his engraving in visual reference to the frontispiece of this master anatomical text. Although Hogarth represents dissection as a (literal) punishment worse than death, his reference to Vesalius places the practice in a lineage of rising medical expertise. Vesalius, himself, offered a repudiation of the static Galenic tradition and served as an advocate for hands-on dissection as the root of knowledge. Under his model, cadavers themselves "become 'the book' to be read by the surgeon rather than the set text sanctioned by traditional learning."[8] Such direct methods of education, however, are necessarily gruesome, and the enduring split between physicians and surgeons finds its root, in part, in the early physician's distaste for getting one's hands dirty by actually touching the patient, whether alive or dead. Hence, the existence of the barber-surgeon and the now-inconceivable move from cutting hair to amputating limbs. In her study of public exhibitions of the body, Elizabeth Stephens argues that the Galenic tradition of speculative anatomy persisted into the late eighteenth century (another two centuries after Vesalius's masterwork) because of a belief that dissection defiles the integrity of the body and what Helen MacDonald calls "a natural aversion to touching the dead."[9] The case for dissection as an important source of knowledge about the body and its ills was not, then, self-evident. These works of art, even when anxious about the grisly elements of dissection, nevertheless argue for the practice as a central tenet of rising medical expertise.

An increased understanding of the value of hands-on experience with anatomy was appropriate to the eighteenth century, with its zeal for classification and experimentation. Art historian Barbara Maria Stafford looks to extend this connection between dissection and knowledge production. She understands anatomy as the Enlightenment paradigm for the study of depths and the unseen, claiming "metaphors of decoding, dividing, separating, analyzing, fathoming permeated ways of thinking about, and representing, all branches of knowledge from religion to philosophy, antiquarianism to criticism, physiognomics to linguistics, archeology to surgery."[10] Medical historian Roy Porter similarly understands the conceptual reach of anatomy: "The anatomist's knife served as a blade of truth in a new and fashionable 'culture of dissection' expressed through poetry, plays, piety, and (not least) the rituals of divine justice."[11] Such comprehensive vision casts dissection and anatomy not simply as valuable practices in and of themselves, but a paradigm for the most exciting and important way to understand the world.

In addition to Stafford and Porter, a chorus of cultural historians agrees that the study of anatomy contributes to the modern concept of self as well as social and political life. As Michael Sappol argues, "In the rituals of the anatomical theater and the anatomy room, ambitious young men learned to dissect, and to regard that operation as a paradigm for the broader mastery of instrumental reason over the body, the lower classes, the savage races, the material world, women, and animals" (169). Elizabeth Stephens similarly sees in anatomical exhibitions "the cultivation of the respectable bourgeois subject" (13). Corinna Wagner extends this argument to the politics of the period, noting the profound ties between concepts of transparency, the interior self, and visibility to the history of revolution.[12] Dissection and display of dead bodies, then, serves as a new site of action and mastery for modern subjects. This notion emerges against enduring belief in the body as inviolable, merely an object of contemplation that carries a strict prohibition against incursion. The anatomy era literally opens the ground for a newly valued practice of bodily intervention. As such, it provides the necessary foundation for the transplant era two centuries later. In order for this advancement to take place, it was essential that we accept rupturing the integrity of the corpse and reusing the interior toward a social good—education in the earlier case, harvesting for transplantation in the latter.

The comparison of Rembrandt and Hogarth's work captures a change from a religious reverence for an intact, interred corpse to placing the body under medical authority. As such, they show to different degrees the acceptance for the use and display of corpses, but they also show the public mistrust and panic attached to the practice. Medical authority over corpses appeals to a popular sense of broad social good and to an increasing value for scientific thinking, but these changes do not happen without fear and skepticism. A more immediate expression of this dynamic appears in organ transplant, where the public sees the practice as the highest expression of twentieth-century medical achievement. The Donate Life America Web site, for example, asserts,

"Transplantation is one of the most remarkable success stories in the history of modern medicine."[13] But, still, voluntary donor rates are low compared to public expressions of approval and medical professionals struggle with how to approach families about the possibility of donation from their recently diseased loved one. The contradictory cultural dynamic that celebrates organ transplants while retreating from donation becomes less perplexing when understood in the context of a long history of conflicting attitudes toward the use of the dead.

Popular resistance toward medical dissection is rooted in our most basic fears, many of which endure in discussions about cadaver donation today. Many Christians believe in a literal rising from the grave on Judgment Day, a belief that was particularly strongly held during the Georgian era. To desecrate a body by separating its parts meant that it could never be whole again during the resurrection. In Judaism, prohibitions against mutilating the dead, benefiting from the dead, and postponing burial have all emerged in debates about organ transplant. Across many religions, violating the sanctity of the grave provokes deep fear and anxiety.

The belief in a future reunion after death, even if distant, speaks to a widespread desire for a lingering self attached to the buried body. Much of the modern funeral industry relies on a confounding "still her/not her" approach to corpses. Both Ruth Richardson, in her history of dissection, and Lesley Sharp, in exploring the anthropology of organ transfer, discuss past and present beliefs in a corpse that retains some kind of sentience beyond death.[14] The use of executed murderers for dissection certainly suggests a public concept of a body that will continue to suffer punishment even after death. This understanding of the body as preserving something of the deceased individual has profound effects on discussions of organ donation. Many donor kin, for example, express fears that further surgeries will prolong the suffering of their brain-dead relatives. This sense of a lingering self or a transmigration of something from the donor to the recipient animates much of our thinking—good and bad—about organ donation, thinking that has roots in centuries-old attitudes about the dead body and its treatment. Even when surgeons did not have the techniques to achieve transplantation, the practice of dissection creates an important pathway toward its conceptual possibility by authorizing a radical new mode of handling the dead.

In addition to religious or spiritual reservations, the process of parting up the corpse through dissection and anatomy also runs counter to foundational beliefs in somatic wholeness. Many historians, including Ruth Richardson and Elizabeth Stephens, capture an understanding of dissection as representing "a gross assault on the dignity and integrity of the body."[15] Where "integrity" means "wholeness," this phrase captures an essential hurdle in coming to our idealized understanding of organ donation not as a violation or assault but as a "gift." Even on the side of the recipient, we must first acknowledge the failed integrity of the body in order to allow for a new part that would "make one whole again." The possibility of the broken-down corpse in anatomical dissection is a first productive challenge to the concept of somatic integrity itself. Dissection is not simply a violation of dignity of a specific individual's body, but a long and rocky move toward rethinking the inviolable integrity of corpses in general.

The fundamental move in overcoming these forms of resistance to both dissection and organ transplant is to relocate the proper authority of the corpse from the sanctified grave to the realm of medicine. As heirs to Rembrandt's *The Anatomy Lesson*, American artist Thomas Eakins's paintings *The Gross Clinic* (1875) and *The Agnew Clinic* (1889) illustrate the anatomy theater as the site of medical authority.[16] These surgical paintings are not uncomplicated demonstrations of medical authority, but they represent a mid-point between the dissecting terror of the eighteenth century and the surgeon-heroes of the twentieth century. In *The Gross Clinic*, Dr. Samuel Gross embodies the confident authority of a world-class surgeon, presiding over an operation viewed by an amphitheater full of students. Like Rembrandt's work in *The Anatomy Lesson*, the painting plays with strong contrasts in shadow and light, again using the supine body as the brightest area of canvas. In this case, the patient's head is not simply cast in shadow, but entirely obscured from view; instead, the viewer is confronted with the bright red, bloody incision on the left thigh with the patient's buttocks and rear flank the only areas of the body that can be seen. This disorienting perspective on the patient emphasizes the total authority of the operating team to manipulate the body to their own ends. Dr. Gross's bloody fingers grip his spectacles—his tools of vision—as he lectures to the amphitheater. By contrast, a diminutive woman in black dress and bonnet (typically identified as the patient's mother) covers her own eyes with upraised arms, a representative of outmoded, sentimental ways of thinking that shrink before the power of medical progress.

The young Eakins created the painting for the 1876 Centennial Exhibition, as a showcase of both his own talents and the scientific progress of Philadelphia. Public reception of the painting, by contrast, ran to shock and horror. But Eakins's celebration of the surgical theater is consistent with the rising power of medicine and science, even if popular tastes lagged behind. Historian Michael Sappol sees anatomy as part of the "victory of the bourgeois medical profession" (12), central to the narrative of mastery celebrated by the medical students who commissioned the Eakins paintings. More broadly, though, anatomy—and the changing understanding of the body that accompanies it—became increasingly common in public education; Sappol chronicles the period from 1840, when only two common schools in New York State taught anatomy, to 1885, when it was a curricular requirement for nearly every state outside of the South (190). In understanding anatomy as central to both medical training and the education of the citizenry, the nineteenth century increasingly brings the body under the authority of the surgeon. Such authority is central to creating the conditions of possibility for organ transplantation. Because the surgical solution to organ failure is so radical, our understanding of medical authority must be total. As Lesley Sharp writes in *Strange Harvest*:

> In a sense, the range of medical expertise associated with the retrieval, preservation, and replacement of human organs represents the zenith of biomedical accomplishments in a nation that celebrates biotechnological solutions to human health problems. When framed by this dominant ethos, the transfer of human parts within disparate bodies is conceived of as a natural progression within medicine. (22–23)

In the cult of medical technology, the transfer of human organs from one body to the other—a paradigm of horror stories—surprisingly comes to be seen as "natural progression" when understood as an extension of the total control assumed by doctors over patients' bodies. In order to achieve this naturalized model of medical intervention, cadavers must first fall under a dual process of dehumanization and depersonalization.

The Depersonalized Corpse

The representative scheme by which we move from "corpse" to "cadaver" performs a series of removals, eliminating both humanity and individuality from the dead body. This process, however, is not total. Something of the person seems to persist in the cadaver. As such, transplant professionals and modern anatomists must grapple with contradictory conceptual interests among the players involved. Transplant professionals attempt to manage recipients' emotional responses by requiring anonymous donors and "insist[ing] that donor bodies should be viewed as mere corpses that generate reusable parts; that recipients should neither identify with nor idealize their donors nor humanize their organs."[17] Donor kin, on the other hand, are often coached to understand an organ donation as a way for their loved one to "live on" after death. The legally required separation among procurement and transplantation teams facilitates this contradictory representation scheme, as the retrieving surgeon is prohibited from contact with the recipient's doctor.

Among the resurrectionists and anatomists of the body-snatching era, the prime method of overcoming resistance to the use of corpses was dehumanization. In *The Diary of a Resurrectionist*, a primary source account of a body-snatching gang active in 1811, numerous entries demonstrate attempts to deny the humanity of the corpses retrieved. [18] Examples of these entries include "got 9 large & 4 small, took them to Barthol" or "me and Butler went to Newington, thing bad." Here, children become "smalls" and "thing bad" denotes a corpse at an advanced stage of decomposition.

Scottish writer Robert Louis Stevenson offered his own contribution to resurrectionist lore with his short story, "The Body-Snatcher" (1884).[19] Stevenson tells the story of two men who have worked as medical assistants for a thinly veiled anatomist Robert Knox; the violent excesses they perpetrated during their employment; and the divergent impacts of these acts to their consciences in the decades since. The story offers a vivid contemporaneous description of the social dynamics of body snatching. Stevenson writes:

> The Resurrection Man—to use a by-name of the period—was not to be deterred by any of the sanctities of customary piety. It was part of his trade to despise and desecrate the scrolls and trumpets of old tombs, the paths worn by the feet of worshippers and mourners, and the offerings and the inscriptions of bereaved affection. To rustic neighborhoods, where love is more than commonly tenacious, and where some bonds of blood or fellowship unite the entire society of a parish, the body-snatcher, far from being repelled by natural respect, was attracted by the ease and safety of the task. To bodies that had been laid in earth, in joyful expectation of

> a far different awakening, there came that hasty, lamplit, terror-haunted resurrection of the spade and mattock. The coffin was forced, the cerements torn, and the melancholy relics, clad in sackcloth, after being rattled for hours on moonless byways, were at length exposed to utmost indignities before a class of gaping boys. (14–15)

In this passage, Stevenson emphasizes a series of important divisions. On one side, we have the pious citizens of rustic neighborhoods, united by bonds of love, blood, fellowship, and natural respect. In violation of these values, we find the body snatcher and the "class of gaping [medical students]" he ultimately serves: both groups characterized as urban, enterprising, and unbound by custom, religion, or community ties. This description captures a familiar battle of values and expresses the strongly felt costs of innovation. In this passage, Stevenson captures the resistant force of popular opinion and reminds us that the growing force of medical authority over death and dead bodies was not unchallenged.

Stevenson's characters find refuge in the same logic of dehumanization employed by the real-life resurrectionists of the day. When one medical assistant is shocked to recognize a local prostitute brought to the medical school as a body for dissection, he turns to his partner in a moral crisis that the violent practices he may have suspected in the past have now been confirmed. He begins, "Suspecting is one thing—" and his partner replies, "'And proof another. Yes, I know; and I'm as sorry as you are this should have come here,' tapping the body with his cane. 'The next best thing for me is not to recognise it; and,' he added coolly. 'I don't'" (9). Instead of talking about "Jane Galbraith," the name of the body known to both of them, the language turns to "this" and "it." The stage direction of tapping the body with the cane completes the process of dehumanization, turning the body into an object to be prodded and used. Earlier in the story, corpses delivered in the dead of night are called "tragic burden[s]" and "the unfriendly relics of humanity" (6). Read together with the "thing bad" from *Diary of a Resurrectionist*, these impersonal pronouns and phrases enact the middle phases of transition from corpse to cadaver.

A conceptual cousin to the practice of dehumanization is depersonalization. The practice of anatomy is predicated on the concept of moving from the individual to the universal. As Barbara Maria Stafford describes in her examination of art and medicine of the eighteenth century, "The idea of 'normative' anatomy had existed since Vesalius. It was customary to urge that the cadaver used for public dissections ought to be as normal as possible (a 'middle' or 'general' form). Thus other bodies might be compared to it with an eye to assessing non-natural deviations from that form" (108). This reverence for a universal norm is a foundational assumption in the modern theory of pathology.[20] Anatomists, then, rejected the individual status of the cadaver by casting it as a universal teaching tool, moving from *this* body to *the* body.

The world of painting offers us several vivid examples of the depersonalizing effects of medical education, illustrating the ways in which the body on the table begins to lose individual status. In *The Agnew Clinic*, Thomas Eakins offers his second representation of the surgical theater. Commissioned by his medical students on the occasion of Dr. D. Hayes Agnew's retirement in 1889, the painting depicts the surgeon directing a medical team performing a mastectomy. As in Hogarth's satiric engraving, the audience of the surgery demonstrates varying degrees of attention, made perhaps more surprising in this case by the fact that the patient's breasts are bared to both the students and the viewer of the painting. In this respect, the painting must be placed in conversation with Henri Gervex's *Avant L'Opération* (1887). In *Avant L'Opération*, the female patient is rendered in even more conventionally sensual form: Her hair curls back over the pillow, and her torso is bare above a sheet draped over her waist, and her skin is rendered in soft pinks. Of the ten additional figures in the room, the only one who directs his or her attention to the patient is the anesthetist, who reaches beneath her bared breasts to grip her wrist and brings a cloth to her face. By contrast, the speaking surgeon draws much greater attention from his colleagues in the room. In both Gervex and Eakins's works, the traditional male gaze first places these partially nude female patients in the objectified position of residual sexual desire. But in the staging of the audiences within the paintings themselves, the artists emphasize the depersonalization of the patient, washing out this presumed intimacy by making the women objects of disregard, reduced to universal teaching tools. As described above, *The Gross Clinic* has already taken this universalizing move even further, rejecting the individuality of the patient by revealing only a patch of incised thigh and buttocks.

This move from the individual to the universal follows the same ideological impulses that govern transplantation. A widespread practice of anonymity enforced by transplant professionals has drawn a heavy curtain between donor and recipient in cadaver donation.[21] Donor organs are universalized through the "gift" rhetoric, and the specifics of a donor's life and death are typically withheld. In the 1980s, the development of cyclosporine as a solution to immune rejection problems represented a massive leap forward in transplant technology and constitutes a practical move toward the fantasy of a universal body capable of total interchangeability. Through these forms of depersonalization, the body and its organs become the raw materials of instruction or transplant; their individual origins are only important in as much as they relate to the goal at hand.

On this path to anonymity, cadavers become useful objects, dedicated to the public good. The belief in the social value of corpses has run so deep in history that William Harvey, credited with discovering the circulation of blood in 1628, dissected his own father and sister after their deaths.[22] While one might see this story as evidence of the anatomists' macabre disrespect for death, it could also be understood as attaching a profound value to the acquisition of medical knowledge, in fact an expression of respect for life. Such a view, however, must rely on a rejection of the personal in favor of the universal.

As seen in visual representations from *The Anatomy Lesson* to *The Agnew Clinic*, anatomy or surgical lectures are typically structured around the specific body part in question. Contemporary anatomy classes continue this practice, often removing whole limbs from the examination table after they've been studied, in part to limit students' exposure to toxic formaldehyde. These literal forms of subtraction and the radical manipulation of corpses in the interests of the anatomist rupture the belief that respect for the body lies in the concept of bodily integrity. Modern medical education understands contact with cadavers as instruction in both "the real" materiality of the body and a conceptual confrontation with death itself.

While many doctors would argue that a level of depersonalization is essential in the practice of medicine, the rising influence of the medical humanities and contemporary students' thoughtful approach to their cadavers illustrates their belief that something of the dead has remained in the cadaver. Modern practices like course funerals for donated cadavers or descriptions of the students' treatment of the cadaver as if it were "merely sleeping" capture the split between necessary dehumanization and the residue of reverence and humanity that has characterized the medical use of cadavers.[23] In his vividly titled article "'I Actually Don't Mind the Bone Saw': Narratives of Gross Anatomy," Douglas Reifler describes how the reflective process of writing deepens medical students' experience of cadaver dissection.[24] Reifler and other pioneers in medical humanities, most notably Rita Charon, describe the role of storytelling, writing, literary analysis, and "parallel charting," as central to the education of ethical and empathetic physicians.[25] These educators work with students and practicing doctors to equip them with a new set of tools for making meaning out of the graphic realities of illness and death.

In order to normalize a range of shocking practices from dissecting corpses to transplanting organs, we must keep in mind the profound sense of value attached to the bodies as material objects beyond the spiritual value of the individual. While dehumanization and depersonalization help achieve this translation at one level, the value of the corpse itself must be brought into public acceptance through language, cultural representation, and economic markets. The use of euphemistic language like "resurrectionist," "transplant," and "harvest" works to mask the gory realities of the practices involved. Instead, radical surgery is recast in the realm of either religion or life-affirming horticulture. This language continues in the transplant campaigns of the twentieth century, as one emblematic slogan exhorts viewers, "Transplant Kidneys/ Don't Bury Them."[26] Such euphemism, as many critics, including Lesley Sharp and Ruth Richardson, have argued, allows medicine to "minimize, normalize, and render unobjectionable" the practice of organ transplantation.[27] Word choice like "harvest" and "transplant" recast donor bodies as part of a natural and socially responsible practice of altruism, an alternative mode that elevates the public value of the "cadaver" over the simple "corpse."

The Valuable Corpse

The accepted social value of dissection comes in the acquisition of medical knowledge that would serve the greater good. Like the "gift of life" campaigns that constitute the overwhelming messages about organ and tissue donation in the USA and Britain, individual cadavers were seen through a lens of altruism. Insights gained through dissection served the population not only by improving medical practice (and, hopefully, health outcomes for patients), but also by advancing general knowledge. Anatomical study was considered an important part of public life in the eighteenth century.[28] Crowds in the thousands thronged to the anatomical lecture circuit during this era. Medicine was a subject of broad interest, transcending class and gender lines. Through lectures, museums, pamphlets, textbooks, satirical engravings, wax models, specimens, and home manuals, America and the UK captured a democratic zeal for the inner workings of the body.

In addition to this specialized knowledge production, however, the tradition of public attendance in anatomy theaters speaks to a broader social value attached to attempts at classification and knowing. The eighteenth-century design for the Paris École de Chirurgie, for example, included a twelve-hundred-seat anatomy amphitheater and thus served not only the medical students, but also a massive audience of the paying public.[29] The motivation for visiting such theaters rests in a passion for understanding the physical world, and by extension, the self. Beyond in-person visits to these sites, art depicting surgeons' theaters "visually exhorted spectators to know themselves through the charnel-house sight of skeletons or decomposing cadavers."[30] Such images were not simply a reminder of death and the fragility of the human form; they expressed a value for anatomizing, classifying, and mastering the diversity of the world. Anatomy was part of a larger zeal to find definitive classification systems, to establish rules and norms of beauty, differences between human and animal, and national or racial origin. A similar impulse continues today in the Human Genome Project, commercial genetic profiling, and the extensive typing of tissue, antigens, and antibodies that serves as the crucial step in organ matching for transplant. Both tissue typing and dissection bring the body under the authority of medicine in the service of social good, both abstract and material.

The value of corpses, of course, is not limited to the spheres of altruism and education. There is a clear commodity value in corpses, an economic reality that requires widespread legal prohibitions against organ brokerage or compensation for donation. In this century, the commodity value of organs is most urgently located in the realm of black market organ exchange. As Nancy Scheper-Hughes and Lawrence Cohen, among others, have argued persuasively, organs have a very measurable commodity value and often produce conditions in which impoverished individuals sell their kidneys to brokers for a fraction of the ultimate cost to the recipient.[31] Even considering legal practices of organ exchange within the USA reveals the tremendous value in both dollars and prestige conferred on hospitals with transplant centers. Some ethicists have argued against the prohibition of paying for organs, arguing that such a policy discourages donation in a time when, according to current US government statistics, around 20 people die each day waiting for an organ transplant.

Transplant scholars may argue about whether the rhetoric of scarcity is inflated, but any brief scan of news coverage about transplantation will reveal a rehearsal of the same set of dire statistics purporting to demonstrate shortage. If we return to the short story, "The Body-Snatcher," we can see how Robert Louis Stevenson uses the same rhetoric. Even over a century ago, he explicitly credits the excesses of the day with a fundamental problem of supply and demand:

> The supply of subjects was a continual trouble to [the medical assistant] as well as to his master. In that large and busy class, the raw material of the anatomist kept perpetually running out; and the business thus rendered necessary was not only unpleasant in itself, but threatened dangerous consequences to all who were involved. It was the policy of Mr. K— to ask no questions in his dealings with the trade. 'They bring the body, and we pay the price,' he used to say, dwelling on the alliteration. (7)

It was exactly this sense of scarcity and the favorable market conditions it produced that made body snatching a lucrative career in the eighteenth and early nineteenth centuries. The dead human body became an object that could be bought and sold, an essential but obscured condition of organ exchange today. Corpses in the body-snatching era were more transparently tied to market forces: "An adult body in the mid-eighteenth century could be bought by surgeons for about one guinea, but the price had doubled by the 1780s and then leapt to as high as sixteen guineas over the next twenty to thirty years. The bodies of children ... were priced by the inch, while a rare medical condition always commanded a premium."[32] Such naked acquiescence to the commodity value of the body may seem distasteful, but it also allowed for a reconceptualization of corpses through a familiar logic that dismissed the deep spiritual and existential resistance of the time.

Of course, the high economic value attached to corpses and the failure of the political system to act to produce new bodies for dissection were contributing factors in the excessive practices among body snatchers of the day. The most extreme and infamous version of this excess came with the mass murderers William Burke and William Hare. Over a period just short of a year in 1828, the two men strangled boarders at a local rooming house and delivered the fresh corpses to Dr. Robert Knox. According to documents from the case, they fell upon the scheme as a method to dispose of the body of their first victim, a lodger they smothered for failure to pay his rent. The public outcry over these events was intense and directed at both the murderers themselves and Knox, the surgeon. Many wondered how Knox could not have questioned the bodies appearing at his back door, especially when their corpses were fresh, not prepared in any way for burial, and showing signs of similar ends. The aftermath of the case was ironically appropriate. Tens of thousands of spectators filed through the anatomy lab to view Burke's corpse and several wallets made from Burke's skin remain on display at the Royal College of Surgeons in Edinburgh. The Burke and Hare case was so notorious that "burking" entered the British vernacular, first as slang for murdering by suffocation and later as a broader term for getting rid of something by indirect methods.

While the notoriety attached to this case was extreme, even legal methods of advancing medicine often involve a mingling of horror and progress. In Wendy Moore's biography of John Hunter (1728–1793), *The Knife Man*, and Ruth Richardson's account of his contributions to transplant surgery, both authors acknowledge Hunter's role as the father of transplantation.[33] In his work on tooth transplants and experimentation with animal subjects, Hunter represents some of the first attempts to transplant human or animal organs. Public reactions to this work, however, were so negative that Richardson argues his predatory practice of tooth transplant "led to a suspension of interest in transplantation for a century or so" (157). Hunter's experiments included successfully transferring a cockerel testicle into the belly of a hen and attempting to transplant a human tooth into a cock's comb. While these seemingly odd surgeries were consistent with the age of experimentation, he also turned his focus to human subjects. Summing up public recoil against the practice, caricaturist Thomas Rowlandson skewered Hunter's human teeth transplants as a predatory robbing from the poor to serve the vanity of the wealthy. In addition to the exploitive nature of Hunter's practice, his dental work was both unsuccessful as a transplant and dangerous because it contributed to the spread of disease from donor to recipient. Rowlandson's drawings helped to cement public opinion against Hunter (and perhaps transplantation), even though the less ambitious practice of using human teeth in dentures continued into the next century.

Such public skepticism continues in our approach to work with cadavers today. In addition to horror tropes of the surgeon with a dangerous God complex, Lesley Sharp chronicles more specialized cases where organ procurement specialists are cast as modern-day resurrection men. These self-described "vultures" and "ambulance chasers" must grapple with the taint of profit motive and, for lack of a better term, creepiness attached to public attitudes of the use of corpses.[34] In his medical school, John Hunter acknowledged the contradiction between the public need for better surgeons trained through hands-on education and the popular desire not to know the particulars of the activity. Each student had to take an oath upon entry to "speak with caution of what may be passing here, especially with respect to dead bodies."[35] Such secrecy again parallels the emphasis on anonymity in organ transplant and a desire for total medical control over information about the cadaver and its deployment.

Public reaction to Hunter, Burke and Hare, and a rash of copycat Burkists in London, spurred the passage of the Anatomy Act of 1832 in Britain. Under this legislation, Parliament acknowledged a political responsibility to deliver corpses to anatomists, but debated over how. The law extended the scope of the Murder Act of 1752 by offering any unclaimed corpse up to the scalpel. Since such corpses were traditionally found in the workhouse, the law intentionally targeted the nation's poor. In the decades before the passage of the law, debates raged over the proper source of corpses for dissection. The terms of this debate ring almost identically with the contemporary ethical arguments around increasing the supply of organs in a scarce market. As Richardson chronicles: "Ideas ranged from the need for prominent exemplars to make body donation acceptable, or fashionable (the exemplary person most often proposed was the King), to the dissection of all suicides, all hanged criminals, all those dying in prisons (where death rates were high), importation from abroad, or the offer of money awards for future donations" (160). Each of these ideas corresponds to contemporary proposals around organ supply. Contemporary reform proposals to the donation system similarly focus on methods to increase voluntary participation, from Facebook public education campaigns (Mark Zuckerberg as modern "exemplary person"), presumed consent or "opt out" policies (like those adopted by Wales in late 2015), and financial incentives short of straight compensation (including payment for funeral costs or charitable donations).

As Richardson goes on to argue, sources of both corpse and organ "donation" have historically, but also continue to, placed a disproportionate burden on the poor, the criminal, and the mentally ill, targeting our most vulnerable populations. These exploitive practices were both direct and indirect. As examples of the latter, the work of anatomists during the eighteenth and nineteenth centuries resulted in two cottage industries. "Mortsafes" were iron cages placed over a buried coffin that promised to keep a loved one's body safe from the body snatchers. These cages can still be seen in cemeteries in Scotland and England. The second example lies in the funeral insurance industry, which took payments from the poor to avoid the risk of one's body being taken under the auspices of the Anatomy Act of 1832. Such insurance, of course, still exists, in part because of the skyrocketing costs of funerals in the USA. Among the compensation proposals currently suggested for donated organs, among the most popular is payment to offset the cost of a funeral for the family.

The history of organ exchange reveals more directly exploitive practices targeted at vulnerable populations. Echoing the dental experiments of John Hunter, in her anonymous novel *The Adventures of a Rupee* (1781), Helenus Scott describes the pressures brought to bear on the poor, describing a twelve-year-old now working as a chimney sweep whose mother had sold all of his front teeth years before. Of his sister, the sweep says, she "has had nothing but her naked jaw since she was nine years of age. It is but poor comfort to her that her teeth are at Court, while she lives at home on slops, without any hope of a husband."[36] The contrast here between the "naked jaw" and the teeth circulating "at Court" emphasizes the disparity in position felt among these social classes. This sense of exploitation persists in the deep residual reservations people hold about transplantation, especially in the form of skepticism about perceived unfair allocation practices that covertly privilege the richest recipients over those most in need. The most persistent ethical argument surrounding organ donation lies in a proposed system of compensation as a way to alleviate the resounding drumbeat of scarcity. The West has staunchly resisted moving away from a strictly altruistic model of legal donation, precisely for reasons described so vividly in the scene above. Principles like autonomy and freedom of choice lack credibility in economic and social systems that produce sharp disparities between the most and least advantaged. Since the chorus of debate on these questions has continued into the contemporary era, it is important to observe that such concerns have structured popular accounts of transplantation from its inception.

The eighteenth and nineteenth centuries establish medicine as the primary authority over the body, laying the essential groundwork that will make transplantation possible centuries later. Even as the government understood the social value of increasing medical knowledge and experimentation, however, fears lingered in the public imagination. Many of the roots of contemporary anxieties about predatory transplantation practices lie in the age of anatomy, most notably expressed in *Frankenstein*. Echoing Mary Shelley's masterwork, we continue to see recurring expressions of fear about the overreaching authority of the medical profession. As we move from corpse to cadaver and come to understand the dead body as a useful object, we understandably find ambivalence and resistance to this evolution. In his short story, "The Premature Burial" (1844), Edgar Allan Poe uses narrative structure to position readers to believe that this will be another horrifying tale from America's first master of suspense.[37] Popular preoccupation with premature burial speaks to anxieties about the boundaries between life and death and insecurities that medical professionals cannot be trusted to locate this boundary reliably. The narrator opens the story: "The boundaries which divide Life from Death are at best shadowy and vague. Who shall say where the one ends, and where the other begins?" (258). He goes on to assert, "I might refer at once, if necessary, to a hundred well-authenticated instances" of premature interments, of which he believes "a vast number" have taken place (259). Taken together, these lines reveal anxieties about the overreaching power of medical authority, especially in light of its apparent fallibility in knowing such a fundamental condition as death. The body, the narrator asserts, is an "incomprehensible mechanism" (258), and he rejects the posturing of medical professionals who would claim mastery over its inner workings. The clever narrative structure emerges as the story reaches its climax: After enumerating several instances of documented premature burial and describing his own profound fear of experiencing the same end (due to a diagnosis of catalepsy), the narrator wakes up in a wooden enclosure, convinced he's been buried alive. The dramatic irony of the piece reveals that he has not been buried in a coffin, but has simply fallen asleep in a small berth aboard a ship and forgotten where he was. The trauma of the simulated burial is enough to prompt the narrator's reform; instead of dwelling in paralyzing fears of death, he embraces travel and exercise. Crucially, as a step in this reform, he "discard[s his] medical books" (268), understanding that medical knowledge can equal a preoccupation with death. These acts cure him of his cataleptic disorder, suggesting that medical pursuits are not the solution to disease, but its cause.

Stories like "The Premature Burial," "The Body-Snatcher," and the familiar figure of Frankenstein document the conceptual push and pull produced by the rising authority of medicine over life, death, and the body. Although many of the narratives under examination here capture resistance or ambivalence to medical authority, those attitudes become increasingly residual as time passes. The emergent and then dominant strains in Western culture present an increasingly unquestioned transfer of power from religion to medicine. This transfer appears in legal measures like a series of increasingly far-reaching anatomical and human tissue acts or in the requirement of a medical pronouncement of death. It also appears in cultural texts from transplant propaganda campaigns to real and fictional accounts of transplantation. In the following section, I look at a contemporary heir to the anatomy age. Such an extended discussion reveals how a specialized case of modern cadavers both evokes and modifies the terms of medical authority. The early anatomists insisted upon a depersonalized model of the cadaver as an object of universal social good. As such, they established the principles of experimentation and a mechanistic view of the body that become the condition for organ exchange over a century later. They were operating in a time, however, when transplantation was only imagined. What do these questions look like when staged for a modern era, an era in which transplantation is not only possible but celebrated as the pinnacle achievement of the century?

The Exhibited Corpse

Happily for our purposes, the twenty-first century has produced a new expression of the eighteenth-century anatomy theater with Gunther von Hagens and his *Body Worlds* exhibition. His series is the world's most popular traveling exhibition, seen by over 40 million visitors in at least 90 cities and spawning sequels by von Hagens himself as well as several popular knock-offs.[38] In *Body Worlds*, von Hagens uses a process called plastination to arrest decay and turn corpses into pliable, colorful figures. In this process, bodies are first preserved in formaldehyde, and then, water and fats are replaced by synthetic resins, which don't have the "canned tuna fish" look produced in embalming. The individual poses of the "plastinates" are often radically manipulated and artistic: dynamic feats of athleticism, flayed muscles to suggest a body in flames, the intricacies of a father and child's isolated circulatory systems. Von Hagens claims that one of his goals is to "democratize anatomy," harkening back explicitly to the age of anatomy and the tradition of public dissection.

The popular exhibition and its bold creator have not been without controversy, however. The ethical debates surrounding consent of the donors and the proper terms under which corpses may be used or displayed are familiar to both dissection and organ transplant. Rather than focusing on whether the show is art or science or if it is disrespectful to display corpses in this manner, I am interested in how von Hagens casts his work under a set of cultural registers that allow him to defeat his critics. Much like organ transplant, the display of corpses violates powerful taboos and must be authorized by translating the experience into suitable, legitimizing discourses. What, then, constitutes what museum theorist Jane Desmond calls "the right to look"?[39] Critics like Desmond and Elizabeth Stephens argue that contemporary exhibitions of human bodies avoid public censure by drawing on the legitimacy of display strategies found in art and anatomy.[40] As we have seen already, a crucial step in accepting cadaver organs for transplant lies in the placement of the body under medical authority, a body that is both dehumanized and depersonalized in the service of a broader social value. A detailed examination of the dynamics of the *Body Worlds* exhibition demonstrates these and similar dynamics in a contemporary context, exposing additional ways that we have come to see cadavers as both "wonderful" (according to visitors' comments) and useful.

A crucial element of the show's appeal is the fact that the bodies on display are "real." The show's subtitle announces itself: "The Original Exhibition of Real Human Bodies." Similar calls to the real resound throughout the promotional material; the bodies are described as "authentic," "intact," "natural," and "real human specimens." The plastination process obviates the need for glass jars and allows for a seemingly "unmediated" approach to the preserved body.[41] But even if the show wants to emphasize the "reality" of the cadavers, it is specifically anti-realist in its formal presentation. The cadavers are not presented supine as if on a dissecting table or in realistic poses drawn from life; they are upright and, usually, strikingly posed in action. To extend Jane Desmond's point about the "anti-taxidermic" elements of von Hagens's work, the exhibition's success in overcoming criticism from religious and human rights groups requires that the plastinates must be without skin and removed from the lifelike context of the taxidermic diorama (371).[42] The paradox here is that visitors are drawn to the aura of authenticity cast over the bodies on display, but they need their reality mediated by the technical process of plastination, the legitimizing setting of the science museum (the most common venue for the exhibitions), and the highly aesthetic nature of the poses. These registers—technology, science, medicine, and art—come together to make approaching dead bodies not only tolerable, but worth the not-insignificant price of an admission ticket.

We might ask, however, if the display of dead bodies is at worst a violation of human rights and at best simply gross, could we not just use models to demonstrate similar anatomical points? As Stephen Bates describes in his article "Bodies Impolitic? Reading Cadavers," from the sixteenth through nineteenth centuries, when medical students outnumbered available bodies for dissection, European sculptors collaborated with anatomists to produce "wax replicas of extraordinary realism."[43] While his British colleagues were snatching bodies from the grave, in eighteenth-century Italy Felice Fontana was among the most famous of a series of artists who produced wax figures for medical education.[44] This visualizing technique—like anatomical illustration, the practice of dissection, and *Body Worlds* itself—is an attempt to fix human knowledge about the messy, variable body hidden beneath the skin. Von Hagens, however, openly rejects the value of models, arguing on the Web site's "Mission of the Exhibitions" that "the authenticity of the specimens on display is essential [to appreciate the body's anatomical beauty and individuality]. Every human being is unique…. It would be impossible to convey this anatomical individuality with models, for a model is nothing more than an interpretation. All models look alike and are, essentially, simplified versions of the real thing."[45] Casting models as mere "interpretation" is odd in the context of a show that directly places itself in the lineage of public anatomy and depends on reference as an essential aesthetic strategy. Consider, for example, *The Runner*, a plastinate whose muscles are peeled away from each other in a strong reference to Vesalius's illustrations in his enduring anatomy textbook (a text we have seen before, recall, in both Rembrandt and Hogarth's art). In Jose van Dijck's study of *Body Worlds* he argues, "We are urged to consider Vesalius's muscle man not as a representation, but as the paper model for an animated representation; and because we are so used to seeing

MRI scans as representations, we don't even flinch at seeing a body slice of a 'real' cadaver. Bodies and body models, bodies and representations, seem to have become interchangeable in Bodyworlds" (119). This interchangeability between the body and the model, the real and the representation, is a crucial mode authorizing von Hagens's work.

Von Hagens continues the tradition of mingling art and medicine in order to draw on the legitimizing effect of both discourses. As part of the exhibition, von Hagens includes banners with anatomy prints from the tenth through nineteenth centuries along with literary quotes on the power of the "new" anatomical science. By placing himself as the technological and artistic apex of an enduring and important tradition, von Hagens seeks to silence his critics. In another example of artistic reference, *The Skinned Man*, a plastinate holds his skin aloft in a reference to Juan Valverde de Amusco's nearly identical anatomical illustration. Referential aesthetics abound in this case: Valverde's illustration is itself a reference to the depiction of Saint Bartholomew's martyrdom from Michelangelo's *Last Judgment*, and Valverde's 1556 anatomical work more broadly was charged by Vesalius as rank plagiarism, with Vesalius casting aspersions that Valverde performed few of his own dissections. In Valverde's illustration, the removed skin retains the presence of holes demonstrating the face and the man clutches a knife in his other hand. Both elements seem to suggest a series of possible interpretations: a confrontation with death; self-examination as possible destruction; and a meditation on the proper location of the self—the hidden inside or visible outside. Von Hagens's version of this figure is more clearly triumphant: The skin is held up higher, individualizing face holes hidden, and the head looks upward. Jane Desmond, Elizabeth Stephens, and Petra Kuppers share an understanding of von Hagens's overt references to art mingled with science as a way to access "the legitimizing power of historical antecedents" (Desmond 369). Kuppers extends this idea by emphasizing the museum setting of *Body Worlds*, writing that von Hagens "creates visions of medicine that reference art historical topoi of the ideal human shape and its display and that align the medical project with the sanctification and validation traditionally bestowed by museal practice."[46] I share these critics' interest in the ways that cultural positioning can authorize practices that should, on their face, be outlawed. *Body Worlds* is interesting in the context of organ transplantation if only for its ability to move cadavers into the realm of popular use. More profoundly, though, a closer examination of von Hagens's strategies reveals close correspondences with the conceptual framing of transplantation. Cadaveric donors fall, like dissected corpses, under medical authority and social good. Although surgeons are not commonly seen as artists, von Hagens's strong use of artistic reference suggests interchangeability of figures and a belief in an essential sameness under the skin. This emphasis on an essential sameness with minor variations drives the practice of tissue matching and transplant more broadly.

Despite arguing for the reminder of "anatomical individuality" conferred by using "real specimens," the educational mission of *Body Worlds* relies on a familiar narrative of the universal body of anatomy. The function of anatomical visualization is to prompt identification between the viewing individual and the dissected object as the universal Body.[47] Because plastination strips away differentiating features like fat and skin, the social positions of a heterogeneous population fall away in favor a slim, muscled, universal ideal. In visitor comments reproduced on the Web site, many use the phrase "*the* human body" (emphasis added) and appeal to a broad, human "we." Von Hagens's exhortation to "discover the mysteries beneath your skin" uses second person direct address to draw individual visitors into the universal story of health and embodiment being told by the exhibition. This turn to the universal body mirrors underlying fantasies in the transplant world of endless matching among a population made same. It is common for visitors to *Body Worlds* to participate in an endless back and forth of looking and feeling their own bodies, trying to root out the pancreas tucked into their own abdomen or to discover veins, muscles, and ligaments protruding from below their skin. These acts of identification suggest that our bodies are a collection of essentially similar parts—a belief that lies beneath many of the earliest conceptions of organ transplant and which relies on a universalizing narrative of the body.

Along with this idea of the interchangeability among an essentially universal body comes a belief in the body as malleable. The plastinates in von Hagens's work are shockingly manipulated, their material forms pushed to seemingly limitless new dimensions of height, separation, and physicality. In his article "On Gruesome Corpses, Gestalt Plastinates, and Mandatory Interment," von Hagens describes the painstaking process of moving from a "crumbled heap of matter" that emerges from the silicone tank to the ultimate fixed specimen.[48] He writes, "all of the dissected structures, every organ, every nerve and every vessel must be positioned anatomically before the plastic hardens.... A whole-body plastinate requires approximately 1000 pins, foam pads and supporting wires until each structure has been fixed and hardened" (261). This difficult labor may have been obscured if von Hagens hadn't taken the next step to develop what he called "gestalt plastinates." He writes that his early plastinates "appeared rigid as lifeless manikins or they looked unnaturally distorted or even grotesque" (261). The paradoxical answer to overcoming this lifeless and unnatural appearance was to showcase distortion in producing plastinates that emphasize beauty and the role of the artist/anatomist. Von Hagens again places himself in the lineage of anatomists, writing "it was the anatomical artists of the Renaissance who were the first to reduce the distance between anatomized cadavers and the living, by imparting poses of motion to whole-body specimens" (262). The continued emphasis on the real, intact, authentic bodies on display in the exhibition is, for von Hagens, paradoxically produced by the heavy hand of the anatomist in posing and manipulating the specimen. In particular, he drew from a technique in architectural drawing called "exploded views," which allows for a complex presentation of three dimensions; this kind of exaggeration and expansion are dominant tools in von Hagens's formal repertoire.

In *Organ Man*, for example, the cadaver is split laterally to suggest a shell of skin and bone surrounding a central core of essential organs. Enhancing the pathos of this choice, the figure is seen holding out his liver in one hand and digestive system in another, suggesting an offering to the viewer. The plastinate serves as a visual metaphor for our cultural fantasies about cadaver donors. Here, the corpse is re-invested with the agency of the living, literally handing over his essential core as an offering to an unknown other. This ideal of the generous donor, however, is only made possible through the structuring hand of the anatomist. It is the technological process that arrests the decay of the corpse and brings death under the authoritative register of medicine. Here, as in organ exchange, the interests of medical authority and the public direct the private interests of the corpse.

Von Hagens's radical posing techniques offer up a vision of the body as endlessly malleable, capable of manipulation in the interests of improvement and education. This vision of the malleable body is a cornerstone of twentieth-century and twenty-first-century medical discourse, particularly in transplant rhetoric. One manifestation of this phenomenon comes in the Visible Human Project, a digital archive completed in the mid-1990s in which 1-mm or smaller slices of both male and female cadavers were translated into electronic images to facilitate anatomy education. These electronic images can be endlessly reconfigured and reoriented to meet the needs of the demonstration. By dialing down to increasing specificity or reassembling parts to the anatomist's specifications, this Visible Human is entirely subject to anatomical inquiry.[49]

This construction of the malleable corpse was prefigured in the earliest forms of anatomical study, in which illustrators took liberties to reproduce isolated sections of cadavers in order to illustrate a specific organ system. One striking example of this strategy comes from William Hunter, the brother of the famed anatomist and tooth transplanter John Hunter. Although John conducted all of the dissections and Jan van Riemsdyk produced the engravings, William Hunter was the publisher of *The Anatomy of the Human Gravid Uterus Exhibited in Figures* (1774). The volume was a huge atlas with thirty-four highly detailed plates taken from dissections of fetal cadavers. One of the most enduring images depicts a Y-shaped maternal torso, with tissue removed to show the fetus in utero. The woman's legs are severed at the thigh with a visible cross section of bone and muscle. This strikingly dehumanizing image rejects the individual identity of the woman in favor of a universal scientific analysis of pregnancy and human development.[50] This desire to peek inside the uterus, of course, continues in the ultrasound technology of today; a zeal for reproductive imaging which, as many critics have described, has profound effects in producing the fetus as a subject independent of the mother.[51] Similarly, the radical manipulation of cadavers in anatomical illustration produces a cadaver wholly subject to medical and public interests. Instead of the spiritual or human rights of the deceased individual, the cadaver falls under the authoritative hand of the anatomist or surgeon, the material effects of the body subject entirely to external interests.

Hunter's atlas of limitlessly malleable pregnant and fetal cadavers resonates with one of the most controversial exhibits in *Body Worlds: Reclining Pregnant Woman*. This piece proves to be a limit case for von Hagens's broader fantasy of the universal human body. The plastinate showcases the cadaver of a woman who died while eight months pregnant. There are several elements that make the exhibit discordant with the rest of the show. First, while the woman's skin is removed as in the other plastinates, the skin of the fetus remains, conferring an odd sense of subjectivity upon the unborn fetus—an imaginative strategy that dovetails strongly with anti-abortion rhetoric in the USA. Second, the woman's come hither pose—hips cocked forward, arm behind her head to emphasize her breasts, and scraps of skin remaining on her lips and nipples—is in sharp disconnect from the dominant cultural exclusion of pregnant women from sexual desire. *Reclining Pregnant Woman* is more pin-up than pietà. By infusing this plastinate with an emotional world of sexual desire, von Hagens violates the universalizing, depersonalizing mandate of cadaver display and produces an uncanny response in the viewer. More broadly, women cadavers often fall into a category of specificity, traditionally used to demonstrate the reproductive system alone while their masculine counterparts stand as the representative human body.[52]

Imagining the cadaver as a choosing, desiring subject is contrary to the anatomist's interest in translating corpses into malleable, universal objects. This fantasy of malleability is similar to mechanistic views of the body, usually discussed within the transplant scholarly community through the "spare parts" analogy. In *Body Worlds*, the role of technology in creating the contemporary body is highlighted in *Tai Chi Man*, a plastinate that showcases orthopedic surgeries and prosthetics. This exposure of the hybrid—or in Donna Haraway's formulation, cyborg—body demonstrates the primacy of medical technology in shaping the contemporary human form.[53] Beyond prostheses, however, a more profound understanding of the body itself as a machine with interchangeable parts is the structuring trope in modern medicine in general and organ transplant in particular. As actor Gary Oldman comments, "I never knew there was so much going on inside—like a silent pink factory" (bodyworlds.com). This machine fantasy is common among transplant patients and their surgeons as well. Pioneering Houston transplant surgeon Denton Cooley told *Life* magazine in 1968, "The heart has always been a special organ. It has been considered the seat of the soul, the source of courage. But I look upon the heart only as a pump, a servant of the brain."[54] *Body Worlds* makes a visual show of this machine logic, emphasizing the body as a series of linked systems subject to tinkering and modification by expert hands.

This vision of a malleable body, of parts that exist independently from a whole, signifies an important crossing over the conceptual barrier of death as an absolute category. As von Hagens describes, he seeks to create a "living anatomy"; this oxymoron reveals an important step in a changing understanding of death and corpses. The first boundary von Hagens crosses is the absolute Western prohibition against proximity among the living and the dead.[55] This move away from proximity, however, goes beyond the physical. As Tony Walter writes in his critique of the exhibition,

> In modern, as in many societies, the bodies of the dead are ritually separated from the living. In a secularized, Protestant society such as Britain, the living and the dead are separated not only physically, but also conceptually, with transgressors across the boundary (ghosts, prayers for the dead, appearances of the dead to the bereaved, spiritualist mediums) treated with suspicion.[56]

In bringing corpses back across the boundary of death, *Body Worlds* reflects an important conceptual change away from death as the absolute barrier that cannot be breeched by man. Instead, the exhibition constructs death as a chronological point that can be understood and, ultimately, hopefully, mastered.

Megan Stern uses Foucault's influential work in *The Birth of the Clinic* in her reading of *Body Worlds*.[57] For Foucault, death is no longer the "privileged point" beyond which we cannot see or know; instead, the rise of medical science and anatomy understands death as a condition to be read, diagnosed, and—in the case of organ transplantation—postponed. By opening up the chronology of the body beyond death, Foucault also paves the way toward the logic of organ transplant, in which death produces raw materials used to prolong life elsewhere. Even in the context of *Body Worlds*, the plastinates are seen in an odd condition of suspended life. In a visitor's comment reproduced on the Web site, "Bree" writes, "Death brought back to life in an immortal and beautiful way. Thank you for a different perspective on Life." In this quotation, the movement from individual death to immortality through recourse to a universal "Life" happens in the space of two sentences. This slippage from death to life similarly animates the ubiquitous "Gift of Life" organ campaigns. The work of these first three chapters lies in demonstrating how it can be possible that we accept this slogan so uncritically; it uncovers the ideological sleight of hand that allows us to accept labeling donated parts from dead loved ones as a gift of "life."

This expressed fantasy of "death brought back to life" is not wholly unlike the motivating force of organ transplant to prolong life at all costs. That donor cadavers provide the material basis to achieve this goal parallels the "living anatomy" paradox of *Body Worlds*. The acts of identification between the visitor and the plastinate described above are predicated on a theory of health and sameness, showing off the now-perfected (if oddly dead) body the viewer wants. Death and technology come together in a utopian impulse that is shared with the logic of organ transplant. In both cases, death and technology become the vehicles for imagining or achieving a new form of life.

In the conclusion to the first edition of *Spare Parts* (1992), Renée Fox and Judith Swazey reflect on the costs of the American refusal to accept the limitations of death and illness. Titled "Leaving the Field," Fox and Swazey describe what they call "participant-observer burnout" and announce their intention to discontinue work in the fields of transplantation and artificial organs. They confirm this departure twenty years later in a new introduction written for the book's paperback reissue. Fox and Swazey offer a direct articulation of a feeling shared by many of the medical anthropologists, sociologists, and ethicists who study transplantation. They write: "we have come to believe that the missionary-like ardor about organ transplantation that now exists, the overidealization of the quality and duration of life that can ensue, and the seemingly limitless attempts to procure and implant organs that are currently taking place have gotten out of hand" (204). In the new introduction, they emphasize that what was "now" and "currently" true in 1992 was even truer upon republication in 2012. For Fox and Swazey, organ exchange is the epitome of a distinctive value in American culture: "our pervasive reluctance to accept" the biological and human limits imposed by illness, aging, and mortality (204). Transplantation, then, becomes the "obdurate, publicly theatricalized refusal to accept these limitations" (205). Fox and Swazey are careful to acknowledge the admiration and gratitude that they have experienced through their intimate proximity to healthcare professionals and families involved in organ exchange. Nevertheless, their sense of the excesses of organ replacement—concerns chronicled throughout *Spare Parts*—mingles with and overwhelms this sense of awe. The rise of medical authority emblematized by the anatomy age expresses a changing Western attitude toward death and the body. The "missionary-like ardor" Fox and Swazey describe is appropriately articulated through religious metaphor; Americans have come to view the goal of prolonging life at all costs as an article of faith and often treat the technical advancements of the past century as miraculous. In the following chapter, we continue on the journey from "corpse to cadaver," exploring how the treatment of corpses reveals an American attitude toward death that makes organ transplantation conceptually possible.

Notes

1. For more on Lippard in the context of nineteenth-century anatomy, see Michael Sappol, *A Traffic of Dead Bodies: Anatomy and Embodied Social Identity in Nineteenth-Century America* (Princeton, NJ: Princeton University Press, 2002), 221–237.
2. Deborah Lupton, *Medicine as Culture: Illness, Disease, and the Body*, 3rd Edition (London: Sage, 2012), 42.
3. Ruth Richardson, "Human Dissection and Organ Donation: A Historical and Social Background," *Mortality* 11, no. 2 (May 2006): 153.
4. Sappol, *A Traffic of Dead Bodies* and Roy Porter, *Bodies Politic: Disease, Death and Doctors in Britain, 1650–1900* (Ithaca: Cornell University Press, 2001).
5. Martin Kemp and Marina Wallace, *Spectacular Bodies: The Art and Science of the Human Body from Leonardo to Now* (Berkeley: University of California Press, 2000). In their reading of this work, Kemp and Wallace place it in the tradition of Surgeon's Guild paintings flourishing in seventeenth-century Holland (14). In their reading, the suite of surviving images from this tradition "are not literal representations of their public acts, but are allegorical proclamations of surgeons as the renowned masters of the secrets of the body" (24).
6. Roy Porter, *Bodies Politic*, offers a history of the dissection of felons following execution, beginning with annual exhibitions in Renaissance Italy during carnival. By 1564, The Royal College of Physicians in England were given a grant to dissect four corpses each year and this question of appropriate number and allocation of corpses—as well as the intersecting practices of punishment and dissection—continues for centuries.
7. With a few notable exceptions, many physicians up to this point would have relied upon "preparators" to do the messy work of preparing bodies for anatomy lessons. These individuals would have been trained to do the knife work, while the respected instructor would use pointing instruments or lecture from above the corpse (as seen in Hogarth's engraving). With an increasing enthusiasm for experimentation, however, and an increasing respect for the more hands-on profession of surgery, more and more doctors performed their own dissections.
8. Kemp and Wallace, *Spectacular Bodies*, 22.
9. Elizabeth Stephens, *Anatomy as Spectacle: Public Exhibitions of the Body from 1700 to the Present*, Representations: Health, Disability, Culture (Liverpool: Liverpool University Press, 2011) and Helen MacDonald, *Human Remains: Episodes in Human Dissection* (Melbourne, VIC: Melbourne University Press, 2005), 4.

10. Barbara Maria Stafford, *Body Criticism: Imaging the Unseen in Enlightenment Art and Medicine* (Cambridge, MA: MIT Press, 1993), 48.
11. Porter, *Bodies Politic*, 49.
12. Corinna Wagner, *Pathological Bodies: Medicine and Political Culture* (Berkeley: University of California Press, 2013), 6.
13. "Donate Life America," accessed July 17, 2015, http://donatelife.net/.
14. Richardson, "Human Dissection and Organ Transplantation," and Sharp, *Strange Harvest*.
15. Ibid., 154.
16. For more on Eakins and the role of these paintings in the context of medicine in the nineteenth century, see Amy Werbel, *Thomas Eakins: Art, Medicine, and Sexuality in Nineteenth-Century Philadelphia* (New Haven: Yale University Press, 2007).
17. Sharp, *Strange Harvest*, 5.
18. James Blake Bailey, *The Diary of a Resurrectionist*, 1811–1812 to Which Are Added an Account of the Resurrection Men in London and a Short History of the Passing of the Anatomy Act, 2010, http://www.gutenberg.org/ebooks/32614. Both Mary Roach, *Stiff: The Curious Lives of Human Cadavers* (New York: W. W. Norton, 2003) and Richardson, "Human Dissection and Organ Transplantation," also offer analysis of *Diary of a Resurrectionist*. Roach reads these passages to explore the psychology of men working in the body-snatching trade.
19. Robert Louis Stevenson, "The Body-Snatcher," in *The Body Snatcher and Other Stories* (New York: Signet Classics, 1988), 1–19.
20. See also Sander Gilman, *Picturing Health and Illness: Images of Identity and Difference* (Baltimore: Johns Hopkins University Press, 1995); Roy Porter, *Bodies Politic*; Michael Sappol, *A Traffic of Dead Bodies*; and Elizabeth Stephens, *Anatomy as Spectacle*.
21. For a more thorough discussion of the anonymous donor "rule" and donor families' work to challenge this widespread practice, see Sharp's *Strange Harvest*; Sharon R. Kaufman, "Fairness and the Tyranny of Potential in Kidney Transplantation," *Current Anthropology* 54, no. S7 (October 1, 2013): S56–66; Robert Steinbrook, "Public Solicitation of Organ Donors," *New England Journal of Medicine* 353, no. 5 (August 4, 2005): 441–444; and Tilney, *Transplant*.
22. Sanjib Kumar Ghosh, "Human Cadaveric Dissection: A Historical Account from Ancient Greece to the Modern Era," *Anatomy & Cell Biology* 48, no. 3 (September 2015): 153–169.
23. Roach, *Stiff*, 39.
24. Douglas R. Reifler, "'I Actually Don't Mind the Bone Saw': Narratives of Gross Anatomy," *Literature and Medicine* 15, no. 2 (1996): 183–199.

25. Rita Charon, *Narrative Medicine: Honoring the Stories of Illness* (Oxford: Oxford University Press, 2006).
26. *NOTA Proceedings*, 342.
27. Richardson, "Human Dissection and Organ Transplantation," 158.
28. Sappol, *A Traffic of Dead Bodies*; Stephens, *Anatomy as Spectacle*; and Wagner, *Pathological Bodies.*
29. "The permanent anatomy theater became an architectural genre in its own right, and a conspicuous feature in a number of European seats of learning." Kemp and Wallace, *Spectacular Bodies*, 24.
30. Stafford, *Body Criticism*, 54.
31. Lawrence Cohen, "The Other Kidney: Biopolitics Beyond Recognition," in *Commodifying Bodies*, ed. Nancy Scheper-Hughes and Loïc J. D Wacquant (London: Sage, 2002), 9–29.
32. Wendy Moore, *The Knife Man: The Extraordinary Life and Times of John Hunter, Father of Modern Surgery* (New York: Broadway Books, 2005), 39–40.
33. Although Hunter is credited by the Oxford English Dictionary as the first person to use the term "transplant," Charles Allen, in fact, used the term first in his 1685 book *The Operator for Human Teeth*. David Hamilton, *A History of Organ Transplantation: Ancient Legends to Modern Practice* (Pittsburgh, PA: University of Pittsburgh Press, 2012), 40.
34. Sharp, *Strange Harvest*, 34.
35. Quoted in Moore, *The Knife Man*, 42.
36. Quoted in Tilney, *Transplant*, 23.
37. Edgar Allan Poe, "A Premature Burial," in *The Complete Tales and Poems of Edgar Allan Poe* (New York: Vintage Books, 1975), 258–268.
38. *Body Worlds* has also spawned significant critical attention, including works by Stephen Bates, "Bodies Impolitic? Reading Cadavers," *International Journal of Communication* 4 (2010): 198–219; Connor; Jane Desmond, "Postmortem Exhibitions: Taxidermied Animals and Plastinated Corpses in the Theaters of the Dead," *Configurations* 16, no. 3 (Fall 2008): 347–378; Petra Kuppers, "Visions of Anatomy: Exhibitions and Dense Bodies," *Differences: A Journal of Feminist Cultural Studies* 15, no. 3 (Fall 2004): 123–156; Stephens Leibodd, *Anatomy as Spectacle*; Megan Stern, "Dystopian Anxieties versus Utopian Ideals: Medicine from Frankenstein to the Visible Human Project and Body Worlds," *Science as Culture* 15, no. 2 (2006): 1–24; Jose van Dijck, "Bodyworlds: The Art of Plastinated Cadavers," *Configurations* 9, no. 1 (Winter 2001): 99–126; and Tony Walter, "Body Worlds: Clinical Detachment and Anatomical Awe," *Sociology of Health & Illness* 26, no. 4 (May 2004): 464–488.
39. Desmond, "Postmortem Exhibitions," 347.
40. Ibid., 367 and Stephens, *Anatomy as Spectacle*, 4.

41. For more on the tension between authenticity and mediation in *Body Worlds*, see van Dijck, "Bodyworlds," 110.
42. Petra Kuppers makes a similar point about the imperfect nature of von Hagens's simulacra, where the plastinates seem to have little to do with the bodies or lives of visitors. Kuppers, "Visions of Anatomy," 134.
43. Bates, "Bodies Impolitic?" 208.
44. For more on wax modeling in the tradition of anatomical exhibition, see Kemp and Wallace, *Spectacular Bodies*; Wagner, *Pathological Bodies*; and Stephens, *Anatomy as Spectacle*.
45. Gunther von Hagens, "Bodyworlds," *Bodyworlds*, accessed June 29, 2015, http://www.bodyworlds.com/en.html.
46. Kuppers, "Visions of Anatomy," 138.
47. The principle of the universal body finds an important exception in medical education. The increasing turn to technological modeling to replace gross anatomy classes has met push back from students and educators who argue that hands-on experience with individual cadavers is an essential preparation for the physiological variation they will encounter in a clinical setting. In this debate, the textbook, wax, or computerized model is the universal standard by which anatomy is still largely taught, but dissection offers the opportunity to explore difference.
48. Gunther von Hagens, "On Gruesome Corpses, Gestalt Plastinates and Mandatory Interment," *Brave New Body Worlds: The Question of the Exhibition*, 261, accessed May 11, 2016, http://www.koerperwelten.com/Downloads/OnGruesomeCorpses.pdf.
49. Catherine Waldby's scholarly work on the Visible Human Project demonstrates its role in broader reconceptions of the medicalized body. Catherine Waldby, *The Visible Human Project: Informatic Bodies and Posthuman Medicine* (London: Routledge, 2003).
50. "This warts-and-all style was particularly characteristic of British illustration. Hunter's abrupt severing of the woman's legs, a standard technique in the preparation of obstetric models and other abdominal dissections, is portrayed with a raw directness that underlies the incisive real-ness of the dissection." Kemp and Wallace, *Spectacular Bodies*, 50.
51. See, for example, Rosalind Pollack Petchesky, "Fetal Images: The Power of Visual Culture in the Politics of Reproduction," *Feminist Studies* 13, no. 2 (1987): 263–292 and Joanne Boucher, "Ultrasound: A Window to the Womb? Obstetric Ultrasound and the Abortion Rights Debate," *The Journal of Medical Humanities* 25, no. 1 (2004): 7–19. Also see Chapter 4 connecting anti-abortion activists' use of ultrasound technology to transplant debates regarding anencephalic infants.

52. For more on the role of women in the history of anatomy, see Stephens, *Anatomy as Spectacle*; Stern, "Dystopian Anxieties"; Waldby, "Biomedicine"; and van Dijck, "Bodyworlds."
53. Donna Jeanne Haraway, "A Cyborg Manifesto: Science, Technology, and Socialist-Feminism in the Late Twentieth Century," in *Simians, Cyborgs, and Women: The Reinvention of Nature* (New York: Routledge, 1991).
54. "The No-Nonsense Heart Man of Houston," *Life* (August 2, 1968): 34.
55. It is relevant to note this prohibition is not transhistorical or universal. During the Ebola outbreak of 2014 in West Africa, public health professionals struggled to halt traditional funeral practices in which washing and touching the body of the deceased family member is common.
56. Walter, "Body Worlds: Clinical Detachment," 472.
57. Stern, "Dystopian Anxieties," 63.

CHAPTER 3

Making the Lifelike Corpse

The tools of the [embalming] trade may also include the hardware necessary for external and internal preparation. Mechanical or electrical lifts assist in moving the body, and special tables with gutters and drains are used during the embalming and restoration. The procedure, which ideally should be done within eight hours of death, takes approximately two to three hours and may be preceded by massage and manipulation to break rigor mortis, if present. The body is first undressed, washed, and sprayed with disinfectant soap, and towel-dried. It may also be sprayed with a disinfectant. It is then arranged on a table using a head rest and limb emollient so that the head is above the chest and the body is tilted slightly to the right. It may be washed a second time with soap or bleach, and solvents may be used to remove any stains on skin. Orifices are swabbed and packed with cotton to prevent leakage, and cream may be applied to the hands and face. The mouth is swabbed, and dentures are removed, disinfected, and replaced. Fluids may be drained or suctioned, and the trachea and esophagus are sometimes tied off internally to prevent further secretions. The mouth is stitched manually with mandibular sutures at the gum line and through the nasal septum, wired closed, or pinned with a needle injector. Tissue builder may be injected into the lips to give them fullness if they have flattened. The throat is packed with gauze. The mouth is padded with mortuary putty or cotton (or a plastic or metal mouth-former), if necessary, and given a pleasing expression. The face may be shaved with an electric razor. The eyeballs may be injected with cavity fluid to restore their roundness and knobbed plastic caps are often placed

E. Russell, *Transplant Fictions*,
Palgrave Studies in Literature, Science and Medicine,
https://doi.org/10.1007/978-3-030-12135-8_3

> beneath the lids so that they do not appear sunken. The lids may be sealed shut with vaseline or eye cement, or the lower ones may be tucked underneath the upper lids to rid the eyes of wrinkles.
>
> —Christine Quigley, *The Corpse: A History*

> Richie looked healthy—to his parents he was indestructible, a kid with a lifetime left to live—but his appearance was seriously misleading, for he was in no way being supported by his own resources. Every vital function was connected to a corresponding machine, a process initiated the moment the ambulance had brought him to Charlotte Memorial.
>
> He had been immediately intubated—a plastic endotracheal tube was inserted partway down his throat into the trachea to open his airways—and ventilated, meaning that the tube was connected to an electronic ventilator that would force a prescribed measure of oxygen into his system. As Dick lingered in the tiny curtained cubicle in the ICU, he could see Richie's heart beating strongly, the boy's chest rising and falling twelve times each minute to the perfectly paced thump-clunk sound of the ventilator, which sustained his breathing. Richie was being fed intravenously a solution of glucose and saline through a plastic tube connected to a plastic bag extending from an IV pole above his bed, while a similar apparatus, called a Foley catheter and Foley bag, below the bed, helped him pass urine.
>
> —Lee Gutkind, *Many Sleepless Nights*

From the colonial era to the end of the nineteenth century, funeral practices in America were quiet, even mundane affairs. During peacetime, death generally occurred at home or bodies were brought home in preparation for burial. Family and friends were responsible for laying out the body, wrapping the winding sheet, procuring the plain pine box, and transporting the coffin to the community burial ground. Today, by contrast, death has been largely removed from the home, moved decidedly into the medical and professional domains. Consider the swarm of strangers involved in many contemporary deaths: Hospital personnel, EMTs, a doctor to pronounce legal time of death, hospice workers, the funeral director, and embalmer are just the most common actors in this cast. The rise of the hospital death has recast the stark scene of the corpse laid out in the back bedroom. Authority over the dead and dying now lies firmly in the hands of medical and funerary professionals. This shift toward a medicalization of death, as we have already seen in the case of dissection and anatomy, constitutes an important step in moving away from the corpse as a sacred and inviolable object toward imagining dead bodies as a rich resource for public good.

This shift toward medical authority over the dead and dying is not the only ideological change necessary to pave the way for organ transplantation. A second, related problem is how it becomes possible to understand a corpse as providing the "gift of life." In *Many Sleepless Nights*, Lee Gutkind offers a journalistic account of the pioneering transplant work conducted by Thomas Starzl and his team during the mid-1980s. In his description of one transplant surgery, Gutkind captures the complicated simultaneity of life and death involved in organ transfer. He writes, "If there is a truly special moment, a triumphant instant through the transplant process, this is it. Richie Becker, a fifteen-year-old boy, who is now dead, and whose funeral will take place in Charlotte within a few hours, is giving the gift of life to a dying mother of four children, Winkle Fulk" (309). The word choice in this second sentence—in which "dead," "funeral," "gift of life," and "dying" nearly trip over one another—reveals a rapid shuttling among our conceptions of dying, death, and living. This phrase—"the gift of life"—is so commonly repeated in transplant rhetoric that has entirely lost its strangeness. But why should that be so? What changing notions of death had to occur for this acceptance to become so commonplace?

In order to find life in death, we had to undergo a series of profound changes in how we think about and handle the dead and dying. With the rise in medical authority, death became something to be managed and (ideally) postponed indefinitely. This management occurred through a diverse array of technologies: from hospitalization, artificial respiration, and monitoring of vital signs to embalming and death photography. The rise in these technologies enacts a new concept of the "lifelike" corpse and the "natural" death, both achieved, rather than precluded, by technological intervention. These concepts provide one key conceptual pathway toward transplantation as the gift of life. In other words, we must have existing traditions of finding life in death and the technological management of both the dying and the dead in order to accept the radical intervention of cadaver organ transplantation.

In order to unpack the weighty concepts supporting the ubiquitous phrase "gift of life," this chapter unfolds in two parts. Proceeding somewhat out of order, the first half examines the question of "life" as it attaches to cadavers. How do we move from the inevitability of death, to death as something to be managed, and finally to the seeming life in death found in artificial respiration, embalming, and death photography? Although less than one percent of all deaths in the USA are brain deaths, the ways we think about funerals and everyday practices surrounding dead bodies lay important groundwork for the way we approach cadaver donation. In fact, many of the same principles, especially the idea that the treatment of a body after death should reflect the values of the person in life, find expression in both funeral and organ donation rhetoric. The second half of the chapter explores how altruism—the central premise of our voluntary donation system—emerges as a special form of much more long-standing notions of dead bodies as public resources. In our system, the "gift" of a dead loved one's organs cannot be directed, but must be offered up to the public for distribution according to politically constructed rules of eligibility. This move from individual will to public good is an essential component in the "gift of life," and conceptions of the body as public object connects practices as diverse as the circulation of medieval relics, the life insurance industry, and the public display of political leaders like Lenin and Lincoln. The texts under consideration here are similarly diverse; I draw from book-length accounts by reporters like Lee Gutkind and Jessica Mitford, but also include anthropological studies on artificial respiration in intensive care units. Another textual jump brings into conversation pamphlets on death photography at the turn of the twentieth-century and high modernist literature by Wallace Stevens and William Faulkner. The unifying element in all of this diversity remains a method of cultural critique that unpacks language and representation to discover shared ideological premises. In order to understand how we have managed the liminal space between life and death on all sides of organ exchange, we must understand how these concepts first found expression in more quotidian approaches to death.

Although it's not always thought of as such, the hospital is perhaps our most far-reaching technology for managing death and dying. In his landmark study, *The Hour of Our Death*, Philippe Ariès studies social rituals surrounding death and notes a striking shift in the mid-nineteenth century when death comes under the authority of the doctor and the site of death shifts from the home to the hospital.[1] This trend increases over time in the West. In 1945, most American deaths still occurred in the home; by the 1980s, that number fell to 17%.[2] Death and dying became increasingly hidden, cordoned off in special wards, hospice centers, cemeteries, or funeral homes.[3] Writing in 1955, in the provocatively titled essay "The Pornography of Death," Geoffrey Gorer describes his sense of death as something that has become "unmentionable," like pornography, a process achieved in part by the widespread loss of personal experience with the death of loved ones: "Questioning my old acquaintances, I cannot find one over the age of sixty who did not witness the agony of at least one near relative; I do not think I know a single person under the age of thirty who has had a similar experience."[4] This sea change in our collective experience with death creates the conditions for what Joseph Jacobs called as early as 1900 "the dying of death."[5]

As scientific and medical authority rose in the decades following the Enlightenment, death itself came to be understood as subject to human control. Social historians of death and medicine agree: Death can no longer be understood outside of medical terms and, as such, becomes a risk to be avoided or a disease to be cured.[6] In her essay, "Reflections on the 'Mortal' Body in Late Modernity," Lindsay Prior traces the logic of conquerable death this way: As theories of disease and its documentation grew, they helped "to generate the illusion that death can somehow be controlled. In other words, since death is caused by disease and since, in theory, all diseases are conquerable through human praxis, then death itself is conquerable."[7] This understanding is echoed across the critical literature. Such consensus emerges in the narrow band of language used to describe modern attitudes toward death; in each instance, repeated terms like "control," "prevent," "manage," "intervene," and "authority" express our belief in death as a thing to be managed and avoided. Always far thinking, even Benjamin Franklin gave voice to this fantasy: "It is impossible to imagine the Height to which may be carried, in a thousand years, the Power of Man over Matter.... Agriculture may diminish its labor and double its produce; all diseases may by sure means be prevented if not cured, not excepting Old Age, and our Lives lengthened at pleasure even behind antediluvian Standard."[8]

This belief that death can be controlled and life should be prolonged at all costs provides important conceptual grounding for the radical intervention posed by organ transplantation. Especially in the early days of the procedure, when almost all recipients would die within days or months of surgery, an unshakeable belief in the noble battle against death itself was essential to sustain the work of transplant pioneers. Describing medical interventions at the end of life more broadly, however, some scholars acknowledge that the physician's fight with disease and death can take on a ritual element that moves beyond a rational belief that the treatment will serve the patient. Echoing the language so central to organ donation campaigns, Jessica Muller and Barbara Koenig describe the way that treatments, "offered as 'gifts of life,' take on symbolic meaning for physicians that extends beyond the individual patient to represent medicine's battle with death" (370). In this study of medical residents' definitions of dying, Muller and Koenig argue that procedures that might give a patient "a chance" often overwhelm other perspectives. They write, "Other considerations—that the procedures might very well be futile, that they may only prolong the patient's life for a short period of time, or that the patient may experience considerable suffering as a result of the procedures—become secondary in face of the physicians' overriding concern with fending off premature death" (Muller and Koenig 368). The familiar phrase "prolong life at all costs" captures some of this ambiguity, reminding us of the costs of radical intervention, costs that often go unacknowledged in triumphant accounts of "medical miracles." As one transplant surgeon recasts the problem: "The question is: Are we extending her life by transplanting her—or prolonging her death?"[9]

Transplant patients themselves express ambivalence about treading the borderlands of living and dying. In the following quote from a transplant recipient, note the verbal gymnastics that betray a complex sense of both regret and gratitude about her prolonged life:

> Two months after the transplant, the cancer reappeared in my hip.... I had to have my hip replaced twice. And now I've got it [cancer] in my ribs and I've got it in my lungs. It's hard to say now that I'm not glad I had it [the transplant] done, because otherwise I would have been dead a year ago. It did give me some extra time, and every little bit of time, I guess, helps. Yet so often I think I would have been better off dead, and that way it would be over with. Sometimes I think that all it's done is prolong the misery. If I would have died because I didn't have the transplant, then I wouldn't have gone through all the pain I'm going through now.[10]

With phrases like "it's hard to say now that I'm not glad" and "every little bit of time, I guess, helps," this recipient captures the ambivalent reality of existing in a complicated space of both living and dying. It is important to note that this patient is speaking in the late 1980s and that transplant outcomes and quality of life for recipients have made great strides in the decades since. The realities of post-surgical complications, pain, recurring disease, and repeat transplantations, however, are still unavoidable for many organ recipients. In nearly every sentence, her word choice captures the ambivalence of patients in late-stage disease for whom the costs of prolonged life are very real. In addition to the pain and repeat procedures described here, the "costs" of prolonged life are often also social, psychological, and economic: including strained relationships; fractured sense of self, especially if return to work or everyday activities is impossible; mounting bills from gaps in insurance; and loss of income for patients and caregivers.

The prevailing biomedical vision of death as something to manage and avoid has created conditions in which families and individuals struggle to make meaning from death when it inevitably happens. In placing nearly all of our hope and focus on death as a battle to be won, we are often left without useful social scripts by which to identify or accept dying. Atul Gawande opens his book, *Being Mortal: Medicine and What Matters in the End,* by reflecting on a quote from a Tolstoy novella he encountered during a seminar in medical school. Offering a touchstone moment of the medical humanities, Gawande powerfully articulates for his readers the value of considering literary representation alongside scientific accounts of death and dying. In Tolstoy's *The Death of Ivan Ilyich*, the titular character struggles with the liminal space of dying—that poorly understood period of both life and death—also captured in the organ recipient's quotation above. Tolstoy writes, "What tormented Ivan Ilyich most was the deception, the lie, which for some reason they all accepted, that he was not dying but simply ill, and he only need keep quiet and undergo a treatment and then something very good would result."[11] In these cases, families often surrender their agency to medical authority, for whom "dying" is also a slippery category, often located in a complex constellation of interpretation. This "lie" that families "accept," this denial of dying, is made possible by the cordoning off of death, by taking it outside of common experience and locating it in the specialized space of the hospital and under medical authority. The rising dominion of the hospital "remove[s] death from the home and render[s] it artificial, arranged, civilization's chief product."[12] But in order to move forward and understand how technologies like artificial respiration and heart rate monitors paradoxically enact a new mode of "natural" death for families, we need to return to the once common phenomenon of the death at home.

In the American literary context, few works capture death at home's peculiar combination of the quotidian and the profound like Wallace Stevens's "The Emperor of Ice-Cream":

Call the roller of big cigars,
The muscular one, and bid him whip
In kitchen cups concupiscent curds.
Let the wenches dawdle in such dress
As they are used to wear, and let the boys
Bring flowers in last month's newspapers.
Let be be finale of seem.
The only emperor is the emperor of ice-cream.

Take from the dresser of deal,
Lacking the three glass knobs, that sheet
On which she embroidered fantails once
And spread it so as to cover her face.
If her horny feet protrude, they come
To show how cold she is, and dumb.
Let the lamp affix its beam.
The only emperor is the emperor of ice-cream.[13]

The poem was first published in 1922 and likely set in Key West, Florida, where a quiet, domestic laying out would have still been common. Both the poem's theme and its basic action are notoriously dense. In the first stanza, the "roller of big cigars" is called to "whip … concupiscent curds," serving girls called "wenches" wear their typical dress, and boys bring flowers to the home. These details set a sensual, even celebratory, tone and the final line offers the famously opaque, even silly sounding: "the only emperor is the emperor of ice-cream." The penultimate line of the first stanza, however, suggests something of the turn the poem will take: "Let be be finale of seem."

This line makes more sense in the context of the next stanza, where the accumulation of details alerts us to the fact that while the sensual flirting is taking place in the kitchen, there is a corpse laid out in the back bedroom. From the plain "dresser of deal, lacking three pine knobs" is taken a hand-embroidered sheet to "cover her face." Then, "If her horny feet protrude, they come to show how cold she is, and dumb." We now understand that this shrouded, supine figure is the corpse of an elderly woman. The stanza concludes by repeating the line "the only emperor is the emperor of ice-cream."

A few correspondences unite the details of the first and second stanzas, demonstrating the unity of both setting and theme in the poem. Where the ice cream can be expected to be cold in the first, the body is explicitly "cold" in the second. The flowers brought by local boys in old newspapers are not romantic, but funeral flowers. The physicality of the muscular roller of cigars, whipping ice cream in the kitchen is transferred to the strikingly physical reminder of the dead old woman's "horny feet." Given these connections between stanzas, the confusing line, "let be be finale of seem," could now reasonably be explicated as "death brings a reminder of stark reality, opposing the romantic illusion of the sensual." The "only emperor" line also suggests a toppling of God and religious meaning in life and death. Stevens's thematic argument about the eventual priority of physical reality resonates with the social meaning of the home death.

The corpse was deeply present in domestic space, and death was a starkly pragmatic reality for Americans into the early twentieth century. While Stevens famously said that his poem contained "something of the essential gaudiness of poetry,"[14] the lines describing the corpse are importantly plain and stark. The poem tells us that material things break down even as they assert their presence, from the pine dresser missing knobs to the corpse's protruding and horny feet. The quotidian nature of these details—dresser, sheet, and old newspapers—remind us that death was a common part of domestic life in America. High rates of child mortality meant that most families had buried one or more children. Multigenerational households saw adults and children caring for dying grandparents. For many women, widowhood was a "primary, lifelong social role" communicated by clothing and social address.[15] As such, dead bodies laid out in the home served as a reminder of the material and social demands of the body and death.

The notion that family have a social responsibility to the dead body is a cornerstone of contemporary organ donation conversations, where procurement specialists harken back to a century before and encourage kin to take a stronger role in decision-making about their loved one's dead body. In her account of eighteenth- and nineteenth-century funeral practices, Ruth Richardson describes the strong sense of social responsibility to the body while at home: "People tried not to leave the body alone. It was considered a duty to 'watch' the body day and night.... Families shared this task, which derived from a sense that between death and burial the body had needs, one of which was to be kept company" (152). This account of nineteenth-century vigils resonates with current practices of keeping watch over a family member while on life support. In cadaver donation, where the vast majority of cases involve brain death after artificial respiration, families must grapple with a return to centuries-old realities where corpses were strikingly present and social responsibilities included dealing not just with mourning the lost loved one but with the practical considerations of the corpse itself.

Artificial Life and Natural Death

The special case of artificial respiration foregrounds an enduring tension between "dead" and "dying," or the difference between conceptions of death as a finite event and death as a process, unfolding unevenly over time. In addition to popular belief in the special social needs of the body described by Richardson above, cultural critic Christine Quigley describes commonplace attitudes which understood life and death existing in a kind of simultaneity: "In the early 1900s, the consensus of theological opinion held that a person was alive for up to a half an hour after apparent death due to lingering illness and at least an hour after a sudden accident. The soul was thought to adhere to the body for some time after the cessation of circulation and respiration."[16] Although these theological debates fell away in the face of rising medical authority, they have been replaced by contemporary arguments about the appropriate timing of organ retrieval. Deborah Lupton draws from Michel Foucault's work to argue, "Following the spread of the dissection of corpses, death became not a single moment in time, but a series of 'partial deaths,' of small changes in parts of the body at different times" (44). This notion of "partial deaths" that can impact "parts of the body" becomes an essential condition for families to grapple with the simultaneous death of their loved one and the possibility of a "gift of life" that follows an extracted body part.

Returning to the case of Richie Becker (the cadaver donor described above from Lee Gutkind's *Many Sleepless Nights*), his parents express the difficulty of making his dire condition real for visiting friends and family:

> "The day after the accident, the phone kept ringing off the hook. It was kids from school, and they kept saying, 'I've heard the horriblest thing, that Richie is dead.'"
>
> I would listen and I would say, "No, not exactly, he's still on the respirator."
>
> "Oh, thank God."
>
> "Wait a minute. You don't understand. Richie is clinically brain dead."
>
> "Well, just so long as there's hope." (76)

The Becker case illustrates the multiple, simultaneous effects of artificial respiration and its impact on our understanding of death. On the one hand, seeing the chest rise and the heartbeat on the monitor makes it difficult to believe Richie is, in fact, brain dead. At the same time, this artificial preservation of organs—a process that relies on Richie's own circulatory system—makes the gift of life possible. Artificial respiration also extends the temporality of "death" and can provide families with a window that allows them to come to terms with the reality of death, creating time to imagine previously unconsidered options like organ donation.[17] Taken together, these conflicting effects of artificial respiration on loved ones' ability to grapple with the meaning of death and organ donation demonstrate the real-life complexities faced by families and organ procurement organizations.

As argued above, one of the gaps of contemporary culture is our inability to meaningfully transition from a medical battle with illness to death as an unavoidable outcome. While we have wholly backed medical technology in the fight with disease, we hold a contradictory viewpoint that the presence of technology is at odds with a "good death." Our notions of humane and dignified dying are deeply enmeshed in our widely held dichotomy between the natural and artificial. In the past half-century, much of the critical literature on death includes a lament about the loss of humanity and familial care that accompanies death in hospital settings.[18] Many of the goals of hospice and palliative medicine include limiting the loved ones' experience of technical intervention as death approaches. The following quote from a widow, recorded five months after the death of her spouse, captures an important ambivalence in lay attitudes toward the role of technology and death. She tells researcher Jane Seymour:

> I knew when he left [the other hospital] that there wasn't much chance, to me he more or less died here.... In the [ITU] they were only keeping him alive there artificially. I realised there wouldn't be much chance you know... I wish now that I hadn't agreed to, er, taking him to [ITU] and he'd just died here... I mean [he] would have loved it, being attached to all that machinery, he loved all that sort of thing you know, but the chances of him pulling through were very small. (1241)

Like the complexity of language expressed by the transplant recipient above, this quote is peppered with ambivalent phrasing. Word choice like "to me he more or less died here" demonstrates an understanding of death that relies on a definition that is both relational—"to me"—and unstable—"more or less." The notion that her husband "would have loved" the technological intervention is similarly important in family decisions about organ transplantation and death more broadly, as we embrace the notion that a "good death" is one that expresses the individual's values and interests in life.

While both scholars and laypersons tend to think of technology and dignified dying in mutually exclusive terms, recent research on the withdrawal of artificial respiration suggests quite the opposite. In practice, clinicians use medical technology to create an experience of death that reflects loved ones' expectations about how dying will occur.[19] A series of studies published between 1997 and 2009 examine the relationship between technology and death in emergency room or intensive care units.[20] These scholars agree that rather than serving as an obstacle to "natural" death, careful regulation of drugs and machine intervention can allow doctors to enact or stage a death that families will perceive as *more* natural and dignified. As Jane Seymour argues, "during death, medical technology becomes *constitutive of* 'the natural' in so far as it frames and determines perceptions and thinking about the way things *should* happen" (1249). Making a similar case, Janet Harvey writes, "there is a procedural attempt to regulate, routinise and produce a *standard* death" (724). Harvey continues, dying trajectories "generally [do] not represent a 'switching off' of technology as depicted in popular mythology and the tabloid media (this applies only to 'brain death') but a *process* of withdrawal, which takes place over time" (724). This process, which is crucially produced by technology, conforms to our expectations of death having a "natural course," one that unfolds over time and registers as peaceful to onlookers. These scholars offer an important intervention in discussions of end of life care, suggesting that we may have been too quick to assume "natural death" meant limited technical intervention.

The ubiquitous hospital practice of monitoring patients illustrates a special and complicated case of the mingling of technology and family experiences of contemporary death. Screen displays of blood pressure, heart activity, and oxygen levels can take on totemic levels of importance for family members struggling to understand the opaque processes of the body. In his observations of a Norwegian intensive care unit,

Hans Hadders found that medical monitoring serves an essential role in enacting death:

> Physicians and nurses attest that it is common that relatives fix their gaze on the monitor screen. Indeed, to some extent relatives learn how to follow a patient's physiological status via the monitor screen. The monitor, which initially may have appeared alienating or scary to them, gradually provides them with some form of security. When they have become accustomed to this technological medium they may shift their gaze from the monitor screen toward the patient and back again within seconds, not unlike the way staff observe patients during their work. Thus, for relatives, observing medical technological enactment of the life of their loved one becomes just as important an ontological mooring for them as seeing or touching him/her. (581)

This scene offers an emblematic example of the twentieth-century shift from death at home to a hospital death highly managed through medical technology. Family members become good disciplinary subjects, trained to reject the alienating elements of the monitor and instead accept it as a channel for the appropriate care of the dying. Holding a hand and watching a monitor achieve a kind of equivalence as family members come to understand real-time status reports as essential to their own experience of the death trajectory. Interviews with nurses, however, reveal continued expressions of ambivalence toward the role of technology at the time of death. Some healthcare professionals find families' focus on bedside monitors to be excessive and make it a point to turn off alarms and screens so that relatives will re-center their attention to the patient (Hadders 581). Others embrace the monitor as an important way to facilitate relatives' understanding of death; says one nurse, "The famous 'flat line' display visible on the monitor can be very significant, but not necessarily in a bad sense, as it can help finalize the death and enable acceptance" (Hadders 583). This ambivalence demonstrates the way that contradictory impulses toward a single phenomenon can coexist. In practice, electronic monitoring can be both dehumanizing *and* reassuring, producing a complex of emotional reactions and competing narratives about death's "natural course."

It is important to remember that families of brain-dead donors will not have an opportunity to participate in these enacted moments of finality and acceptance. Since artificial respiration must persist through the procurement surgery, relatives will say good-bye to a loved one who they understand to be brain dead, but who is still registering heart and lung function on the monitor. This disjunct between the evidence of their eyes and the diagnosis they've been told reveals the heights of medical authority in cases of organ procurement. While donor families won't get the psychological benefits of this technological enactment of death, these scenes of removing artificial respiration are nevertheless relevant to our concept of transplantation. Death in the intensive care unit provides an important reframing of the relationship between medical technology and "the natural." By uncovering this paradoxical understanding of technology as a producer of a dignified and natural death, we can make sense of the radical surgical interventions necessary in organ procurement.

Once we put pressure on the axiomatic belief in "natural death" as being free from medical intervention, we find numerous examples of technology serving as a long-standing mediator in our most common modern experiences of death and dying. In her study of transplant memorials, Lesley Sharp describes a related phenomenon she calls "the greening of the donor body."[21] From illustrations of trees signifying death as new growth or slogans like "go recycle yourself," donation and transplant are recast as natural processes, more "natural," in fact, than traditional death and funeral practices. Even before artificial respiration techniques were widely adopted, the funeral technologies of embalming and death photography were advertised using the language of "natural" and "life-like." In this way, the conceptual groundwork is laid for organ transfer as the "gift of life." Organ "harvesting," then, becomes not the dystopic vision of science fiction, but a celebrated and natural transfer of life from death.

Seeming Life in Death

From its simple domestic beginnings, the USA has seen two important pendulum swings in funeral practice over the past one hundred years. Each of these swings is essential in making cadaver donation conceptually possible. The first swing brings us toward lavish, expensive funerals with almost universal embalming. The second lies in the backlash toward these perceived excesses and opens the door for funeral alternatives like cremation or organ donation. Jessica Mitford's groundbreaking exposé of the funeral industry, *The American Way of Death*, was published in 1963, the same year in which the first kidney, lung, and liver were recovered from deceased donors. This timing meant that just as many Americans were reconsidering the status quo in funeral practice, medicine offered a new alternative, one that seemed to embrace many of the values of the funerals Americans had experienced, but which replaced the exposed commercialism of the funeral industry with the possibility of expressing altruism and social responsibility. Like the sister practices of anatomy and dissection, each important phase in American funeral practice—from domestic simplicity, to highly managed funeral events, to the current diversity of options including space burial and human composting—is a crucial step in establishing the key ideological tenets of organ donation.

Along with Mitford, social historians have explored practices like embalming, death photography, wakes, professionally staged funerals, and commercialization of cemeteries to account for a new American "way of death" that emerged after the Civil War. These studies provide fascinating windows into elements of American life (and death) that are often seen as unseemly or pathological. In his study of professional pamphlets and advertisements from photographers in the nineteenth century, Jay Ruby discovered discussions of taking photographs of the deceased that were both frank and practical. In one striking example, a photographer offers the following advice:

> Place your camera at the foot of the lounge, get your plate ready, and then comes the most important part of the operation (opening the eyes), this you can effect handily by using the handle of a teaspoon; put the upper lids down, they will stay; turn the eyeball around to its proper place, and you will have the face nearly as natural as life.[22]

Although this photographer allows that it is probably best to send the family from the room as some of the practices described might offend their sensibilities, he seems to take for granted the hands-on requirements of the job. Consider this frank description in contrast to the highly euphemistic world of funerals today in which the term "death" is almost never used. We have caskets, not coffins; the deceased or Mrs. X, instead of corpse or body; funeral directors, not undertakers; coach, not hearse; preparation room, not morgue (Mitford 52).[23] We can imagine how today's funeral directors might cringe at this photographer's frank discussion of teaspoons and eyeballs.

The grotesque elements of the above description, however, should not obscure the crucial final phrase in the photographer's advice: "you will have a face nearly as natural as life." The first great pendulum swing toward the typically elaborate funeral of the twentieth century came with the advances in embalming techniques at the turn of the century. The first goal of embalming was preservation in the interests of travel. Soldiers who died during the Civil War were typically sent home in caskets by train and all involved understood the value of fending off decomposition for as long as possible. As America's living population similarly took to the rails and became increasingly far-flung, families wished for the ability to delay funerals to allow for mourning relatives to return for the service.

In *Inventing the American Way of Death: 1830–1920*, James Farrell argues that American acceptance of embalming at the turn of the century was consistent with a host of related factors. Americans "were unconsciously impressed by a concurrence of events—an increased concern for appearances in a consumer culture, a strong and widely publicized sanitary movement, surgical pretensions in an age of respected medicine, a privatization of the home, etc.—which disposed them to accept embalming" (Farrell 7). By placing embalming in a conceptual lineage with more mundane principles like consumerism or sanitation, Farrell demonstrates how a practice that could have been received with shock and revulsion became normalized. The first half of this volume charts a similar pathway toward the widespread acceptance of cadaver organ transfer, revealing a diverse web of practices and concepts that serve as a foundation for later deviations from the norm.

From this first desire for preservation in the interests of travel came a second interest in making the corpse appear as "lifelike" as possible. All of the early advertisements for new chemicals and techniques in embalming touted the ability to restore the look of life to the newly dead. In his study of the ideological effects of embalming, John Troyer describes a 1902 entry called "Bigsa Man" at the Chicago College of Embalming exhibition. Crowds of funeral professionals marveled, in "a testament to how striking it was at the time to see a corpse looking so incredibly *alive*."[24]

Although the Bigsa Man was exhibited primarily to other funeral professionals, the elements that authorized this presentation were similar to strategies used in anatomical exhibition more broadly. Cabinets of curiosity and museums advertise the reality of the specimens on display, but it is a highly modified "real" that halts decomposition and replaces the wet, smelly, unstable body with clean, fixed, and odorless material. Technological intervention offers a path by which death becomes palatable for viewers, a "drying out" similar to popular museum shows of mummies and other anatomical specimens.[25] In the embalming process, the body is drained of its own fluid, which is then replaced by chemicals (typically formaldehyde and water or alcohol) including a drying agent to make the body appear more lifelike. Embalming offers a safe confrontation with death by suggesting a kind of life in death. The fearful or gruesome aspects of death become primarily attached to decay, but by arresting decomposition, embalming isolates the body in a temporary state withheld from the harshest material realities of death.

These presentations of the corpse are in fact highly mediated, but the language of "lifelike" and "natural" obscures the mediating hand of technology. Preserved corpses—from the extravagant setting of *Body Worlds* discussed in Chapter 2, to the anatomy theater, to the open casket at the funeral—offer not a direct confrontation with death, but an approach that is highly structured in the interests of psychic safety and comfort. The corpse at a funeral, after all, is not simply embalmed, but wearing its best clothes, presented as "merely sleeping" in a comfortable casket, and surrounded by flowers, soothing music, religious ritual, and nourishing food. It is this possibility of technical and conceptual management that provides a model for how we might reconceive of cadaver organs in registers contrary to death. As John Troyer argues, "The corpse was no longer controlled by biological death in the late nineteenth century; rather, human control of the corpse and the 'death' it presented became mediated by human actors" (35). Like the medicalization of the corpse so central to the practice of dissection, increasing human control over the corpse in the everyday circumstances of death extends the hope of managed death and paves the way toward bolder forms of control. This opening for greater intervention includes the fantasy of prolonging life for as long as possible through practices like organ transplant.

Controlling time becomes a fundamental theme in both embalming practices and organ transplant. The practical demands of corpse preservation drove technological advancements in the field of embalming, but these practices in turn delivered a new conception of decay as a measure of time that could be arrested or slowed. Here, technical intervention produced the seeming ability to halt the passage of time, to isolate the dead body from the moment closest to life. In transplantation, too, time serves as the structuring trope in the lives of those seeking transplant and in the moments after death for donors and their families. Nearly, every human interest or news story covering transplantation begins with statistics covering the number of people needing new organs and the number of people who die each day while still waiting. At times, the UNOS Web site has included a ticking clock, counting off a live, to-the-minute tally of candidates joining the national transplant list, visually driving home the seemingly urgent gap between supply and demand.[26] The duration of time spent on dialysis, time spent since joining the candidate list, and life expectancy are all important ways that potential organ recipients account for their experience.

Time is important for cadaver donors, too. Organ deterioration happens in a matter of minutes when blood and oxygen are no longer delivered biologically or artificially. Major debates have emerged among clinicians and medical ethicists who have struggled to define appropriate guidelines for the proper interval between "death" and organ retrieval. The importance of time across these very different positions in the transplant world is made possible, in part, by an increasing sense of human control over time. It is useful to recall in this discussion that the development of artificial respiration—colloquially, "life support"—was essential in allowing doctors to prolong a "lifelike" condition for patients; it opened the door to new sources of organs for transplant and prompted the definition of a new category of death that we know as "brain death." Even before the mid-century advent of life support, however, embalming techniques allowed lay individuals to both imagine and experience a corpse that was no longer wholly subject to the biological demands of death and decay.

In a specific expression of the medical fantasy of controlling death entirely, organ transfer requires a series of technologically choreographed deaths. In addition to the brain-dead cadaver whose cessation of artificial respiration is carefully orchestrated, the organ recipient will typically lie dead on the operating table, waiting for his or her new lungs or heart. These technological interventions will continue to take an emotional toil on the organ recipient. Even after "the gift of life," patients can struggle with the change in outlook involved in transitioning "from the point of inevitable death toward an elusive but considerably more optimistic outlook—especially while bedbound, surrounded by a maze of tubes, wires, machinery."[27] Caught in the sustaining web of medical technology, patients must understand their new lease on life as being contingent on an extensive system of drugs, checkups, and (often) repeat hospitalizations.

In the more common experience of the funeral, the work of the embalmer and the reconstruction of the corpse—even those severely damaged in death—change American ideas of how "normal" and "natural" dead bodies should appear.[28] This buffering from even known material realities—as in the restoration of severed limbs, crushed bones, or bullet wounds—produces a new expectation for the corpse as the product of technical intervention. The next step away from the tyranny of decay in death allows for even greater intervention in breaking down cadavers, extracting parts of value to others, and reconstituting the body for a funeral. In fact, one of the frequently asked questions often included on donor brochures reads, "Can I still have an open casket funeral for my loved one?" Procurement specialists are quick to answer: yes. This reassuring notion that parts of the cadaver can be removed but the body can be restored to a seeming wholeness in an open casket is an important psychological hurdle to overcome for many donor families.

The importance of a seemingly whole dead body, even after parts have been removed, in fact, has a long tradition in both embalming and death photography. The goal in each case is to produce an image as lifelike as possible. The two technologies have crucially entwined histories. Critics of film and photography will be familiar with André Bazin's famous remark that "the photograph embalms time." But as Margaret Schwartz elaborates, "Photography is not only like embalming … embalming is like photography."[29] When embalming became widespread in the 1890s, death photography had already emerged almost three decades earlier.[30] As such, the aesthetic of the death photograph, with its emphasis on seemingly sleeping corpses, influenced the stylistic choices of embalmers. The two forms of technological preservation, then, reinforced each other in look and theme.

Just as with embalming, both professional advertisements and documented responses to death photographs repeat the key terms "natural" and "lifelike." Jay Ruby's sociocultural study of the practice of death photography reveals how these photographs and relatives' reception of them reveal important attitudes about death and dying in America. In one typical example, a letter reads, "I am glad you could get so good a picture of the little darling dead Mabel as you did, the fore head and hair look so natural."[31] In some pictures, the corpses are posed sitting upright as if alive; in another example, a mother painted open eyes onto the framed image of her dead daughter.[32] The most common and natural-seeming pose for the recently deceased is what Ruby calls "the last sleep," in which the body seems to be simply sleeping on the couch. Such images correspond to a dominant ideology that turned from direct confrontations of death and replaced it with euphemism, especially in terms like "sleep" and "at rest." Death becomes an unnatural state, and the look of lifelike sleep or rest, paradoxically achieved through technical intervention, becomes *more* natural.

This concept of the lifelike and natural corpse opens the door to explore one of the tricky contradictions in procurement rhetoric about corpses. On the one hand, families of brain-dead patients must reject the visual evidence of a breathing, heartbeating loved one to understand him or her as truly dead. On the other hand, they are told to understand the donation as a gift of life (not death) and, often, to imagine something of the deceased moving on to the new body. This expression of altruism—typically cast as heroic—requires a complex conceptual tension between the fact of death and the seeming of life.

This seeming life in death becomes the dominant aesthetic in death photography. One of Jay Ruby's major contentions is that death photography is a common, but underground, practice during a century in which Americans have participated in a society-wide denial of death. With this claim, Ruby offers an important counter-argument to more common critiques of death photography as a morbid or exceptional practice. The most famous commentary in this line is Michael Lesy's *Wisconsin Death Trip* (1973), which suggests that death photography is symptomatic of a deeper pathology in Midwestern America. In contrast, Ruby argues that these photos served as a common means for families to mourn and preserve memories of their dead.

The rise of social media in the early twenty-first century may be proving Ruby right. While it is beyond my scope to calculate their frequency, Facebook posts and blogs memorializing stillborn or dead children through photographs are not uncommon. One public Facebook group called "Heavensbook Angels" describes its mission as "giving others the space to grieve on social media through pictures, quotes, and gifts."[33] Its founder, Sandra Homer, created the group after receiving harsh comments when she posted online pictures of her son, stillborn at 38 weeks. The site's related. com page and Etsy shop offer bracelets and other memorials for parents in similar positions. This and similarly public exchanges of images of dead children may parallel a growing change in the transplant donor community. As Lesley Sharp documents, families are increasingly pushing back against anonymity requirements and seeking more public acknowledgment of the cadaver donor. This backlash against anonymity highlights the dynamic of denial that structures many stories told about transplantation. While many in the transplant community will acknowledge that "some must die" in order for others to live,[34] these deaths are typically obscured by symbols of life, rebirth, and transformation; donor literature is littered with trees, leaves, water, and butterflies. Contemporary death photography can challenge more traditional, sanitized memorial practices, by puncturing the fantasy of death as a clean recycling. In this sense, technologies of death are importantly ambiguous. Artificial respiration, embalming, and death photography may produce a "lifelike" image, but the mediating suffix "like" is essential here. The seeming life in death that is created in these technological interventions offers a reminder of the complex and sometimes contradictory ideology of organ donation.

As a sideshow cousin to the death photograph, the nineteenth century also saw a rise in spirit photography. Tom Gunning argues in his essay "Phantom Images and Modern Manifestations," that the spiritualism movement rejected the Calvinist emphasis on faith and sought scientific and technological verification of supernatural forces. Again, we see the theme of technological control over death. Some photographers of the era, most notably William Mumler, who was eventually prosecuted for fraud, would sell pricey "spirit photographs." These portraits would feature the sitter "in the company of ghosts,"[35] usually transparent images of famous dead persons or deceased relatives. As in artificial respiration and embalming, technology serves as the vehicle for breaching the absolute boundary of death; here, the figure of the deceased can return in limitless reproduction. Gunning employs the dual concepts of the uncanny and the double to understand the effects of this photography. Both ideas are relevant to organ transplant, where the cadaver donor is understood as existing in a postmortem state of separation and replication in the bodies of new recipients. The Web site for UNOS announces triumphantly, "one organ donor can save eight lives." Donor families typically emphasize the multiplicative potential of the retrieval surgery, expressing hope that their loved one will help or even "live on" in up to a dozen imagined recipients. These organs and tissues cross the boundary of death to create an uncanny state of "dead but living on."

For many donor kin, spirit photography has an even more direct resonance with their experience. In *Strange Harvest*, Lesley Sharp includes examples of ghost stories in her study of how people memorialize organ donors. She writes, "All donor family counselors have stories about how various parties read peculiar events as evidence that donors can assert themselves beyond the grave."[36] Rather than discounting the veracity of these stories, Sharp argues, "I view ghost stories told by donor kin as a key component of the complex narrative structure so intrinsic to organ transfer."[37] Given the intense psychological weight resting on the notion that something essential of the donor will follow the organs, it is not surprising that families would find supernatural evidence of life persisting beyond death.

Funeral as Values Statement

By focusing on altruism and appeals to what the deceased "would have wanted," hospital discussions and media campaigns represent organ donation as an expression of personal values. In the USA, funerals serve a similar function. In the current pendulum swing in funeral practice—away from lavish services with lifelike corpses and toward diverse alternatives—America has retained a fundamental understanding about what funerals as a "way of death" are supposed to communicate about the deceased and their families. For funeral directors and their clients, funerals are intended to be an expression of the values and status of the deceased. This form of expression has been so important that for decades in the twentieth century, funerals constituted the third most expensive household purchase behind a house and a car. According to the National Association of Funeral Directors, the average cost of an American funeral in the early twenty-first century is between $7000 and 10,000. For our purposes, it is important to note that the massive expenses associated with modern funerals have some roots in the history of anatomy as well as contemporary offshoots in transplant policy. One effect of Britain's Anatomy Act of 1832 was increased sales of burial insurance among the poor; fear of dying in the workhouse and being subject to the anatomist's scalpel was reason enough for Victorians to buy into penny-a-week policies that would save them from that fate.[38] The broad social stigma attached to a "pauper's funeral" contributed to the social currency attached to a more elaborate funeral as a public display of financial security. In the modern context, the continuing high cost of funerals influences current discussions about revisions to transplant policy that might address concerns about organ scarcity. Some suggest that one way around the prohibition against paying directly for organs would be to offer relatives money to offset funeral costs. Funerals, as we can see, have important social and economic dimensions that condition the choices made by surviving relatives.

In her typically engaging prose, Jessica Mitford, scourge of the funeral industry, captures how funerals emerged as an expression of personal status and values: "over the years the funeral men have constructed their own grotesque cloud-cuckoo-land where the trappings of Gracious Living are transformed, as in a nightmare, into the trappings of Gracious Dying" (14–15). What is fascinating for the context of transplantation, moreover, is the way that this treatment of corpse as status symbol becomes redeployed among Organ Procurement Organizations (OPOs). Once we generally agree that what happens to the body immediately after death should be an expression of a person's identity and position, then we have laid the groundwork for discovering better, more appropriate ways to express individual values.

In a consumer and image-driven society, however, personal values can be channeled through expensive caskets, flowers, and cosmetics. Consider another passage from Mitford:

> Alas, poor Yorick! How surprised he would be to see how his counterpart of today is whisked off to a funeral parlor and is in short order sprayed, sliced, pierced, pickled, trussed, trimmed, creamed, waxed, painted, rouged, and neatly dressed—transformed from a common corpse into a Beautiful Memory Picture. (43)

Here, the excessive nature of Mitford's language parallels the perceived excesses of the industry. In documenting the profit-centered nature of the funeral industry, however, Mitford does not disagree that our treatment of the body in death should express our values. Funerals *can be* an expression of values, she argues, but instead of extravagance, she advocates for the value of simplicity. By most accounts, Mitford's book worked. In 1961 (two years before publication), 3.75% of American dead were cremated (Mitford 111); in 2013, according to the National Funeral Director's Association, that number had risen to 45%. In the western United States, current rates of cremation top 70%. Of course, savvy funeral directors were quick to reassure families that one can still hold a funeral for a cremated relative and to find other profit opportunities. In addition to cremation, organ donation and willed body programs have risen in popularity just when Americans were looking for funeral alternatives.

Organ and cadaver donation represents a particularly attractive alternative because the ideology underlying these practices asserts them as a better expression of individual choice, generosity, and community values. Donors are cast as heroes, and the special kind of death required for cadaver donation is even cast as exceptional, a lucky circumstance for altruistic individuals. Taking over the role of the funeral director, Donate Life tells families "all major religions in the United States … see [organ donation] as the final act of love and generosity toward others." A T-shirt for sale on their Web site includes an image of a heart nestled inside a tree with the tagline: "be kind. love hard. remember." The use of "love" here and the more-typical call upon "life" involves a powerful recasting of the choices made immediately following certain kinds of death. Here, OPOs argue, the parody of "transformation" that Mitford describes above assumes its proper form as a laudable act of altruism.

In *The American Way of Death Revisited*, Mitford describes the response to the first edition of her work among funeral professionals. She describes one memorable incident in which florists held a "Symposium on Sentiment": "the announced purpose of the symposium was to 'combat the forces which are attacking sentiment, memorialization and the rights of the individual in freedom of expression'" (Mitford 78). Advertising for the symposium continued, "The final rites, memorial tributes, the hallowed pageant of the funeral service all speak for the dignity of man.… Memorialization is love. It records a love so strong, so happy, so enduring that it can never die" (quoted in Mitford 79). Today, OPO professionals have recast this sentiment in the terms of cadaver donation as the gift of life, a gift that more properly expresses an enduring love. OPOs do not deny the above principles by insisting that the deceased is gone forever and the body is an empty vessel, but instead argue for organ donation as the better path to achieve these goals for those lucky enough to have loved ones die in a way that allows for donation.

Interviews with families confirm that this values-centered approach to death is a powerful motivator in decisions about donation. Returning again to the case of Richie Becker, we can see how his family understood their choice to donate his organs as an expression of Richie's character in life:

> We are all put on this earth to accomplish one thing or another … that's what I truly believe. And perhaps, you never know, this was Richie's purpose—to give life to others. We do know that Richie would have wanted us to donate; Richie was a truly generous and compassionate young man, and our decision was ultimately based on our strong sense that this is what he would have wanted, had he himself been given the choice.[39]

These words from Richie's father illustrate how the social values of altruism—"generosity and compassion"—and autonomy—"what he would have wanted"—find expression in the donation decision. Another donor mother expresses this principle more succinctly: "He was a good boy … and his body should also do good. We'll give the organs."[40] The florist symposium's elevation of the "hallowed pageant of the funeral service" may seem hyperbolic, especially when quoted in the larger context of Mitford's work, but the notion of a love "so enduring that it can never die" is a compelling concept for families. Since brain death is often characterized by a sudden and unexpected injury, the idea that the qualities of their loved one can "live on" in another body, continuing the expected life span of their child in a new form, is particularly important.

These quotes from family members are emblematic of more foundational assumptions in donor ideology. Both medical ethicists and lawmakers in the USA have consistently reinforced an organ donation system rooted in the principles of altruism. These ideas have been variously described by individuals from transplant coordinators to President Ronald Reagan as an expression of "neighborliness" or "that small town idea" that governs how to behave toward others.[41] In the 1980s, when many of the legal principles governing organ transfer were established, a federal task force acknowledged the problems of scarcity produced by a voluntary gift system, but rejected commercial alternatives. In their critical examination of what they call "the tyranny of the gift," Renée Fox and Judith Swazey study the report of the National Task Force on Organ Procurement and Transplantation (1986), written by James Childress. They write,

> For Childress, these concerns [about departing from an altruistic for a market model] were not only grounded in basic ethical principles, such as

> 'the dignity of the individual,' 'respect for persons' and their bodies, and 'the obligation to benefit others.' They also rested on theological precepts such as the person's 'transcendence' and 'stewardship' obligations to our bodies and to the community. (Fox and Swazey 67)

Fox and Swazey's work offers an important caution to the widespread embrace of the voluntary donor system and I explore their argument more fully in the later chapter on sentiment. In the context of this discussion of funeral practices, however, Childress's language offers a succinct articulation of the values tying decisions about dead bodies to community. In the following section, I will argue that as Americans consider alternative ways of handling corpses, we have found new expressions for long-standing beliefs. What Childress calls "'stewardship' obligations to our bodies and to the community" demonstrates a fundamental link between social demands toward both the dead body and to the community at large. Death, then, forms an important pivot point between the individual and the community. Several long-standing traditions—perhaps most notably the circulation of religious relics—mark the transfer of meaning granted to organs or corpses from the domain of the individual to the property of the community.

Public Death

This transfer from individual to public makes visible key elements of the donation system. In the USA, the rule of anonymous cadaver donation means that donor families do not direct their "gift," but instead offer it up to the ill public. The organ, then, is best understood as the property of the community at large, to be distributed according to public policy, not according to the wishes of the individual.[42] Along with religious relics, the emergence of life insurance, the public display of embalmed political leaders, and policies like the repatriation of Native American remains all converge as examples of cultural practices that express a belief in community possession of dead bodies or parts. Each of these seemingly disconnected practices addresses the fundamental question: How can we make peace with the distribution of an individual's organs to the possession of the body politic? We should first remember that these practices share the fundamental truth of the other cultural phenomena under examination in this book, in that they do not represent an uncomplicated or totalizing ideology—there are fissures and contradictions everywhere.

But as scientists, clinicians, and patients sought new and radical solutions to dire health problems, we can see how cracks in the dominant cultural logic provide fertile ground for alternative approaches. The extent to which these alternatives can find supportive holds in existing, even seemingly unrelated, practices is the key to opening up consideration of medical possibilities like transplantation, which violate basic concepts like self/other, individual/public, and life/death.

While personal fears about one's own death or the death of loved ones tend to dominate people's thinking, there are important strains in Western thought that suggest a counter-notion of death as a collective phenomenon. In his 1980 book, *Inventing the American Way of Death 1830–1920*, James Farrell argues for a once-emergent "species perspective of death" that mitigates some of the personal fears associated with dying by redirecting attention away from the individual. In the late nineteenth century, changes in popular thinking, including the profound influence of Darwin's theory of evolution, provided a channel away from a narrowly personal perspective of death. Farrell writes, "Evolutionary naturalism also shifted the focus of death from the individual to the species. Consequently, in assessing the place of death in evolution, many naturalists preferred to stress the immortality and improvement of the race rather than the mortality of the individual" (51–52). Evolution paired with the philosophy of sympathy as the structuring logics of American life into the next century. As Farrell notes, even Nathaniel Southgate Shaler, author of *The Individual* (1901), saw the increasing influence of sympathy in "American institutions near the turn of the century. Shaler himself noted that the family, the church, the state, corporations, clubs, and benevolent societies all institutionalized sympathy and transcended the life of individuals" (Farrell 64). At the same time, the rising concepts of public health and demography shared in this project of reframing death away from the individual.[43] Each of these conceptual systems—evolution, sympathy, and public health—asks us to relocate individual tragedy under the banner of the collective.

More specifically, James Farrell's account of the life insurance industry offers a special case in our discussion of the intersection of collectivism, altruism, and finding value in death. Each of these principles forms an essential plank supporting our system of voluntary cadaver organ donation—the "gift" in the "gift of life." For Farrell, life insurance expresses a move away from the death of the individual to a species perspective that focuses on survivors. He charts the rapid and astronomical growth of the life insurance industry as evidence of this successful reframing. In roughly the century spanning 1830–1920, the dollar value of the industry increased from $600,000 to over forty billion and the number of companies offering insurance increased from just nine to 335.[44] Farrell also cites two nineteenth-century contemporaries who emphasize the collective orientation of the growing life insurance industry:

> [Nathaniel Southwick] Shaler felt that "the moral advantage of the life insurance system" was its ability to bring men "to face death in an unselfish manner; to face it as men who consider their lives not as their own, but as part of the larger life of their kind." Similarly, Josiah Royce argues that "the greatest social power for life insurance was 'the fact that man does not in general purchase an insurance policy merely for the transient creature of today called "himself,"' but for beneficiaries. "His linkage with such beneficiaries," said Royce, "may join him to the whole social order". (67–68)

Shaler's language of facing death in an "unselfish manner" is particularly revealing as it suggests a new morality of death in which the decedent strives for generosity and attention to the needs of survivors. Where the individual is "transient," the "whole social order" is enduring; gifts—from inheritance, to insurance benefits, to anatomical gifts—offer a way to "transcend" the self by participating in the timeless collective. Life insurance, in its very name, accomplishes the same conceptual move found in organ donation, in which death confers a benefit—named a benefit of "life"—upon others.

Where life insurance typically serves a named, individual beneficiary, other practices surrounding dead bodies make a larger leap from the individual to the anonymous social body. A brief look at the centuries-spanning example of religious relics offers insight into the ways we both transfer individual remains to the property of the public and how we invest those remains with meaning. Both Christine Quigley and Anneli Rufus offer engaging accounts of the tradition of turning human remains into relics that are then circulated or displayed. The Crusades was an important historical flash point for this practice; given the difficulties of transporting a body home for burial, Crusaders serving thousands of miles away would remove and preserve organs and then boil bodies to separate flesh from bone. While prompted by logistical necessities, these practices reinforce a tradition of conferring different measures of importance on different parts of the body. By constructing some parts of the dead body as noble, revered, and crucial for burial and other parts as eligible for disposal, the transportation of religious relics provides a foundation for the logic of organ donation. Instead of understanding the dead body as an incorruptible whole—as is common in most religious traditions, including Christianity—relics offer a counter-narrative in which a dis-integrated corpse is a proper object of religious reverence, perhaps even more holy than those buried under normal circumstances. The practice of keeping relics to honor those of high status led to some radical and bizarre departures from the usual. In just one striking example, after the execution of Sir Walter Raleigh in 1618, his widow kept his preserved, severed head by her side in a red bag until her own death years later.[45] If we acknowledge that removing organs from cadavers and relocating them to different bodies marks a radical departure from the norm, it is useful to find these examples through the centuries of body parts that were removed and kept from burial in acts of love and reverence.

Part travelogue, part narrative history, Anneli Rufus's 1999 book *Magnificent Corpses* offers insight into centuries of relic veneration. Although she writes of visiting almost three dozen reliquaries, her account of St. Chiara's heart—an object of reverence since the fourteenth century—speaks most directly to the logic of cadaver donation. As Rufus tells it, Chiara had announced in 1308 that the crucified Christ was "in my heart."[46] Upon her death and amid calls for her sainthood, surgeons investigated the literal extent of this claim through a dissection of the corpse. Rufus writes:

> Witnesses reeled.
>
> Chiara's was strikingly larger than an ordinary heart. Surgeons slit it open to reveal, it was widely reported, images naturally occurring in the tissue. A pale crucifix the size of a thumb was said to have stood out, with a red spot denoting the wound in Christ's side. Another protrusion was hailed as representing a lance. Dark and pointed strips of tissue were identified as representing nails. A ring of spiky outgrowths effected a crown of thorns. Yet another protrusion, said to be harder than the surrounding tissue, evoked the marble column against which Christ was flogged. Yet another recalled the scourge itself, down to the knots in its thongs. (69)

At one level, this religious account of a miracle proved through a close reading of human anatomy would seem to contradict the prevailing scientific rationalism of the organ transplant era. Modern readers are unlikely to be as credulous as the reeling witnesses of the time. We do, however, have a contemporary tendency to mingle religion and science, perhaps best illustrated in the common phrase "medical miracle." We also understand donation decisions as an interplay between the symbolic and the material. We turn to the material organ to manifest more abstract values of goodness, generosity, and life. When a donor mother says, "He was a good boy … and his body should also do good. We'll give the organs,"[47] she captures an important conceptual pattern in which the son and his body are connected, but not identical. Organs, then, become a manifestation of the goodness of the individual and the "gift of life" operates on both a metaphorical and material level.

For many, these dual registers will evoke the materialist-discursive debate that has dominated theoretical discussions of the body for decades, most notably following Michel Foucault, Judith Butler, and an answering tide of phenomenologists. We can look to exceptional bodies and body parts as a reminder that the material and discursive exist in a constant relation without beginning or end (for which Elizabeth Grosz powerfully uses the metaphor of the Möbius strip).[48] In order to make organ exchange conceptually possible, we need to conceive of organs as both strictly material—mechanistic "spare parts" that are interchangeable—while also constructing compelling stories about organs as carrying something of the donor—sometimes rendered broadly as "life" or "love," sometimes imagined in stories of tastes, skills, or attachments transferring from donor to recipient. For the purposes of this cultural study, and a methodology grounded in textual close reading, it is important to note that both the material and symbolic conceptions of donor organs are articulated through metaphor. As the image of the Möbius strip reminds us, the material and symbolic are not in pure opposition; we may isolate or arrest these concepts and speak of their dominance in one frame or another, but holistic understanding must account for both sides of the strip.

Preserved Heads of State

This tie between the material corpse and its abstract significance finds further expression in the several political leaders whose bodies have been preserved for public display after their deaths. Like the religious reverence inspired by holy relics and pilgrimages, embalmed political leaders signify the enduring nature of the body politic. The list of leaders who have been displayed in this way includes Lenin, Stalin, Mao Zedong, Kim Il-Sung and Kim Jong-Il, Eva Perón, Ferdinand Marcos, and Hugo Chávez. In a popular example, Vietnamese leader Ho Chi Minh lies under guard in a refrigerated tomb in Hanoi, visited by more than 15,000 people each week.[49] If we consider the tremendous cults of personality attached to these leaders—and the extent to which they served as modern expressions of the "king's two bodies"—we can understand how the preserved corpse could properly exist in the public domain. The formulation of the king's two bodies—and from it, the "body politic"—comes from medieval historian Ernst Kantorowicz.[50] This influential analogy of the nation being like a body in its organization and unity resonates with questions of organ distribution as doctors, ethicists, and families work to figure out the relationships between parts and whole, individual and community. In the case of embalmed political leaders, or, meaningfully, "heads" of state, this complex interweaving of part and whole is already prefigured in the ways we locate meaning in the power and person of the politician. Visiting the embalmed corpse as a tourist or pilgrim is an act of encounter with both the individual and the nation. This simultaneity of meaning offers an important model for how we understand cadaver organ donation in which the transfer of the body's parts is understood simultaneously as both continuing and ending the life of the loved one.

This simultaneous encounter with the exceptional individual and the embodied collective is nowhere more striking than in the embalmed corpse of Vladimir Lenin. Since his death in the winter of 1924, Lenin's body has been lying in state in a mausoleum on Moscow's Red Square. In order to avoid association with religious relics, Soviet leaders emphasize the role of science and technology in preserving and maintaining their founder's corpse. Over time, the group of half a dozen anatomists, biochemists, and surgeons who are responsible for this preservation have become known as the "Mausoleum Group" and their expertise has also been sought for Ho Chi Minh, Kim Il-Sung, and Kim Jong-Il. The work of the Mausoleum Group differs from typical preservation techniques intended to last a very long time; where common preservation focuses on preventing decay of the physical matter but allows for changes in the exterior form (e.g., in mummification), this group focuses on maintaining the body's form—shape, color, look, flexibility—while allowing sacrifice to the original matter of the body. As such, skin and flesh are substituted for plastics or other materials that will achieve the lifelike "look" of the corpse, but disregard the value of original matter.

In his comprehensive research on the subject, Alexei Yurchak describes the many trials experienced by the Mausoleum Group over the years. They have had to contend with wrinkles and mold growing on the body, with a missing patch of skin on the left foot, and to reconstruct the nose and face to restore its lifelike look and feel. One Russian minister, arguing that a burial for Lenin was long overdue, recently told colleagues, "Do not fool yourselves with the illusion that what is lying in the mausoleum is Lenin. What's left there is only ten percent of his body."[51] As the continued stream of visitors to Lenin's tomb suggests, however, the lifelike look of the body—as achieved through technology—is deemed more important than strict material purity. In contrast to our assumption that purity and authenticity would be necessary for such an object of reverence, the case of Lenin's extensive physical restoration showcases a competing value of *seeming* fidelity to the corpse's look in life. While the choice to embrace appearance may seem counter to the logic of authenticity that governs "the incorruptible" religious relic, it in fact harkens back to mourners' positive responses to embalmed or photographed dead relatives. In those cases, the "natural" condition of the corpse is understood as the one that most closely resembles life, not the reality of unavoidable decay. As such, it expresses a fantasy of control over death and illness, a desire that animates radical life-extending procedures like organ transplantation.

The anxiety to arrest decay in the recently dead has pragmatic, psychological, and ideological roots. In the case of embalmed political leaders, their corpses are also often invested with the political concerns of the public. When Abraham Lincoln was assassinated in 1865, his embalmed body became a kind of traveling exhibition as it made the journey to burial in Springfield, IL. Hundreds of thousands of mourners waited in cities like Washington, Philadelphia, New York, Buffalo, and Chicago to view the fallen president. The Lincoln Special—his dedicated funeral train—passed through seven states and generated an outpouring of national grief; people who could not view the coffin on display in select cities lined the railroad tracks by the tens of thousands to watch the train go by. As Margaret Schwartz argues in *Dead Matter: The Meaning of Iconic Corpses*, "Mourning Lincoln coincided for many with their grief over the millions of war dead and served also as a rededication of the reunited but still shaky nation. Thus Lincoln's embalmed body plays a central role in a secular hagiography wherein the fallen leader redeems the injured body of the nation" (30). In this scheme, Lincoln's death, and the circulation of his corpse, brought life to another body: the newly reunited states. Again we see a material enactment of finding life in death. Lincoln's public display also served to showcase the new technology of embalming to a broad swath of the American public. As a remarkable public event, this three-week period of national mourning accepted technology—most notably, in the "Lincoln Special" train car and the embalmed body—as a properly mediating force in the treatment of dead bodies. Such public displays recall arguments made above about the role of technical interventions like intensive care monitoring, embalming, and death photography in producing a (paradoxically) "natural" death.

Where Lincoln's funeral train serves as an emblematic example of how technological intervention and circulation can promote community feeling, the strange case of Jim Thorpe demonstrates how notions of a body as public possession can go awry. Jim Thorpe has often been called the world's greatest athlete. He was a 1912 Olympic decathlon and pentathlon gold medalist, Hall of Fame football player, and major league baseball player. When he died in 1953, his body entered an itinerant chain whose contestation has continued into this century. Although he died in California, his body was transported to Oklahoma where members of the Sac and Fox tribe began their traditional three-day burial ceremony. Oklahoma was the site of the former Indian Territory where Thorpe's lineal tribe had been relocated during the Indian Removal Act; Thorpe, however, spent much of his boyhood at the Carlisle Indian Industrial School, where he was coached by "Pop" Warner. Before the concluding interment of the burial ceremony, however, Thorpe's widow, who was not Native American, got a police escort to remove his body to a temporary tomb. She was interested in the commercial possibilities of her legendary husband's body, envisioning everything from a sports museum to a motel named "Thorpe's Tepees."[52] Ultimately, the widow found an unlikely buyer in the form of two Pennsylvania towns. Thorpe had likely never visited the towns of Mauch Chunk and East Mauch Chunk, located near the Lehigh River and Pocono Mountains in eastern Pennsylvania. But the towns were in search of a new identity and were enthusiastic about the tourist potential for a town renamed Jim Thorpe, PA. By all accounts, the town has been sincere in honoring its acquired namesake. But Thorpe's surviving sons and members of the Sac and Fox tribe have argued all the way to the Supreme Court that Thorpe's remains should be disinterred and returned to Oklahoma for the proper completion of their traditional burial rites. The plaintiffs have cited the Native American Graves Protection and Repatriation Act, a piece of federal legislation from 1990 which seeks to relocate control and ownership of human remains and funerary objects from museums and federal agencies to lineal descendants or tribes.[53] NAGPRA offers an important intervention to the understanding of Native human remains as artifacts to be discovered, and especially to the practice of removal or exhibition of these remains. The act attempts to mediate the tension between public scientific interest in human remains and their study with enduring cultural rights to honor the dead according to tradition. In what many saw as a hit to NAGPRA, the Supreme Court ultimately refused in 2015 to hear an appeal of the case, meaning that Jim Thorpe's remains will stay in the town of Jim Thorpe, PA.

The recurring themes of relocation in Thorpe's biography remind us that circulation of people and their remains are political acts. The embodied history of Thorpe and his tribe includes Indian Removal, native boarding schools, itinerancy prompted by economic instability, and profit motives reflecting an understanding of human remains as objects. The public exhibition of leaders like Lincoln and Lenin is an affirmative enactment of political unity, a category that the townspeople of Jim Thorpe, PA, may see themselves occupying as well. The broader history in this case, however, evokes many of the same cautions offered by bioethicists who worry about coercion, exploitation of vulnerable populations, and dehumanizing commercialization in organ exchange. While it is important for our current system of altruistic donation that we understand organs as part of the public good, it is also important that we consider the enduring wrongs perpetrated in the so-called public interest.

Death in the Family

Transplant coordinators and physicians understand that decisions about a family member's organs can be fraught and contested. In 1987, revisions to the Uniform Anatomical Gift Act included provisions for "routine inquiry," in which patients are asked about organ donation upon admittance to the hospital, and "required request," where medical personnel are required to ask relatives or surrogates about donation upon death. These policies speak to a continuing hesitation among medical personnel to raise questions that might seem challenging or unorthodox during times of extreme stress.[54] In making decisions about one's own or a relative's organs, the conceptual frames of control over death; funeral decisions as an expression of values; finding life in death; and technological intervention are all important avenues toward an affirmative decision of donation. They offer a series of maps by which families and medical personnel can make sense of unfamiliar terrain. As this chapter demonstrates, we come to these conceptual frames through a series of seemingly disparate historical practices, like embalming, public exhibition, corpse photography, and repatriation.

In American literature, familial decisions about a corpse are nowhere more central or more strange than in William Faulkner's 1930 novel, *As I Lay Dying*.[55] When Addie, the matriarch of the Bundren family, dies, her husband and five children tie her coffin to their wagon and set off across the county to keep a promise to bury her in her hometown. As in Wallace Stevens's "The Emperor of Ice Cream," the rural Southern setting of *As I Lay Dying* means that although embalming technology had existed for decades, it would have been uncommon and expensive for a family like the Bundrens to pursue the practice.[56] As days go by on the journey, Addie's corpse begins to decompose, mirroring or prompting disintegration among her family members. As critic Erin Edwards argues, "Where culture would define the body through, for instance, the medical diagnosis, the anatomical model, the illustrative cadaver, or the discrete image, the novel erodes such certainty, showing that which escapes inscription—the body's dimensionality, its densities and volumes, the 'terrific hiatus[es],' to use Darl's phrase, that comprise bodily existence."[57] When brought into conversation with our cultural attitudes toward organ exchange, these gaps and excesses around simple definitions like diagnosis or anatomical illustration create an opening for unconventional approaches to the body. The corpse at the center of *As I Lay Dying* rejects straightforward accounts. Like the bodies of both organ donors and recipients, Addie's body is strikingly present and requires new models of affiliation among those in closest proximity.

The disastrous consequences of the family's plan to bury their mother in her native soil prompt reexamination of seemingly secure concepts like life and death, self and other, home and alien. It is exactly these concepts (among others) that organ exchange troubles. Close reading of scenes from *As I Lay Dying* can offer touchstones for understanding how revised approaches to corporeality might lead to radical experimentation in modes from the medical to the literary. Certainly, Faulkner's modernist novel celebrates experimentation—most notably in its narrative structure and point of view, with over a dozen narrators, including a pivotal section narrated by Addie after her death. In extracting a promise from her husband to bury her in her hometown, Addie conforms to a common and enduring practice. As Tom Weil writes in *The Cemetery Book*, "Death and burial at home, snug in one's native soil, seems so much cozier than reposing in some far land. The enfolding sod and clods of familiar earth coddle us more than can any alien terrain."[58] Addie dies in her bed with her son, Cash, building her coffin outside the window and her children and neighbors surrounding her. Her husband Anse's insistence that the family travel for days to remove her body from one home and bury it in another does not suggest the comforting "sod and clod of familiar earth" cited by Weil, but instead calls out the fraught nature of domestic space. Rather than express a fantasy of the simplicity of death at home, Faulkner's novel showcases the impossibility of rendering death familiar.

In one section, Cash narrates his rationale for his coffin-building method, beginning "I made it on the bevel" and proceeding through a numbered list of considerations, including everything from "1. There is more surface for the nails to grip" to (the opaque) "8. Animal magnetism" (48). While the form of the numbered list suggests an attempt to control death, the increasingly oblique considerations reveal the difficulty of that project. Although the coffin is well made—"I made it to balance with her. I made it to her measure and weight" (52)—Addie's body in its wedding dress must be placed in it upside down to account for her voluminous skirt; what results is a constant imbalance, a material weight that the family has to always adjust and account for. These attempts to manage death, to make it familiar according to the common means of handling bodies, result in disruption for the living and a troubling of common practice. By making the typical seem strange, or even perverse, Faulkner uses the material demands of the decomposing body to explore a series of more abstract considerations.

The dead body, in *As I Lay Dying*, is not an absence, but a striking presence. Several critics have noted that Addie is approached by the characters as though she were a corpse before her death—"she is no more than a bundle of rotten sticks" thinks her doctor (Faulkner 26)—and as a "strangely living entity afterwards."[59] Rather than become increasingly distant through the course of the novel, Addie's corpse is more and more demanding. The most significant example of her presence after death comes in her narrated section. These four pages serve as a key by which to understand the novel as a whole. Her physical decomposition is similarly impactful, prompting both internal musings among her children and dramatic changes to the family structure. Her sons become consumed with imagining Addie in her coffin, "within which now and then she talks in little trickling bursts of secret and murmurous bubbling" (123). Here, in this strangely lyrical description of decomposition, Faulkner seems to anticipate Foucault's description of the corpse as a "teeming presence."[60] Foucault goes on to argue, "long after the death of the individual, miniscule, partial deaths continue to dissociate the islets of life that still subsist."[61] Both writers emphasize death as a discursive force and the corpse itself as a catalyst for action. Organ exchange is marked similarly by a number of these "partial deaths" and "islets of life" that confound clear cut definitions of life and death. Descriptions of these moments of life and death are woven through this volume, but include most notably: artificial respiration used on brain-dead donors up to and through the retrieval surgery; removing transplant recipients from life support during heart/lung surgery; and the very notion of "the gift of life."

Despite the lyrical dimensions of Faulkner's above description of decomposition, the uncontainable reality of the corpse, most notably in its increasing smell, foregrounds the social nature of death—"And when I went to supper it still seemed like I could smell it. And the next day I met the marshal and I began to sniff..." (118–119). Death is not merely the absence of the dead individual, nor, at the next level, a burden on the immediate family; it carries a broader social weight that draws in the community. Reversing the formulation of altruism and therapeutic public mourning, *As I Lay Dying* agrees that the corpse has crucial social dimensions, but catalogs the harrowing effects of these public demands. Tanya Slankard argues, "Strangely, through her necrotic relationships with other characters—particularly with her sons—Addie becomes the unifying figure of the novel; but it is a progressively putrefying unification."[62] Addie's dying and decomposition produces a series of new relationships, both among members of her family and with the communities they pass through.

Scholars of organ exchange, especially those in medical anthropology, focus on the new forms of affiliation that transplantation creates. New modes of fictive kinship emerge to classify a whole range of relationships—from donor families to savior siblings, and human-interest stories of a recipient walking his donor's daughters down the aisle at her weddings. Most fundamentally, though, organ exchange challenges our foundational split between self and other. What might it mean for one's concept of the individual and the self to radically incorporate parts of another person? *As I Lay Dying* takes up precisely these questions of existence and identity. For both Darl and Vardaman, two of Addie's sons, her death prompts intense meditation on the nature of their own lives and how their lives intertwine with others.

The novel opens with Darl as a kind of organizing consciousness. He narrates many of the early sections and takes on forms of omniscience, often describing scenes where he is not present. Many transplant recipients describe experiencing a dual or altered consciousness after transplantation, or express worries about the influence of their new organ before surgery. Darl's confusing early meditation in the novel gives language to some of these anxieties about the boundaries between self and other:

> I dont know what I am. I dont know if I am or not. Jewel knows he is, because he does not know that he does not know whether he is or not. He cannot empty himself for sleep because he is not what he is and he is what he is not.... And since sleep is is-not and rain and wind are *was*, it is not. Yet the wagon *is*, because when the wagon is *was*, Addie Bundren will not be. And Jewel is, so Addie Bundren must be. And then I must be, or I could not empty myself for sleep in a strange room. And so if I am not emptied yet, I am *is*. (46–47)

Darl's meditation here is famously opaque, but its shuttling confusion between binary categories suggests the inadequacy of conventional thinking. For Faulkner, language cannot account for the fraught multiplicity of human experience. As Addie narrates after her death: "words dont ever fit even what they are trying to say at" (99). The simultaneous tumbling between "is/is not/was" in Darl's passage demonstrates that dying and decomposition require new modes of both corporeality and affiliation and that ordinary language cannot properly fit these changes. By the end of the novel, Darl is committed to an asylum, his speech reduced to a repeated affirmative: "yes yes yes yes yes" (146). It cannot be said straightforwardly that Darl's apparent madness is caused by his mother's death or even his hallucinations of her speech after death (those "secret and murmurous bubblings"). Faulkner does not reject his meditations as simple incoherence or insanity. Rather, his turn from rationality and his replacement as central narrator by his more-organized brother Cash suggest the difficulty posed by the kinds of deviations from the norm that Darl considers. Death in the novel is not a simple or bounded condition. Both Addie's body and something of her consciousness persist after her death and her family must consider their own identities in a relational landscape changed by death.

Organ exchange requires similar reconsiderations. For example, the construction "donor family" follows a similar pattern in which the transfer and persistence of the decedent's organs brings into being an entirely new identity for the surviving family. In this new form of kinship, both recipients and donor families are left to puzzle out an entirely modern model of affiliation, a model with competing layers of grief, altruism, hope, medical technology, and complex expectations. Placed in this conversation, Darl's confounding exploration of is/is not/was seems appropriate to the simultaneous registers evoked by thoughts of death.

Darl's very young brother, Vardaman, expresses similar anxieties about the boundaries of life and death, self and other. In a single-line chapter immediately following Darl's meditation before sleep and Cash's "I made it on the bevel" list, comes Vardaman's line: "My mother is a fish" (49). This naïve confusion of the major events of the day—catching a large fish, watching it killed for his family's supper, and his mother's death—can be partly attributed to Vardaman's youth. Taken together, though, these three pages capture the three brothers' attempts to understand, control, or rationalize death and its meaning for their lives. Vardaman most expressly considers the implications of violating physical boundaries between self and other, imagining the fish-as-mother taken into the bodies of his family: "Then it wasn't and she was, and now it is and she wasn't. And tomorrow it will be cooked and et and she will be him and pa and Cash and Dewey Dell and there wont be anything in the box and so she can breath" (39). Critics have offered competing readings of this scene; some argue that the family consumes Addie's figurative body as a symbolic death, or to free Addie from her material body, or as a kind of totem by which to distribute her power.[63] Read in conversation with organ exchange, however, this scene offers an imaginative frame for literal acts of parting dead bodies and distributing organs into new bodies. Instead of an attachment to an inviolable body in death, Vardaman offers a new model, one in which, after consumption, "she will be him and pa and Cash and Dewey Dell." While we might recoil from the plain way in which Vardaman talks about his fish/mother being "cooked and et," he expresses a strange and important mingling of harsh realities and symbolic fantasies of life continuing after death. In order to fulfill donor families' belief in some continuation of life or self after donation, we need the rupturing technology of surgery. While we might deny the harsh realities of the surgical process, Vardaman's naïve understanding of the dead continuing in his siblings through the process of parting and consumption has uncanny, if uncomfortably explicit, parallels to the way we understand organ transfer.

Whole undergraduate discussions and online grammar articles have been written about the complexities of Faulkner's title. If we assume that Faulkner is being grammatically correct and means "lay" as the simple past tense of "lie," then we face an entirely new strangeness in a first person talking about their "dying" in the past tense. If they were dying then, what are they now? The phrase "as I lay dying" is an allusion to *The Odyssey* and is spoken by the shade Agamemnon while Odysseus visits the underworld. Thus, Faulkner establishes a literary precedent for his inclusion of Addie's post-death narration in the novel. But I would also argue that the strangeness of the phrase puts pressure on the much more quotidian term "dying." Most legal, medical, and lay definitions of death understand it as an event, with a finite and specific time. In an influential 1971 article for *Science*, however, Robert Morison asks "Death: Process or Event?"[64] How does our collective belief in death as "a sharp end to life" create a host of complications in matters both practical and conceptual? In the following chapter on the invention of brain death, I explore how, in the late twentieth century, committees appointed by both Harvard Medical School and the federal government created a sea change in the way we understand and treat death under a special set of circumstances. Although both committees insist that they are not redefining death, only refining its diagnosis, the implications of these new rules form a watershed moment in the history of organ exchange. It is difficult to imagine the widespread adoption of organ transplantation as a life-saving technology without this foundational change in the way we understand death. I examine how highly philosophical questions about death and its declaration script new deathbed scenes, creating effects that are both abstract and profoundly personal.

Notes

1. Philippe Ariès, *The Hour of Our Death: The Classic History of Western Attitudes Toward Death over the Last One Thousand Years*, trans. Helen Weaver, 2nd edition (New York: Vintage Books, 2008).
2. Atul Gawande, *Being Mortal: Medicine and What Matters in the End*, 1st edition (New York: Metropolitan Books, 2014), 6.
3. Lupton, *Medicine as Culture*, also argues that "the sequestration of dying" is an expression of our need for control over death (45).
4. Geoffrey Gorer, "The Pornography of Death," *Encounter* 5, no. 4 (October 1955): 51.
5. Joseph Jacobs, *The Dying of Death* (Tucker Publishing, 1900).
6. For more on the intersection of death and medicine, see James Farrell, *Inventing the American Way of Death, 1830–1920* (Philadelphia: Temple University Press, 1980); Gorer, "Pornography of Death"; Lupton, *Medicine as Culture*; Jessica Mitford, *The American Way of Death Revisited*, Rev. edition (New York: Alfred A. Knopf, 1998); Lindsay Prior, "Reflections on the 'Mortal' Body in Late Modernity," in *Health, Medicine, and Society: Key Theories, Future Agendas*, ed. Simon Williams, Michael Calnan, and Jonathan Gabe (London: Routledge, 2000), 186–202; and Sappol, *A Traffic of Dead Bodies.*
7. Prior, "Reflections of the 'Mortal' Body," 193.
8. Quoted in Farrell, *Inventing the American Way of Death*, 25.
9. Gutkind, *Many Sleepless Nights*, 143.
10. Ibid., 246.
11. Quoted in Gawande, *Being Mortal*, 2.
12. Alan Warren Friedman, *Fictional Death and the Modernist Enterprise* (Cambridge: Cambridge University Press, 1995), 23.
13. Wallace Stevens, "The Emperor of Ice-Cream," in *The Collected Poems of Wallace Stevens*, Reissue edition (New York: Vintage, 1990), 64.
14. Alex Davis and Lee M. Jenkins, eds., *The Cambridge Companion to Modernist Poetry* (Cambridge: Cambridge University Press, 2007), 61.
15. Jay Ruby, *Secure the Shadow: Death and Photography in America* (Cambridge, MA: MIT Press, 1995), 7.
16. Christine Quigley, *The Corpse: A History* (Jefferson, NC: McFarland, 1996), 51.
17. In his study of resuscitation technology in emergency room settings, Stefan Timmermans argues that while most social science literature places technology and "dignified dying" at odds with each other, the prolongation of time and control offered by resuscitation might allow for a different kind of dignity, one in which the dying person's wishes are

honored and family and friends are included in the final moments. Stefan Timmermans, "Resuscitation Technology in the Emergency Department: Towards a Dignified Death," *Sociology of Health & Illness* 20, no. 2 (1998): 144–167.

18. See Ariès, *The Hour of Our Death*; Gawande, *Being Mortal*; Hans Hadders, "Enacting Death in the Intensive Care Unit: Medical Technology and the Multiple Ontologies of Death," *Health: An Interdisciplinary Journal for the Social Study of Health, Illness, and Medicine* 13, no. 6 (2009): 571–587; Janet Harvey, "The Technological Regulation of Death: With Reference to the Technological Regulation of Birth," *Sociology* 31, no. 4 (November 1997): 719–735; Jane Elizabeth Seymour, "Negotiating Natural Death in Intensive Care," *Social Science & Medicine* 51, no. 8 (2000): 1241–1252; and Timmermans, "Resuscitation Technology."
19. Harvey, "Technological Regulation," 721.
20. Seymour, "Negotiating Death"; Timmermans, "Resuscitation Technology"; Harvey, "Technological Regulation"; and Hadders, "Enacting Death."
21. Sharp, *Strange Harvest*, 124.
22. Quoted in Ruby, *Secure the Shadow*, 58.
23. Organ Procurement Organizations describe a similar reliance on euphemistic jargon in their line of work. Lee Gutkind, *Many Sleepless Nights*, quotes from a newspaper column written by Ginny Smith, who worked at the Pittsburgh Transplant Foundation: "We didn't talk much about death.... The terminology we used avoided that word. The coordinator who is with a grieving family is 'on a donor.' A patient in an intensive care unit sliding into brain death is a 'referral.' Until brain death is declared and the organs recovered, the coordinator is 'working on a donor.' Transplant surgeons anxious for a donation tell us they're 'strong' and call often to ask if 'anything's going on'" (107).
24. John Troyer, "Embalmed Vision," *Mortality* 12, no. 1 (2007): 23.
25. For more on the wet/dry distinction in museum exhibitions of corpses, see Walter, "Body Worlds: Clinical Detachment"; Kuppers, "Visions of Anatomy"; Bates, "Bodies Impolitic?"; and Desmond, "Postmortem Exhibitions."
26. Sharp, *Strange Harvest*, 18.
27. Gutkind, *Many Sleepless Nights*, 320.
28. Troyer, "Embalmed Vision," 34.
29. Margaret Schwartz, *Dead Matter: The Meaning of Iconic Corpses* (Minneapolis: University of Minnesota Press, 2015), 16.
30. Ibid., 18.

31. Quoted in Ruby, *Secure the Shadow*, 59.
32. Ruby, *Secure the Shadow*, 73.
33. Sandra Homer, *Heavensbrook Angels*, accessed July 12, 2017, http://heavensbookangels.com/.
34. See, for example, ethicist Stuart Youngner's article of the same title as well as Lesley Sharp's anthropological studies of organ transfer.
35. Tom Gunning, "Phantom Images and Modern Manifestations: Spirit Photography, Magic Theater, Trick Films and Photography's Uncanny," in *Fugitive Images: From Photography to Video*, ed. Patrice Petro (Bloomington: Indiana University Press, 1995), 48.
36. Sharp, *Strange Harvest*, 153.
37. Ibid., 154.
38. Richardson, "Human Dissection and Organ Transplantation," 161.
39. Gutkind, *Many Sleepless Nights*, 103.
40. Ibid., 106.
41. See Sharp *Strange Harvest* 170 and Reagan "Radio Address to the Nation" (1983).
42. Dr. Richard I. Cook, emphasizes the importance of community and perceived fairness in a system of voluntary donation: "Equity is also important to sustain the flow of donated organs into the system. Organ donation is voluntary, and donor families, who control access to the potential donor's organs, are financially uncompensated. At the time of the donation, the donor family does not know which patients will receive the organs. Instead, the donation is made to the transplantation system. The appearance of equity in this system is an important incentive to donate one's own organs and also for one's family to confirm (as they must do) that donation when the moment comes." Richard I. Cook, "Hobson's Choices: Matching and Mismatching in Transplantation Work Processes," in *A Death Retold: Jesica Santillan, the Bungled Transplant, and Paradoxes of Medical Citizenship*, ed. Keith Wailoo, Julie Livingston, and Peter Guarnaccia (Chapel Hill: University of North Carolina Press, 2006), 58.
43. For a fuller account of the intersections of public heath, death, and the individual, see Lupton, *Medicine as Culture*; Prior, "Reflections on the 'Mortal' Body"; and Stern, "Dystopian Anxieties."
44. Farrell, *Inventing the American Way of Death*, offers the following statistics: "The growth of life insurance in American occurred almost entirely after 1830. In that year, nine life insurance companies held policies worth only $600,000. By 1850, there were forty-eight companies with policies valued at $97,000,000. In 1900, eighty-four companies held fourteen million policies worth $7,573,000,00, about one life insurance policy for

every five Americans. By 1920, three hundred thirty-five companies held sixty-five million policies worth $40,540,000,000, roughly two policies for every three Americans" (67).

45. Quigley, *The Corpse*, 253.
46. Anneli Rufus, *Magnificent Corpses: Searching Through Europe for St. Peter's Head, St. Chiara's Heart, St. Stephen's Hand, and Other Saints' Relics* (Da Capo Press, 1999), 69.
47. Gutkind, *Many Sleepless Nights*, 106.
48. Elizabeth Grosz, *Volatile Bodies: Towards a Corporeal Feminism* (Bloomington: Indiana University Press, 1994), xii.
49. Quigley, *The Corpse*, 66.
50. Ernst Hartwig Kantorowicz, *The King's Two Bodies: A Study in Mediaeval Political Theology* (Princeton: Princeton University Press, 1957).
51. Alexei Yurchak, "Bodies of Lenin: The Hidden Science of Communist Sovereignty," *Representations*, no. 129 (Winter 2015): 116.
52. Benjamin Hochberg, "Bringing Jim Thorpe Home: Inconsistencies in the Native American Graves and Repatriation Act," *Rutgers Race and the Law Review* 13 (2012).
53. Morris Udall, "H.R.5237—101st Congress (1989–1990): Native American Graves Protection and Repatriation Act," Legislation, November 16, 1990, https://www.congress.gov/bill/101st-congress/house-bill/5237.
54. For more on policy proposals around consent and donation, see Laura Siminoff and Mary Beth Mercer, "Public Policy, Public Opinion, and Consent for Organ Donation," *Cambridge Quarterly of Healthcare Ethics* 10, no. 4 (October 2001): 377–386. For more on attitudes by medical personnel regarding approaching donor families, see Maloney and Wolfelt, *Caring for Donor Families* and Youngner "'Brain Death' and Organ Retrieval."
55. William Faulkner, *As I Lay Dying*, ed. Michael Gorra, Norton Critical Edition (New York: W. W. Norton, 2010).
56. Tanya Slankard writes, "In a more nuanced reading of Southern death practices, James K. Crissman notes that although embalming began being used in the South out of necessity during the Civil War and gained popularity when Lincoln's body was toured through the country, in most rural areas the practice was not used until at least the 1930s (35–36)." Tanya Slankard, "'No Such Thing as Was': The Fetishized Corpse, Modernism, and As I Lay Dying," *The Faulkner Journal* 24, no. 2 (Spring 2009): 12.
57. Erin E. Edwards, "Extremities of the Body: The Anoptic Corporeality of As I Lay Dying," *MFS Modern Fiction Studies* 55, no. 4 (2009): 741.
58. Quoted in Quigley, *The Corpse*, 80.
59. John K. Simon, "The Scene and Imagery of Metamorphosis in *As I Lay Dying*," *Criticism* 7 (1965): 20.

60. Foucault, *Birth of the Clinic*, 142.
61. Ibid. For more on the intersections of Foucault and *As I Lay Dying*, see Erin Edwards, “Extremities of the Body.”
62. Slankard, “No Such Thing,” 10–11.
63. Ibid., 19–20.
64. Robert S. Morison, “Death: Process or Event?,” *Science* 173, no. 3998 (1971): 694–698.

CHAPTER 4

Mortal Signs: Transplantation and the Invention of Brain Death

"Death is the one great certainty." This statement, coming on page 3 of a report called *Defining Death: Medical, Legal, and Ethical Issues in the Determination of Death* (1981), may be forgiven for its status as an obvious lie.[1] As members of the presidential commission authoring that report certainly understood, while the public, courts, and doctors may want to insist that "death is the one great certainty," much ink was spilled in the last quarter of the twentieth century trying to establish and fix that certainty. After the 1960s, changing medical technology in the form of artificial respiration and organ transplantation meant that practices involving death were increasingly divergent from notions that were comfortably and easily understood by the public. Hearts, lungs, kidneys, and livers could be retrieved from bodies whose hearts had been beating moments before. Fearing prosecution for murder, doctors pressed family members to turn off ventilators instead of doing it themselves. As *Defining Death* argues, "a *choice* about the 'definition' of death was at issue" (46). The choice made by the legal and medical communities was to adopt a concept of "brain death," now law in all 50 states. Although there has been little public debate about this new determination of death since its emergence in the late 1960s—a surprising fact that deserves and receives more attention below—examination of the concept and practices surrounding brain death illustrates that much like the circulating relics discussed in the previous chapter, "death" is not stable or fixed. In fact, death and its determination are arbitrary, a choice, relying on language and the reading of signs.

E. Russell, *Transplant Fictions*,
Palgrave Studies in Literature, Science and Medicine,
https://doi.org/10.1007/978-3-030-12135-8_4

For centuries, the prevailing sign of death was the absence of a heartbeat. Family members did not typically require a doctor to know when a relative had passed away; they listened for a stopped heart and the consequent loss of respiration. Mirrors could be held to the nose to check for breath or, if a doctor was involved, the use of a stethoscope to measure heartbeat could be readily understood even by lay bystanders. The cardiopulmonary, or, as it came to be known, "heart-lung," definition of death had the advantage of both popular and long-standing acceptance. While fears of being buried alive and false declarations of death found cultural and economic expressions, these anxieties were nothing compared to the sea change of thinking prompted by the emergence of artificial respiration and organ transplant. The redefinition of death was not simply a practical matter, but spoke to profound philosophical questions about the seat of individual identity in the body, the definition of personhood, and our confidence in death as a unitary phenomenon. Even before the medical and legal communities convened to propose new definitions of death from the late 1960s to the early 1980s, the nascent practice of transplantation forced a rethinking of self and other, living and dead. As the authors of *Defining Death* argue, "the importance customarily accorded to a person's beating heart in differentiating the living from the dead is challenged when a 'dead' person's heart can beat in the chest of a 'living' person whose own heart has not merely stopped but has been removed from his or her body" (4). The twists captured in the preceding sentence are not just cleverness on the part of the presidential commissioners—they touch on very real and practical problems connected to our notions of life and death. These problems have played out in courtrooms, legislation, and bioethics conferences, but they are experienced most deeply at hospital bedsides as families and medical practitioners confront the difficulties that come with being unable to read the signs of death with confidence.

In 1968, confusion around these questions was broad enough that the Harvard Medical School convened an ad hoc committee to address the issue. The committee established new criteria for determining death, an alternative to the heart-lung definition, that they called "irreversible coma" and that we know as "brain death."[2] The new definition was prompted by the burden placed on hospitals, patients, and families by continued artificial respiration; physicians' fears of lawsuit or prosecution for turning off ventilators; and increasing demand for organs for transplant.[3] The report lays out three tests for the diagnosis of irreversible coma: (1) unreceptivity and unresponsivity, (2) no movements or breathing (when the respirator has been turned off for 3 minutes), and (3) no reflexes, especially measured by a fixed, dilated pupil. These tests should be repeated after a period of 24 hours and should be confirmed by a flat electroencephalogram where possible. These measures—known collectively as the Harvard Criteria—offer a clear and reliable method for doctors to diagnose brain death in their patients. These cases are relatively uncommon, less than 1% of all deaths in the USA (about 15,000–20,000 per year), but they serve as the most common supply of deceased donor organs. Brain death is most often caused by direct trauma to the head (as in a car accident or gunshot wound), stroke, or lack of oxygen to the brain. These patients require intensive medical management, not just through ventilation, but also with feeding, hydration, catheterization, and temperature regulation. And, as many sources are quick to point out, even with proper care, "the organs of these potential donors will deteriorate" and "the heart usually stops beating within 2 to 10 days."[4] Total organ failure may be inevitable in these cases, but it can be a trying and labor-intensive vigil, one which results in the unrecoverable deterioration of needed organs for donation. The interest in establishing criteria for death that can be met more quickly centers on the burdens and demands cited by the Harvard Committee—notably, scarcity of donor organs and resource demands on hospitals. Given that the vast majority of transplanted organs come from brain-dead bodies, the difference of days (or minutes) is essential for the health and success of transplant medicine.

Despite the confident clarity of the 1968 Harvard Criteria and a similarly declarative tone found in the hundred plus pages of *Defining Death* (which crafts and supports the Uniform Declaration of Death Act in 1981), I am not so certain. I hope I can be forgiven if the famous line from *The Princess Bride* keeps creeping through my head: "It just so happens that your friend here is only *mostly* dead. There's a big difference between mostly dead and all dead."[5] The legal and medical communities concur in publically insisting that death is a unitary phenomenon, that there should not be a qualified form of death or different definitions of death that apply in different circumstances. But even our public discussion of brain death *as* "brain death" and not simply "death" suggests that the active choice to extend the definition of death has cultural and conceptual seams that are visible in common cases and fraying at the limits.[6] This chapter examines those seams to understand how organ transplant contributes to writing a massive new legal and medical fiction of brain death: A fiction that is relatively uncontroversial, serves as the law of the land, and yet has impacts from the highly abstract (after all, what boundary question is more fundamental than the line between life and death) to the highly practical (directing decisions about medical care on a daily basis).[7]

One of these fraying seams between life and death comes in the Harvard Committee's attempt to script a moment of hospital bedside drama. Twice in their four-page report, the group insists, "Death is to be declared and *then* the respirator turned off" (86, emphasis in original). This attention to timing reflects two interesting elements in our concept of death. First, we understand death as an event, not a process. Our adherence to "time of death" reinforces this notion. Even where experience seems to stray from such a strict insistence on death coming at a single moment, medical practice and a vast body of legal cases rely on a specific time of death. Second, death is something to be *declared* by a medical practitioner. In an emblematic example of the performative utterance, the declaration of death makes death so. In the case of patients in an irreversible coma, over a day of tests are necessary to confirm a diagnosis of brain death. Then, while the patient is still breathing, the physician is instructed to declare him dead and then turn off the respiration: "this declaration should not be delayed until he has been taken off the respirator and all artificially stimulated signs have ceased" (Beecher et al. 87). For Henry Beecher and the co-authors of the Harvard report, this order of events offers greater legal protection to physicians. One could, however, speculate about the effect of this timing on the patient's family; at what point is the loved one "dead" for them? When the doctor declares it? When the "signs of life" (even if artificially stimulated) have ceased? As the report goes on to describe, the declaration of death should not be delayed, since "otherwise, the physicians would be turning off the respirator on a person who is, under the present strict, technical application of law, still alive" (87). This chapter will circle back in greater detail on many of the issues raised here. But even a brief, introductory discussion of the earliest formulation of brain death raises a powerful series of questions. Can there be more than one kind of death? We have a new definition of death, but do we also have a clear, underlying concept of what it means to be dead? How does death relate to other concepts central to life, like personhood? How do elements like time and language shape death? Each of these questions forms the conceptual ground upon which our understanding of organ transplant plays out. After all, in the bedside drama described above, for an organ donor, the respirator is not turned off in the presence of family. Instead, the body is taken to an operating room, resuscitative measures are continued, pain medication may even be administered to a dead body, and a skilled team of medical practitioners works to sustain the organs as well as possible through their removal from one body and transfer to another. Given the absolute requirement of the "dead donor rule," which states that vital organs can only be taken from those who are dead, brain death is perhaps the most foundational ideological shift in a series of cultural changes that have made organ transplant possible in the public consciousness—a requirement that is related to, but distinct from strict technical capability.

Social definitions of death correspond to lay concepts of language and its origins. In the same way that many believe that things exist and we simply attach words to them, we tend to believe that death exists as a straightforward state whether it is named or not. In this view, legal or medical wrangling over terms is largely academic, speaking to esoteric questions of philosophy and exceptional medical circumstances. While such a perspective is certainly comfortable, it fails to correspond to actual practice in hospitals or the prevailing law of the land. Death is not a transparent physical condition, but must be declared according to a complex of socially constructed definitions. The self-contradictory ways in which even medical personnel speak of patients declared brain dead reveals the ways in which we have gerrymandered the definition of death to meet social needs, including the financial bottom line of hospitals and the always-growing demand for organs for transplant. While the charge of gerrymandering seems to suggest ethical disdain, it can also be read more neutrally to demonstrate how contingent our foundational concepts of life and death truly are.

Language used by clinicians in the early years of transplantation reveals not just ambiguity in how medicine understood death, but also the power of naming to make something real in the world. The oxymoron "living cadaver," often used with scare quotes, signals the hazardous ground transplant professionals occupied before the passage of the Uniform Determination of Death Act in 1981. Heart transplant research, in particular, relied on donations from comatose patients, and the obvious contradictions of "living cadaver" invite skepticism toward the entire enterprise. In her foundational anthropological study of brain death in North America and Japan, Margaret Lock enumerates the verbal gymnastics physicians undertook in the years after 1966:

> several physicians invented cumbersome, sometimes graphic terms for patients suspended between life and death: 'dead but in a state of artificial survival' (Hamburger and Crosnier 1968:42); 'living cadaver' (Starzl 1967:70); 'heart-lung preparation' (Alexandre 1966:156); 'potential cadaver' (Revillard 1966:70); 'reanimation patient' (Bessert et al. 1970); 'respirator brain' (Korein 1978:9; Moseley et al. 1976), and 'neomort' (Gaylin 1974:23). (94)

Not only did physicians struggle over how to name the condition of patients on artificial respiration, they lacked consensus over how to locate that condition within existing and essential categories of life and death. Mita Giacomini, in her archival research on the work of the Harvard Committee, reminds us that the language used in these cases has highly pragmatic implications. Word choice has the power to change the jurisdiction of the potential donor; after all, "live 'patients' were legitimate wards of physicians, while 'corpses' belonged solely to next of kin. Once death was declared, physicians could no longer manipulate the body at their own discretion."[8]

The special case of brain death offers an occasion to rethink how we understand life, death, and medicine, but it also brings weight to philosophical discussions of social construction. When I teach the concepts of performative utterance and semiotics in the undergraduate English classroom, I try to distill it all into a clarifying, single-page handout, drawing extensively from Jonathan Culler's work in *Literary Theory: A Very Short Introduction.*[9] I go over "I now pronounce you man and wife" and the arbitrary nature of signs. We talk about how chairs and stools could be divided into other classes. I startle students by informing them that the French have no word for "pet," despite the fact that they certainly keep cats and dogs. In the end, the insights of a century of theory can feel like a party trick: interesting, but removed from students' daily lives under layers of abstraction. In cases of brain death, however, how and when we name life and death matters deeply. The development of brain death as a concept relies on sorting out a series of conflicting signs of life and death and giving them new meaning. This chapter explores how the interests of good stewardship of resources and making organs available for donation have prompted new ways of thinking about death that are often uneven and contradictory.

Dead For Transplantation, But Not Dead Otherwise!

On March 13, 1981, Melanie Bacchiochi died. Months earlier, on January 30, this 23-year-old woman from Connecticut became comatose during a routine procedure to remove her wisdom teeth. In the middle of her two and a half months spent on artificial respiration, doctors at Johnson Memorial Hospital performed tests, including electroencephalography, and concluded that she had suffered irreversible loss of total brain function. Her family requested that she be removed from the respirator, but her physician was unwilling to do so without a court order, fearing consequences arising from a legal uncertainty in Connecticut's law on brain death. After hearing testimony from physicians and the family, Judge Hammer ruled that Bacchiochi had suffered brain death, but refused the request to remove her from the respirator. Citing the gravity of the step and claiming, "it would be almost reckless at this point to render a decision,"[10] Hammer requested additional briefs on the case. Despite the ambiguity of the judicial decision—yes, she is brain dead, but no, do not stop life support—the attorneys, hospital administrators, and medical examiners met and decided to turn off the respirator that evening. She was pronounced dead at 8:07 p.m., March 13, 1981.

Perhaps the most obvious question in this case is: When did Melanie Bacchiochi die? When she was pronounced dead on March 13? When she slipped into an irreversible coma on January 30? When that irreversible coma was diagnosed through clinical tests on February 11? For the legal community, the answer seems secure: Death occurs when it is pronounced. But even the security of such pronouncements, which come from medical professionals on the scene, is undermined by a broader confusion in language regarding such cases. Consider the complexities captured in the following statement on the case by the chief medical examiner for Connecticut. As reported in the *New York Times*, Dr. Catherine A. Galvin states that when the "rigid criteria for brain death have been met," it is the customary practice "to terminate extraordinary life-sustaining measures for an incurably ill patient." In what sense is a dead patient having her life "sustained"? Is it meaningful to describe a dead patient as "incurably ill"? Although the former state medical examiner commenting on the case connects Connecticut's lack of a legal definition of death to also not having statutory prescriptions about euthanasia, proponents of brain death insist that the two concepts are not the same. In fact, the open public debate about euthanasia has not so far extended to a broad call for repeals of brain death statues. For advocates of brain death—which, remember, has largely been a closed issue since the Uniform Determination of Death Act in 1981—there should be no ambiguity in the condition of the former patient; she is dead when irreversible coma has been diagnosed.

Connecticut's laws on death were ultimately more confusing, not because they did not have a legal concept of brain death, but because this definition was contained within a statute governing organ donation. As Bacchiochi's doctor commented: "It is ironic that if the patient had been a donor, she could have been pronounced dead on February 11 and the respirator could have been withdrawn. Dead for transplantation, but not dead otherwise!" (qtd in *Defining Death* 268). This legal quagmire is exactly the kind of murky water that the 1981 presidential commission on the determination of death wanted to clarify. Fundamental to their proceedings was a strongly held belief that their recommended statute "ought not to reinforce the misimpression that there are different 'kinds' of death, defined for different purposes, and hence that some people are 'more dead' than others" (*Defining Death* 60). Both the commission and the earlier Harvard Committee insist that death is a unitary phenomenon. The prevailing legal situation of the late 1970s, however, contributed to this "misimpression" of two kinds of death, as statues like those in Connecticut and Kansas connected brain death only to organ transplant.

Policy advocates for brain death and organ transplant were very aware of public fears regarding medical abuses in such cases. From the beginning, policies on organ donation have insisted on a total separation in the medical team tending to the donor and the team caring for the recipient. But over three decades later, public awareness campaigns still commonly speak to very real concern over diminished standards in medical care for prospective donors, insisting that all life-saving measures will be employed, no matter what box is checked on one's driver's license. As I will discuss in Chapter 6, many of these fears are manifested in familiar horror tropes of organ-hungry doctors killing patients for science. Given these concerns, beginning with the dawn of brain death statues, policy advocates were emphatic on death as a single, underlying condition.

In addition to the complications arising from the sense that there may be two different kinds of death for different classes of patient—donor or not—early advocates needed to grapple with another form of doubling in having two criteria for measuring death: the new diagnosis of brain death and the long-standing heart-lung definition of death. As the authors of *Defining Death* understood, it would be a confusing and excessively radical move to toss out the heart-lung definition in favor of criteria requiring a doctor's diagnosis. In the vast majority of cases, they remind us, artificial respiration will not be necessary and standards of death should conform to common sense. Consequently, the text of the 1981 Uniform Determination of Death Act reads: "An individual who has sustained either 1) irreversible cessation of circulatory and respiratory functions, or 2) irreversible cessation of all functions of the entire brain, including the brain stem, is dead. A determination of death must be made in accordance with accepted medical standards." The commissioners go on to insist, however, "the use of two standards in a statute should not be permitted to obscure the fact that death is a unitary phenomenon" (7). But the use of multiple, either/or criteria in the determination of a question as profound as death—about which we desire zero ambiguity—may not be as straightforward as the committee wants to believe.

The 1968 Harvard Committee casts their work in similar terms, claiming that they are offering new diagnostic criteria for a "more accurate" pronouncement of death, not inventing a new category or kind of death. As stated in their report, published in the *Journal of the American Medical Society*:

> Our primary purpose is to define irreversible coma as a new criterion for death. There are two reasons why there is a need for a definition: (1) Improvements in resuscitative and supportive measures have led to increased efforts to save those who are desperately injured. Sometimes these efforts have only partial success so that the result is an individual whose heart continues to beat but whose brain is irreversibly damaged. The burden is great on patients who suffer permanent loss of intellect, on their families, on the hospitals, and on those in need of hospital beds already occupied by these comatose patients. (2) Obsolete criteria for the definition of death can lead to controversy in obtaining organs for transplantation. (85)

A few elements of this text deserve closer attention as we work to understand how it would be possible for a committee of physicians to redefine a concept as foundational as death itself. Perhaps the most crucial answer to that question lies in the first sentence, and found repeatedly through the report, that they are *not* redefining death, merely offering a new criteria for its determination. Whether their insistence is sufficient to make it so will be considered below. The second interesting feature here is the claim that improved resuscitative measures have led to "increased efforts to save those who are desperately injured" and that "sometimes these efforts have only partial success." Much of the persuasive strategy of the report lies in a manipulation of time, in citing increased efforts on patients who would have died and patients who, based solely on heart-lung criteria, will soon be dead. The gap between "irreversibly" injured and "dead" is the troublesome period for the physicians, who are concerned with the burden on families and hospitals and the loss of possible organs for transplant. In naming heart-lung criteria "obsolete" for these cases, the Harvard Committee announces its new criteria and declares the prevailing understanding obsolete in a single stroke.

Defining Death

The Uniform Determination of Death Act succeeded in ironing out legal discrepancies across state definitions; in reassuring physicians they were secure from prosecution or civil suit; and in expanding the base for organ donation. Less clear, though, is whether the definition adequately offers a unitary understanding of what it means to be dead. Bioethicists, led in the field by Stuart Youngner, have sought to understand whether a new definition of death is the same as a new concept of death. The authors of the Harvard Criteria and of *Defining Death* say no. Ethicists, typically, are not so sure. Into this unsure camp, however, we can also add jurists, at least in the early days of brain death. In their opinion for the landmark case, *In re Bowman*,[11] the Supreme Court of Washington State was careful to acknowledge that death was not simply a settled matter of medical consensus. They write, "It is, in part, a philosophical decision about what conditions define human life, combined with an empirical determination that those conditions are absent and not latent in a given case. The determination involves differentiating between human life and biological life, marking the dividing line between what constitutes human life and what is merely mechanical." This line, between the human and the "merely mechanical," is a further step away from the experientially obvious condition of death that prevailed to this point. As often cited in these legal cases, death was formerly defined by Black's Law Dictionary as "the cessation of life, the ceasing to exist; defined by physicians as the total stoppage of the blood, and a cessation of the animal and vital functions consequent thereon, such as respiration, pulsation, etc." *In re Bowman*, however, effectively captures a case where the break between "a cessation of … vital functions" and continued respiration can last for days or months. What is understood as "vital," then, becomes a question not just for medicine, but for philosophers, courts, legislators, and the public. Much of the literature surrounding brain death would argue that while the debate has effectively concluded with a clear set of tests for determining death, there is no corresponding, broadly held understanding of what constitutes life (or "vitality") and *why* brain-dead patients are dead.[12]

For philosopher Giorgio Agamben, brain death offers an emblematic case by which to understand not just how we define death, but how we define life in modernity. Just as death has split into a second category of "brain death," life can be understood as existing in multiple forms. In his work, Agamben draws from Aristotle in highlighting an early conceptual split between bare life (*zoē*, the biological fact of life) and political life (*bios*, the potential to pursue a good life)[13]—a distinction also echoed in *In re Bowman's* split between "human life and what is merely mechanical." For Agamben, "The hospital room in which [brain dead patients] waver between life and death delimits a space of exception in which a purely bare life, entirely controlled by man and his technology, appears for the first time" (164). He examines the French classification of *coma dépassé* (beyond coma), the Harvard Committee report, and the conflicting legal, medical, and familial decisions surrounding Karen Quinlan in the mid-1980s. Each of these, he argues, provides an extreme example of his central interest: the exercise of sovereign power through the exceptional figure of the *homo sacer* (defined as a life that may be killed without being considered either murder or sacrifice). In placing the power to define death in the hands of the state—through court acts and medical authority—modern biopolitics finds its emblematic expression. This modern democratic structure draws together, for Agamben, seemingly disparate cases such as the concentration camp inmate and the brain-dead patient. These spaces that "waver between life and death" reveal a fundamental lack of distinction between the biological and the political; there is no body that is not always already a biopolitical body (187). Agamben concludes by highlighting these "zones of indistinction" as the terrain upon which a new politics must be thought (187). In the indistinct cases of organ transplantation and brain death, these ideas provide a lens through which we can see the expression of biopolitical sovereignty in our public policies and ethical choices.

Revealing the political and insecure nature of our most fundamental categories, however, does not mean we have escaped the fantasy of a natural and fixed split between life and death. In an editorial published in 1968, the *Journal of the American Medical Association* laments, "When all is said and done, it seems ironic that the end point of existence, which ought to be as clear and sharp as in a chemical titration, should so defy the power of words to describe it and the power of men to say with certainty, 'It is here.'"[14] In drawing on the simile of chemical titration, these medical professionals express their bias for the seeming facts of science and their desire for secure diagnostic tools. While we have accepted the Harvard report as reasonably certain criteria for death, the reliance on tests, technology, and reconfirmation in this method trades on the comforting terrain of medical authority. It sidesteps deeper questions of whether these tests actually mean, "it is here."

Without a clear and broad understanding of what constitutes death, doctors, hospitals, courts, and patients' families can find themselves at odds about a declaration of death. In the winter of 2014, US national news media erupted with the case of Jahi McMath, a 13-year-old Oakland, CA girl who was declared brain dead following complications from a series of operations to remove her tonsils and some sinus tissue. The case garnered national attention because despite the fact that the hospital and a court had found her brain dead, McMath's parents rejected the diagnosis and sought to move her out of state to another medical facility that would not remove artificial support. At six months after her declaration of death, McMath was relocated to New Jersey, a state that allows families to reject a diagnosis of brain death and places the decision to continue medical support in the hands of the family. In 2018, an attorney for the family released a statement that "Jahi died [on June 22] as a result of complications associated with liver failure," a declaration of death that occurred 5 years after her initial diagnosis of brain death.[15] In the early months, the case resurrected some debate over definitions of death, but has also coalesced through public comment the broad medical and legal consensus around brain death *as* death. In fact, the dominant trend among experts interviewed has been to express concern over the misleading modifier in the term, allowing, after all, "if someone dies from a heart attack, we don't call it 'cardiovascular dead.'"[16] Ethicist Robert M. Veatch contributed an OpEd to CNN in which he argues for a "conscience-based" approach in which public policy stays largely the same, but where "people like Jahi's parents should have the option to record their conscientiously held positions and allow pronouncements of death to be based on those beliefs."[17] If, as Veatch advocates and New Jersey law allows, pronouncements of death can be based on familial, non-expert belief, then the McMath case confirms what the court argued with *In re Bowman* nearly 25 years ago: Death is in part a philosophical decision, not a bare medical fact.

Conceiving of death as more than mere biology recognizes that the philosophical decisions involved are also historically contingent. Much has been made of the fact that the heart-lung definition of death made sense during centuries in which the heart was understood as the central organ of the body. But, as *Defining Death* argues, "People's attitudes toward death evolve, and changes in medical capabilities certainly come to be reflected in public as well as professional circles: heart transplantation, for example, cannot help but alter the romantic notion of the heart as the seat of soul or personality" (59). The public acceptance of brain death as a legitimate definition of death is consistent with the cultural movement from the heart to the brain as the seat of individual identity.

This transfer of importance from heart to brain suggests an emergent, but still unsettled, understanding of the underlying concepts linking the brain to death. In 1989, Stuart Youngner and a group of colleagues conducted a survey of 195 physicians and nurses likely to be involved in organ transplantation.[18] The team interviewed these individuals to discover what they knew about the definition of brain death and what personal attitudes they held about brain death and organ donation. While the survey yielded a number of interesting results—including significant variation in the definition and implementation of a diagnosis of brain death among practicing health professionals—perhaps the most revealing result was the lack of consensus and consistency about the underlying concept of death. While some respondents rejected brain death altogether and others articulated a whole brain concept, results were generally split between the higher brain and lower brain concepts. Phrases like "consciousness and cognition," "capacity for social interaction," and "personhood" were key identifiers of death for the higher brain group (2207). The lower brain group focused on the "ability of the organism to function as a whole" and "ability to regulate/integrate bodily functions" (2207). The law is clear in adopting a whole brain definition of death, but it does not explain *why* the brain should have this elevated status. The inward turn of the twentieth century to problems of the psyche and consciousness suggests a new concept of personhood that turns away from the heart or the soul. But as I will discuss below, debates about abortion and the disability rights "Not Dead Yet" movement have exposed the lack of public consensus about the seat of personhood. Others argue for the integrative function of the brain for its place at the apex of our organ system, but is the skin less necessary? The liver?[19]

A second fascinating result of Youngner et al.'s study is the number of respondents who understood the prevailing definition of brain death and who stated that the patients described in the study were dead, but who used language indicating they believed the patients were still somehow alive. The doctors and nurses gave responses like: "'The patient's quality of life is not acceptable,' 'the patient is hopelessly dying,' and 'the brain cannot be replaced'" (2207). These turns of phrase reveal that there is not only a split between the definition of death and our underlying concept of what makes death so, but there is an internal dissonance for individuals about when and how death occurs. While Youngner et al's survey is the most commonly cited work on medical attitudes toward brain death, Margaret Lock cites several other studies conducted between 1970 and 1989 that reveal similar lack of consensus about among medical professionals. Her own interviews with physicians in intensive care units in North America confirm a broadly held belief that brain death does not signal the end of biological life, even if they all believe complete biological death is inevitable in these cases (121–123, 243).

As Youngner explores in a later essay, provocatively titled "Some Must Die" (1996), the continued care required for patients who have been declared dead and the hospital personnel's attitudes toward these patients often reveals a deep gulf between a secure definition of death on one hand, and the limbo state of brain death on the other. For example, Youngner relates that even though legal time of death occurs when the patient is determined to be brain dead, health professionals often record the time the heart stopped beating (after "life support" has been removed) on the death certificate.[20] Perhaps more profoundly, hospital staff describe the intense care required to sustain brain-dead patients before transplant and the emotional jolt that occurs when that care follows the organ and the patient is left to "die again" on the operating table, their surgical incisions hastily stitched back together.[21]

The foundational literature on brain death tries to establish not just the definition of death, but to prescribe language that will shape and reconstruct the experiences described above. *Defining Death* leads in this attempt, offering several linguistic interventions in current legal statutes and criticizing the Harvard Criteria for similar slips of the tongue. First and foremost is the replacement of the perhaps euphemistic Harvard term "irreversible coma" with the term "brain death," since "'coma' is a condition of a living person, and a body without any brain functions is dead and thus beyond any coma" (25). Later, the commission asserts the importance of accuracy in language by pivoting within a single sentence between discussing unnecessary prolongation of treatment for "bodies that have died" to useful treatment for "patients still alive" (48). For doctors, nurses, and families, however, the slow descent from "living person" and "patient" to "body" cannot be as clear or easy as *Defining Death* wants it to be.

The report similarly seeks to excise any qualifying language from the statutory code. Early laws used phrases like "medically and legally dead" or "dead for all legal purposes." The presidential commission rightfully points out the confusing and sinister implications of such qualifiers; after all, what does "legal purposes" leave out? Are there other purposes for which a person might be considered not dead? They also change the phrase "shall be considered dead" to "is dead" in the Uniform Determination of Death Act. This rhetorical sleight of hand again offers a profound example of the power of the performative utterance. In moving from the social condition of being "considered dead" to the ontological declaration "is dead," the statue reminds us of the power of language to structure our most profound experiences and conditions.

Continuing in this semiotic vein, *Defining Death* argues, "But breathing and heartbeat are not life itself. They are simply used as signs" (33). Although they go on to argue that these signs are "windows into a deeper and more complex reality," they also acknowledge that how these signs are read and *which* signs are meaningful is a matter of historical contingency, technology, and choice. The security of the "deeper reality" of death only exists beyond an impenetrable screen of mediation. They acknowledge, "Medical technology has forced us to choose which signs of life are sufficiently important that their loss constitutes the death of the patient, while other signs of life persist" (*Defining Death* 45). The acceptance of brain death offers a fascinating shift in our culture, in which our elevation of some vital signs over others came without a corresponding acknowledgment that such a shift marked a reconstitution of what it means to be alive and dead.

The Harvard Committee and presidential commission share attempts to obscure this shift: in insisting they were simply identifying new *indicators*, without touching underlying realities. But this insistence seems inconsistent with their desire that lay individuals would understand the new definition of death as the same as the old. Both reports insisted that previous methods of diagnosing death did not equate death with loss of heartbeat, but that loss of heartbeat was simply the easiest measure of the failure of "interrelated systems with the brain at its apex" (*Defining Death* 33). Jerry Menikoff, in an undergraduate bioethics textbook, offers a rhetorically convincing rejoinder to this obfuscation:

> In fact, the committee that announced the Harvard criteria stated that it was not in fact changing the definition of death, but rather recognizing that even the traditional criteria of death were followed only as a means of determining whether a person's brain still functioned. Is that conclusion obvious to you? Do you think, if we went back several hundred years and asked the average woman-about-town, she would have said, "Sure, the brain is the only thing that matters when a person is declared dead"? If we had shown that woman a person with a dead brain, but the rest of the body functioning quite nicely, would she be comfortable declaring him dead? As opposed to saying, "This person—with a dead brain in a living body—is not dead until you turn off the machines, and the entire body is dead."[22]

Menikoff's question—"Is that conclusion obvious to you?"—is important not just for students of bioethics, but for medical practitioners who must explain to families why their loved one is dead despite her continued breath and heartbeat. In a nice demonstration of both the power and slippages of social construction, the legal and medical choice to redefine death has been easily adopted, but the full extent of its meaning and implications has not always fully taken hold. We are participating in the obfuscations of these committees, allowing that brain death shall count for death and then using qualifying terminology and phrases like "life support," "patient," "irreversibly dying," "quality of life," and "brain death" itself.

Three Limit Cases

It can be tempting to see these discussions of death as mere navel-gazing, abstract philosophical debates that have no clear answer and no real importance. It may seem typical that a professor of English would be enchanted by stories that hinge on idiosyncrasies of language, signs, and coding. But, as I've claimed already, these slippages in language have very real material and affective consequences for the physicians and families involved as well as in policies governing the life-saving and life-ending practices impacting tens of thousands each year. Three kinds of medical conditions serve as important limit cases at the intersection of brain death and organ transplant and can further clarify (or complicate) our thinking of these questions. Donors after cardiac death, brain-dead pregnant women, and anencephalic infants reveal real attempts to gerrymander the definition of death to open up new sources of organs for transplant. In addition to challenging the definition of death, these cases also speak to problems of time of death and recourse to language of "personhood" as it structures debates about the beginning and end of life.

The use of donors after cardiac death for organ transplant marks an odd return to the heart-lung definition of death. Called Non-Heart-Beating Donation (NHBD) prior to 2003, Donation After Cardiac Death, or DCD, is an end-of-life option for patients who have suffered severe brain injuries but who do not meet the criteria for brain death. Before the introduction of brain death laws, DCD was the method of procurement for all organs for donation. The quick pace of deterioration to organs, however, meant that DCD organs were often of poor quality and limited to kidneys. After the introduction of brain death statues, nearly all organ procurement organizations (OPOs) stopped pursuing DCD donors. But thirty years of medical advances and continued shortages in organ supply have lead to a renewed interest in DCD organs. In these kinds of donations, a family decides to withdraw treatment in consultation with a physician. Then, after a process of evaluation and matching on the part of OPOs, the patient is typically transferred to an operating room, life-sustaining treatment is withdrawn, the patient's physician declares cardiac death, and the organs are surgically recovered.

While brochures describing DCD seek to make this process seem as straightforward as possible, there are several seams in the timeline described above. The deepest fissure can be found in questions surrounding time of death and the definition of the term "irreversible cessation." As discussed at length above, The Uniform Determination of Death Act includes both the irreversible cessation of heart-lung function as well as brain function in its two-part definition of death. The heart-lung definition was kept in place to cover the vast majority of cases in which lay individuals could clearly identify the death of another without recourse to a medical degree or specialized equipment. Recently, however, this notion of cardiac death has been coupled with removal of life support to open up a new class of organ donors. The key problem in these types of donations is to identify the precise moment at which the requirement of irreversibility has been met without excessive deterioration of the organs for transplant. This question must be resolved within a scale of less than 5 minutes. So, what is the definition of "irreversible"? When function cannot be restored with current medical technology? Given our capabilities, such a definition would seem to preclude the use of these donors. Or, should "irreversible" refer to a morally defensible position in which the decision has been made by the patient or family not to restore function even though it may be medically possible? For individuals who have made their wishes clear to family or for families who choose to remove life support, desire is the determining factor in the "irreversible cessation" of their heart. Since the viability of organs would be too severely compromised in waiting for the point of medical and technological irreversibility, doctors have returned to cardiac death (which produces the earliest sign), even in the presence of some continued brain function, in the pursuit of organs for donation and in the enactment of families' wishes.

DCD promotional material places a strong emphasis on choice and familial control in the donation process. Key phrases from organizations like LifePoint, Inc. and Donate Life include "additional *option*," "families who have already *decided* to remove life support," and "advanced *directive*" (emphasis added).[23] Deeply embedded in the ethos of these organizations is the notion of individual and familial control over the end of life. The frequently asked questions sections of these brochures and Web sites reveal a significant amount of anxiety over death; in their often-circular responses, OPOs deploy the many shades of meaning around death to reassure patients' families. Anticipated questions include: "When organs are removed, is the patient really dead?," "Are medical professionals hastening the death of the patient?," and "Does the patient suffer pain during organ recovery?." The phrase "really dead" in the question above puts in colloquial terms something that many suspect: That patients may be considered dead enough for organ donation, but that there is probably a deeper definition of death that they don't quite meet. The response to these kinds of questions hinges on the phrase "declared dead," which may be legally and medically accurate, but feels a bit like skirting the question behind the question. To the question about whether the patient suffers pain, the Southwest Transplant Alliance brochure on DCD responds: "After a patient dies, he or she no longer feels pain. Organ recovery occurs only after a patient is declared dead." Despite the firm nature of these claims, bioethicists including Stuart Youngner and Jerry Menikoff describe a common practice of giving patients pain medication when removing life support because without cessation of all brain function, they may feel some pain.

Perhaps asking whether DCD donors are "really dead" is the wrong question (although it is understandable why families might not think so). Perhaps the question, and one that has been animating much of this chapter, is whether there is something wrong with our definition(s) of death more generally. The focus on timing in DCD retrieval is complicated, in part, because of our insistence on death as an event, not a process. Black's Law Dictionary insists, "death is not a continuous event and is an event that takes place at a precise time." But as Melanie Bacchiochi's case—in which different criteria for death were met over a period of months—demonstrates, a confident break between death and dying is a compelling social fiction. This clear dichotomy is a fiction that may be reassuring, but is it still useful? Some scholars have argued for a public policy that allows for finer gradations in our definition of death, allowing for different responses at different points. In these cases, a patient may be considered far enough along the spectrum of death for cessation of treatment, but not dead enough for burial or, perhaps, for organ retrieval.[24]

In 1971, Robert Morison published an oft-cited article in *Science* critiquing the "misplaced concreteness" attached to our notion of death. His article explores how the literary representation of death is contrary to "the problem of dying under modern conditions" (694). Consistent with his interest in death's move from conception to abstraction to concrete thing, Morison peppers his writing with a series of lively metaphors. He writes, "Death is not only reified, it is personified, and graduates from a mere thing to a jostling old woman in the marketplace of Baghdad or an old man, complete with beard, scythe, and hourglass, ready to mow down those whose time has come" (694). For Morison, the power of language is complicit in convincing the world of an artificial distinction in what he argues is essentially a continuous process. Death as metaphor, then, gives form to abstract and arbitrary splits between life, dying, and death. He argues that, while challenging, even abstractions can be revised to meet new social demands and sees the new (in 1971) definition of brain death as a weak work-around a more fundamental problem.

As Jahi McMath's family was struggling with California courts and hospitals to reject their daughter's diagnosis of brain death, two other cases of brain death found national attention in the winter of 2014. Marlise Munoz and Robyn Benson, over 3000 miles apart in Texas and British Colombia, offer a striking contrast in approaches to women who are, as one media headline put it, "brain dead and pregnant" (ABC). In the Benson case, her husband, Dylan, made the decision to continue artificial support after his wife was declared brain dead in order to give their 22-week-old fetus the greatest chance of life. Dylan told news media "She is doing so much to grow our son. Her brain is not alive, but she still is." A CNN story reporting on the case includes the line: "He's counting down the days to the birth of his son—and the death of his wife." Such rhetorical flourishes in discussing brain death are not just a writerly impulse on the part of reporters; they reveal the always-present difficulty in describing bodies held in the limbo stage between declaration of brain death and removal of artificial "life" support. As we've seen in the cases described here, this limbo stage can go on for months. Dylan's belief that his wife is actively "growing" their son, reveals a special complexity in the case of brain-dead pregnant women and calls attention to our cultural understanding of motherhood more broadly.

In a 1991 essay titled "Containing Women: Reproductive Discourse in the 1980s," Valerie Hartouni offers one of the few scholarly analyses of cultural rhetoric surrounding brain death and pregnancy. Linking the phenomenon to a diverse set of issues including handling frozen embryos and political uses of ultrasound technology, Hartouni sees a cultural trend that dislocates the fetus from the mother and casts motherhood as a biological condition, rather than an experiential one. In her close reading of the 1986 *San Francisco Chronicle* headline, "Brain Dead Mother Has Her Baby," Hartouni sees a form of motherhood that is "literally mindless—a state of being" (30). She jostles our casual acceptance of such notions of motherhood by imagining increasingly disruptive headlines: "Thirty-Two-Week-Old Fetus Extracted from Corpse," "Eight-Month-Old Fetus Extracted from Dead Woman's Body," "Deceased Delivered," "Trapped Fetus Lives" (32). Hartouni's close reading and imaginative play with alternative headlines demonstrate the constructive power of language to reflect and shape our notions of biological processes. By re-animating brain-dead corpses as mothers who "grow" and "have" their babies, our cultural discussion of these cases reveals an ambiguity in our treatment of brain death, but also how we think of motherhood and pregnancy as well.

The contrasting case of 2014 staged a battle between Marlise Munoz's husband, Erick, and doctors' reading of state law in Texas. In late November, Erick found his 14 weeks pregnant wife unresponsive on their kitchen floor. Doctors declared her brain dead and Erick asked to have her removed from artificial support. Marlise had worked as a paramedic and both her husband and her family were in agreement on her wishes not to be kept on artificial support. Her fetus was months from viability. Doctors, however, refused to remove support because, they claimed, state law prohibited them from removing "life-sustaining" treatment from a pregnant woman. On January 14, Erick Munoz sued the hospital, arguing that doctors were misinterpreting the law. The statute in question relies on the Texas Advance Directives Act, which defines "life sustaining treatment" as that which "sustains the life of a patient and without which the patient will die." Munoz's lawyer was able to argue successfully that the statute should apply only in cases of a living pregnant woman, not one who had been declared dead. Two months after her collapse, Munoz was removed from artificial respiration.

In order to properly view this case, it is helpful to take a slight detour into how we understand the notions of part and whole, mother and fetus. Feminist scholarship on pregnancy and technology—most notably by Rosalind Petchestky—has argued convincingly that voiceover and the propaganda use of ultrasound images have conflated medical evidence and politicized belief in the debate over abortion. Typically, technology is used as an apparently straightforward tool in the narrative construction of medical "fact." In her analysis of the anti-abortion video *Ultrasound: A Window to the Womb* (a more recent successor to the immensely popular *Silent Scream* video of the 1980s), Joanne Boucher argues that "when the video is examined closely it becomes evident that it is a complex combination of ultrasound images, photographic images, verbal argument, written text, and emotional appeal which are mobilized to 'prove' that life begins at conception."[25] In the next paragraphs, I will discuss how debates around fetal personhood may or may not be connected to the special case of brain death and anencephalic infants, but before moving on, I am curious to explore how this use of technology functions to imbue fetuses and, perhaps organs, with identity and personality. Boucher goes on to argue, "In the video, this religious or metaphysical position [that the fetus *is* an unborn baby] is presented as scientific fact with reference to the development of human organs, features, functions, and, crucially, personality" (10). In these constructed narratives of fetal development as personality development, fetuses are imbued with characteristics like shyness or friendliness ("Look, he's waving at you!"). These narratives are consistent with both long-standing and more contemporary cultural metaphors that place human emotions in physical organs—think of early concepts of spleen, but also more colloquial phrases like "he's all heart."

Much of the visual rhetoric in post-ultrasound anti-abortion campaigns relies on representing the fetus as fundamentally detached from the gestating "vessel" of the mother. Since the 1980s, posters, videos, and billboards have included free-floating fetuses as an affirmation of the "independent" life of the fetus. This elevation of the status of the fetus over the state of the mother conforms to the mindset of the Texas doctors who believed it would be unlawful to remove Marlise Munoz from life support because she was pregnant, even though she had been declared dead. This imaginative separation of fetus from mother—and the reliance on technology and visual culture to achieve it—offers an interesting analogy to similar ideological moves in exchanging organs from one individual to another. While images of free-floating hearts and livers would be too grotesque for most OPO brochures, the ubiquitous image of the plastic coolers used in transplantation pushes the notion of organs as innocuous, portable, even family friendly. This family-focused vocabulary continues in the commonly used photographs of beaming, healthy recipients with their families. By underscoring portability and successful delivery, these transplant images emphasize the possibility of separation, dislocating organs from one (now absent) owner to another.

Images of fetal separation are motivated by the desire to discover personhood earlier and earlier in fetal development. Fetal personhood is a crucial legal and philosophical tenet for the anti-abortion movement, but the terms of personhood have failed to gain much traction in debates over the definition of death. Where these debates do exist, they have failed to impact medical or public policy. In 1981, the presidentially appointed authors of *Defining Death* even got the endorsement of Dennis Horan, then president of the American Citizens United for Life, who agreed that the proposed definition of brain death "is beneficial and does not undermine any of the values we seek to support" (11). How, then, is personhood so controversial in conversations about the beginning of life and so benign at its end?

Perhaps the difference lies in our drive toward the future and a sense of what will be. Among many of the physicians Margaret Lock interviewed, brain death was a sufficient opening for organ donation, because, in the words of one intensive care doctor, even though "it's not death, ... it is an irreversible diagnosis, which I accept" (243). There is an interesting shared teleological reasoning behind fetal personhood and both brain death and donation after cardiac death. In each case, the status is conferred because the cells, then embryo, then fetus *will be* a person and the irreversibly brain-damaged individual *will be* dead. Anencephalic infants offer a curious combination of this logic because, as articulated at an international meeting of transplant surgeons in 1987, the child "can never develop even the semblance of personhood."[26] One attendee suggested that anencephalic children fall into a new category of "living but brain absent." Categorization is the central difficulty surrounding anencephalic infants—are they alive, but not persons; dead according to some new, third definition; or acceptable exceptions to the dead donor rule?

Anencephaly is a relatively rare fetal anomaly in which major portions of the brain and skull do not develop after the growth of a brain stem. The condition is often diagnosed through prenatal testing and many of these pregnancies are terminated. Some parents, however, decide to carry the pregnancies to term, often with the expressed hope that their newborn can serve as an organ or tissue donor to another child. In an interesting expression of broader organ donation rhetoric, these parental activists couch their interests under the banner of the "purposeful gift." Currently, however, organ donation policies and the definition of brain death exclude anencephalic infants as donors in most cases. Because they are often born with a functioning brain stem, they fail to meet criteria for total cessation of all brain function and if doctors wait for brain death to occur before transplant, it typically means that organs will have deteriorated beyond the point of viability (similar to the circumstances in donation after cardiac death). There are a few possibilities in preserving anencephalic infants as a source for donation. One choice would be to place these newborns on artificial life support until they do meet the criteria for brain death. This process, however, could take weeks or months, and would differ from the typical medical course by potentially prolonging the life of these infants. Another choice would follow the logic of "living but brain absent" to revise the Uniform Anatomical Gift Act to include donations from these living donors. Or, finally, we might redefine death to include this category. Major medical professional organizations are split on this question. The American Medical Association recommends making a special exception to the dead donor rule, arguing that these infants "have never experienced, and will never experience, consciousness." The AMA does not, importantly, recommend revising the more general definition of death to include these infants, acknowledging that their use as donors would mean taking organs from live bodies. The American Academy of Pediatrics has come to the opposite conclusion, siding with every US court in which a case of anencephalic donation has been heard, that there is not a compelling enough need for these organs to justify such a dramatic step as making an exception to the dead donor rule. Slippery slope arguments prevail among both jurists and activists like those in the Not Dead Yet movement. The AAP bioethics committee on this question argues forcefully that to amend the transplant law to allow for retrieval before total brain death would be "to authorize actively causing death," a prohibition that serves as a guiding light in the often murky experience of caring for patients at the end of life.

It is interesting to recall, however, that many of our attitudes toward proper subjects for organ retrieval have changed over time and are contingent upon broader cultural attitudes toward medicine. Donation after cardiac death was once the norm until the definition of brain death opened a new class of donors; now that technology has ameliorated some of the difficulties of retrieval from DCD patients, they are again sought by organ procurement centers as a possible source. Similarly, anencephalic infants are excluded from major organ donation because they would violate national policies around death and donation. But in 1967, the first US heart transplant was from an anencephalic infant to an adult. Some bioethicists argue that the definition of brain death was so uncontroversial because of its emergence in a particular moment in American cultural history. The stamp of university prestige for the Harvard criteria coincided with an era of "almost unprecedented belief and trust in medical science."[27] Stuart Youngner and Robert Arnold go on to argue that "the introduction and early acceptance of brain death preceded *Roe v Wade* and the national debate about physician-assisted death—two issues that have galvanized the religious right to protect life and reject arguments about its quality."[28] It may be that brain death has fallen outside of these crusades not because of a fundamental difference in how life is measured and valued, but because its emergence as a concept came to be accepted before it could be caught up in the sweep of social activism.

The dead donor rule is represented as sacred in court cases and rhetoric about organ retrieval, but a closer examination of how brain death is unevenly understood and the case of donation after cardiac death reveals how deeply scripted declarations of death can be. In 2001, Youngner and Arnold write, "perhaps, after decades of *de facto* violations of the dead donor rule, our society is willing to openly discuss whether or not it is acceptable to take organs from patients who are beyond harm and protected by a rigorous consent process" (535). Over a decade later, however, there is little evidence that we are pursuing such a conversation. Instead, a gerrymandered definition of death creates a jagged line that moves to include or exclude individuals with little clear understanding of what death really means. Ventilators are removed from still-living patients who wish to die. Parents carry fatally ill fetuses to term in the hope of transferring their organs to another child in need, only to be stopped by courts. Pregnant women are held in suspended states of death in the political interests in fetal life. Doctors debate how many minutes constitute "irreversible cessation" of heart function. And medical professionals lament the "poor quality of life" for their brain-dead patients. Each of these choices, made in courtrooms and at hospital bedsides, points to a deeper, collective choice that we have made as a culture: to allow the social need for organs and protection of hospital resources to open up a murky and contingent definition of death.

Notes

1. President's Commission for the Study of Ethical Problems in Medicine and Biomedical and Behavioral Research, *Defining Death: Medical, Legal, and Ethical Issues in the Determination of Death* (Washington, DC, 1981), http://bioethics.georgetown.edu/pcbe/reports/past_commissions/defining_death.pdf.
2. Henry K. Beecher, Adams, and Barger, "A Definition of Irreversible Coma."
3. Mita Giacomini identifies competing historical accouts for the primary factors driving the work of the Harvard Ad Hoc Committee: (1) as a demand of technical progress or (2) a defensive response to skepticism about the ethics of heart transplant research. She concludes that transplantation was not only an early motivating factor in establishing the committee, but that "the degree to which transplantation technologies' ethical and medical needs dictated some clinical features of brain death has not been fully appreciated." Giacomini, "A Change of Heart and a

Change of Mind? Technology and the Reinvention of Death in 1968," *Social Science & Medicine* 44, no. 10 (1997): 1479.

4. *Defining Death*, 21, 17. Although the vast majority of patients who have lost all brain functions will typically suffer cardiac arrest within days, or at most several weeks, there are cases where respiration and heartbeat have been maintained even longer. Youngner and Arnold cite a case in which a patient "lived" for fourteen years with continued artificial respiration. They argue that such variety "undercut[s] one of the reasons for public acceptance of brain death—that is, that brain-dead patients [suffer] traditional death (by cardiac arrest) within hours or days despite aggressive intervention." Stuart J. Youngner and Robert Arnold, "Philosophical Debates About the Definition of Death: Who Cares?" *Journal of Medicine and Philosophy* 26, no. 5 (2001): 530. If cardiac death is inevitable, the public reasons, why not embrace diagnostic criteria that would help others live?
5. *The Princess Bride*, directed by Rob Reiner (1987, Twentieth Century Fox).
6. Mita Giacomini's archival work on the development of the Harvard criteria in 1968 reveals that this caution about the modifying use of "brain death" existed from the very beginning. Upon reading a draft of the article, transplant surgeon Joseph Murray wrote to Beecher arguing, "The term 'brain death' should be eliminated. Death is what we are talking about, and adding the adjective 'brain' implies some restriction on the term as if it were an incomplete type of death." Giacomini, "A Change of Heart,"1477.
7. Of course, the presidential commission would reject this characterization, and in fact insists: "the statute … must accurately reflect the social meaning of death and not constitute a mere legal fiction" (31). Such a perspective, however, relies on a narrow concept of fiction, one not shared by this book. In looking at "transplant fictions," I am exploring precisely these moments in which definitions change and ideology shifts through the work of discourse.
8. Giacomini, "A Change of Heart," 1471.
9. Jonathan Culler, *Literary Theory: A Very Short Introduction* (Oxford: Oxford University Press, 1997).
10. United Press International, "A Connecticut Woman, Taken Off Respirator, Dies," *The New York Times*, March 14, 1981, sec. N.Y. / Region, http://www.nytimes.com/1981/03/14/nyregion/a-connecticut-woman-taken-off-respirator-dies.html.
11. *In re Bowman*, Supreme Court of Washington 617 R2d 731 (Wash. 1980). In this tragic case, 5-year-old Matthew Bowman was admitted to the hospital after sustaining massive physical injuries inflicted by a

care giver. When his parents could not be immediately found, a guardian ad litem was appointed to make medical decisions on the young boy's behalf. After the parents were located, they concurred with the medical personnel that Matthew was brain dead and sought to remove life support. The guardian ad litem, however, resisted the termination of Matthew's dependent position, stating that the consequence would be the termination of life support systems. The Supreme Court of Washington State ruled that the state law must conform to "prevailing medical opinion" and that under Washington law, "William Matthew Bowman is dead."

12. As Youngner and his co-authors put it, "irreversible loss of all brain function has been widely accepted as a *criterion* for determining death, without a corresponding, widely accepted *concept* explaining exactly why brain dead patients are dead" ("'Brain Death' and Organ Retrieval" 2206).
13. Giorgio Agamben, *Homo Sacer*, Meridian (Stanford, CA: Stanford University Press, 1998).
14. "What and When Is Death?" *JAMA* 204 (1968): 219–220.
15. Debra Goldschmidt, "Jahi McMath, California Teen at Center of Brain-Death Controversy, Has Died," *CNN*, June 29, 2018, https://edition.cnn.com/2018/06/29/health/jahi-mcmath-brain-dead-teen-death/index.html.
16. Jacque Wilson and Jen Christensen, "Why Brain Dead Means Really Dead," *CNN*, January 6, 2014, http://www.cnn.com/2014/01/06/health/brain-dead-basics/index.html.
17. Robert Veatch, "Let Parents Decide If Teen Is Dead," *CNN*, January 2, 2014, http://www.cnn.com/2014/01/02/opinion/veatch-defining-death/index.html.
18. Stephen Youngner et al., "'Brain Death' and Organ Retrieval: A Cross-Sectional Survey of Knowledge and Concepts Among Health Professionals," *JAMA* 261, no. 15 (April 21, 1989): 2205–2210.
19. It seems significant to note here that the brain (despite our cultural fantasies) represents a final frontier of transplant medicine. Beyond the perhaps insuperable technological complexities of the operation, the notion of brain transplantation troubles our current notions of identity and triggers ethical prohibitions. For more on the strange case of brain transplant, see Chapter 6.
20. Stuart J. Youngner, "Some Must Die," in *Organ Transplantation: Meanings and Realities*, ed. Stuart J. Youngner, Renée C. Fox, and Laurence J. O'Connell (Madison, WI: University of Wisconsin Press, 1996), 45.
21. Ibid., 46.
22. Jerry Menikoff, *Law and Bioethics: An Introduction* (Washington, DC: Georgetown University Press, 2001), 452.

23. LifePoint, Inc., "Donation After Cardiac Death," accessed May 29, 2014, http://www.lifepoint-sc.org/facts_cardiac.htm.
24. For more on the critique of death as a singular event, see Linda Emanuel, "What Is Wrong with 'Dead'?" in *Brain Death*, Proceedings of the Second International Conference on Brain Death (Amsterdam: Elsevier, 1995), 47–56; Robert S. Morison, "Death: Process or Event?"; and A. Halevy and B. Brody, "Brain Death: Reconciling Definitions, Criteria, and Tests," *Annals of Internal Medicine* 119, no. 6 (1993): 519–525.
25. Joanne Boucher, "Ultrasound: A Window to the Womb?," 8.
26. George J. Annas, "From Canada with Love: Anencephalic Newborns as Organ Donors?" *The Hastings Center Report* 17, no. 6 (December 1, 1987): 36.
27. Youngner and Arnold, "Philosophical Debates," 533.
28. Ibid.

CHAPTER 5

"The Gift of Life": Sentiment and the Family

It is July 1983 and President Ronald Reagan has taken to the airwaves in his weekly radio address. He is issuing a life-saving plea for a baby in need of a liver transplant. That baby is Ashley Bailey. She is a "little 11-month old girl from Texas … and all 11 pounds of her are in critical condition."[1] Reagan describes the extraordinary measures that have been taken to make transplantation a possibility for Ashley, from the financial rallying of local community members and businesses to his personal pledge to have an "Air Force jet standing ready" to transport a suitable organ. He calls on the sentiments of an imagined "pair of stunned and grief-stricken parents" who, knowing "their baby could make it possible for Ashley to live, … would have no hesitation in saying, 'Save that little girl.'"

This presidential address is emblematic of the political response to the new science of organ transplantation and its attendant problems of distribution of scarce resources. Anecdotal appeals, ad hoc fund-raising efforts, competition for publicity, and rhetoric grounded in care, family, and emotions are all characteristics of our national discussions of organ exchange, then and now. Although public policy on transplantation no longer relies on offers of Air Force jets, the seeds of sentimental appeal, planted from the earliest days of tissue exchange, persist as the dominant mode in discussions from the local to the national level.

Reagan's plea expresses a particular valence of national identity, one rooted in a long-standing sentimental vision of the nation as a

E. Russell, *Transplant Fictions*,
Palgrave Studies in Literature, Science and Medicine,
https://doi.org/10.1007/978-3-030-12135-8_5

network of essentially similar families. Reagan tells the nation, explicitly: "Americans are giving people" and "We live in a country where people truly care for one another" and "That kind of caring should make us all proud to be American." These assertions are perhaps so commonplace as to seem unremarkable, but they are essential to understanding the ideological groundwork lying beneath our public policy, individual medical decisions, and organ donation campaigns. Because this model of citizenship has such deep roots, Reagan can reasonably place organ donation in a lineage of Americans rallying in broadly dissimilar circumstances. He says, "America has faced shortage in the past of everything from nylons during World War II to oil in the 1970's. But modern medical science has provided us with a new shortage—a shortage of living organs: livers, hearts, lungs, eyes, kidneys. I urge all Americans to fill out donor cards, little cards you carry in your wallet or purse that, in the event of your death, offer the hope of life to others." In Reagan's scheme, individual acts, minimized as the "little cards you carry in your wallet," add up to a heroic effort to overcome both national problems and to "save that little girl."

Critics of Reagan have been quick to point out that this kind of sentimental public appeal is not, in fact, a public policy. Even after the passage of the National Organ Transplant Act in 1984—which Reagan initially opposed—the law was slow to receive funding. Supporters struggled for the resources to develop a national network that could match donors and ensure that organs were distributed according to medical criteria. Writing in 1987, Ellen Goodman from the Washington Post Writers Group laments, "By now we have grown used to these gaps between Reagan sentiments and actions." She continues, "Without this national system for gathering and fairly distributing such a scarce human resource, we are back in the game of wait and waste. Desperate families will again compete for publicity. Their best hope will be to become the anecdote of the week." Goodman is, of course, right. An anecdotal appeal is not a public policy or an appropriate criterion for the distribution of life-saving organs. Sentiment is, however, at the heart of our national policies of organ exchange. Our ideological investment in life, family, and love as "universal" values is part of why we understand organs to be so valuable in the first place.

This chapter looks at sentimental narratives of organ exchange, arguing that while the systems of distribution have changed in the decades since Reagan's address, the foundational rhetorical appeal has not.

Drawing from public campaigns, news stories, and fictional texts, I demonstrate the cultural work done through these sentimental stories. The recurring tropes of family, feeling, and romance found in organ donation narratives construct entirely new categories of subjectivity and affiliation, including: donor families, savior siblings, surgical altruists, donor chains, and live donors. These new categories have emerged as organ transplantation moved from fringe, risky medicine to a common, life-saving practice. How have we come to near-universal acceptance that one person's sudden death can mean "a gift of life" to another? Or that it is appropriate to create a sibling for the express purpose of donating tissue to a dying child? Or that it is not a mark of mental illness to want to donate a kidney to a complete stranger while still alive? In order to believe these things to be true, we must overcome a host of lingering conceptual reservations about the nature of life and death and our responsibility to each other as citizens or family members. While many of the texts explored here fall into melodrama—including those drawn from real life—they all share recourse to the essential terms of family and feeling to imagine a new set of relationships that support our medical possibilities.

A random but reasonably representative selection of international news headlines from August 23, 2015, illustrates the ways in which popular conversations about organ exchange continue to draw from the sentimental well: "My Brother is Going to Die Without an Organ Transplant" (*The Argus*); "Queensland's First Heart Transplant Mother" (*Courier Mail*); "Harlee-Jae Proctor's Mum Makes Plea for More Organ Donors" (*Lancashire Telegraph*); "Haworth Teen Receives Scholarship for Organ and Tissue Awareness" (Northjersey.com). The characters populating these headlines are typically defined by their familial roles, an illustration of the stakes of their potential loss. They encapsulate two essential features of sentimental literature, defining characteristics that scholars of the genre identify over and over: the family and emotional connection.[2] In her article "Reclaiming Sentimental Literature," Joanne Dobson defines this mode clearly: "Sentimentalism envisions the self-in-relation; family (not necessarily in the conventional biological sense), intimacy, community, and social responsibility are its primary relational modes" (267). She goes on to discuss a second valence of sentimentalism, one less commonly cited, but important for the context of organ exchange. In her reading, the other side of the coin celebrating connection is separation: "in the sentimental vision, the greatest threat is the tragedy of separation, of severed human ties" (267). This separation can include the death of a child, lost love, or a "distorted or unsympathetic community" (267). A second look at the headlines above demonstrates this reciprocal logic, tying family, community, and loss together.

As the "reclaiming" in Dobson's title suggests, sentimentalism is still largely a marginal and maligned genre, despite concerted efforts over the past decades to demonstrate its importance in the American imagination.[3] The criticisms are familiar: disposable tearjerkers, poorly written, feminine, formulaic, manipulative, and simplistic. Such negative claims are especially common to contemporary popular novels aimed at women—sold in airports and supermarket checkout lines—these novels are the modern expression of their similarly popular sisters published in the eighteenth century and nineteenth century, but without the mantle of history to lend them respectability. In this chapter, I explore both high and low cultural examples of sentimentalism, a spectrum perhaps best marked by Jodi Picoult on one end and Booker Prize winner Kazuo Ishiguro at the other. Such a span does not intend to suggest equivalence between the aesthetic contributions of these authors, but to argue for the power of popular cultural forms to reflect and shape broadly held attitudes. These attitudes, in turn, direct decision-making at very real moments in our lives. In *The Female Complaint*, Lauren Berlant argues that the modes of sentimental realism that structure most mass-market "women's culture" create a domain in which women's lives are thought of as broadly shared and understood by other women. Sentimental fictions, then, in both high and low forms, create a road map by which we can understand the conceptual underpinnings of family and the ethical demands of love in the face of loss.

In this chapter, I argue that it is not simply emotionally expedient to turn to sentiment as the structuring trope of organ campaigns, but in fact an organic connection borne from the defining values of the genre. The roots of sentiment in eighteenth-century moral philosophy remind us that sociability and emotion do not have to be treated as manipulative appeals that undermine "higher" values of reason and autonomy. Instead, philosophers like Adam Smith, John Locke, and David Hume understand experience, sympathy, and sensation as central to humankind. These foundational principles of sentiment, in turn, serve as a primer by which to read emerging modes of transplant-specific subjectivity and affiliation.

Sentimentalism also stages an important intervention into traditional discussions of bioethics that tend to emphasize autonomy. As Bruce Jennings argues, bioethical literature tends to take the form of "a quest narrative in which the individual, seeking autonomy, struggles against limitations, constraints, and inhibitions imposed by forces (rules, roles, institutions, interference by others, customs, traditions) from the outside."[4] In sentimental narratives, however, autonomy is not the highest value. Instead, achieving connection to others, typically through emotion and intimacy, represents the goal and the external forces challenging our protagonists are often inescapable realities of illness or death. By contrast, then, sentimental stories of bioethical problems tend to focus on the genuine emotional and ethical binds produced by the threat of loss. As such, they serve as a much more appropriate script for narratives of organ exchange; the set pieces of these stories, in both life and fiction, are death bed vigils, sharing tragic news, mourning, and the rediscovery of connection post-transplant or donation. Rather than seeking a way to resist threats to the individual characterized by narratives celebrating autonomy, sentimentalism offers a pathway for relation and reinvention in the face of death.

The Donor Family

The concept of the "donor family" represents a profound example of the ways in which sentimentalism structures not simply rhetorical appeals made on behalf of organ donation, but creates new categories of affiliation and subjectivity. In testimonials from family members of donors—called, commonly, "donor families"[5]—we can see recurring examples of sentimental tropes, including loss, emotion, search for meaning, and self-reinvention. *Caring for Donor Families* is a handbook for health professionals written by Raelynn Maloney and Alan Wolfelt. The book uses a lens of compassionate care to offer practical suggestions for how to navigate donation discussions, questions around consent, and grieving. Maloney and Wolfelt weave comments from donor families throughout the work, grounding their own professional experience with the direct commentary of grieving families. In a fairly typical sentimental formulation, one parent says, "realizing that our fight for life would not be won, our focus changed to another fight for value, that some good might come from our tragedy."[6] Another family quoted in the same volume says, "When our son died, our world fell apart and we were changed forever. … [The wonderful people at the donor network] have patiently helped us realize that through all of our pain and loss has come a renewal for living" (105). These quotes express key dynamics in the creation of a new social formation called the "donor family." Essential to their concept of loss and reinvention is the reconciliation of seemingly opposed terms: most commonly, life/death and tragedy/miracle. As discussed in more detail below, the paradoxical reconciliation of these concepts lays out the tricky navigational terrain of the periods before, during, and after donation.

Best emblematized in the iconic "Give Life" campaign, this imaginative shift from death to life represents the enormity of the conceptual move required to secure organs for donation. Where Chapter 3 explores the conceptual foundation of the "gift of life" as it is laid in the decades before transplantation is achieved, this chapter focuses on how such rhetoric is employed in actual organ exchanges. It is worth bearing in mind that donation decisions are typically made in a family's darkest hour; cadaver organs are drawn from healthy individuals who have usually died suddenly, either through vehicle accident, violence, overdose, or suicide. Families have little time to reconcile themselves to the fact of their loved one's death, a dynamic often complicated by brain death, for all of the reasons discussed in the preceding chapter. In contrast to Ronald Reagan's call to those "little cards we all carry around in our wallets," donation in practice does not always adhere to the previously made choice of the individual donor. Consistently, studies demonstrate reticence among transplant physicians to remove organs from a donor without the express, written consent of next of kin, *even when the donor has signed an anatomical gift form*. This reliance on families over the wishes of the individual finds another expression in the disparity between high public rates of support for organ donation, but low rates of consent among donor-eligible families. In 1995, only about half of those families who were asked agreed to donate.[7] This break between public opinion and family choice at the time of death requires that we look beyond autonomy as the bioethical value structuring medical decision-making. If we take seriously the fact that sentiment undergirds these moments, we can understand that appeals to family and emotion are not a misguided departure from the principle of rationalist autonomy, but instead the necessary terms by which these discussions must be held.

Families of potential donors are making decisions during an important time of transition, in which each person's sense of himself or herself is in flux. *Caring for Donor Families* reminds health practitioners that relationships with others form foundational pieces of our self-identity and that loss requires a revision of this sense of self (99). Upon the death of a loved one, wives and husbands become widows and widowers, children may become orphans, and parents are now "bereaved parents." Organ donation adds the term "donor family" to these more long-standing social categories and brings new scripts by which to understand the experience of loss.

Over and over again, families talk about their experiences in terms that resonate with sentimental novels and films. In particular, families tend to valorize the sacrifice of the donor, typically seeing donation as an expression of the person's praiseworthy characteristics while alive. A 2016 story of organ exchange from Kellen Roberts (22) in West Seattle to Connor Rabinowitz (17) in Minnesota sounds nearly every note of sentimentalism in this "Valentine's Day Tale." First, Kellen's mother characterizes her son's donation as heroic: "We were so grateful that Kell's organs were able to be donated, and thrilled, as we know Kellen would have been, that he was able to save six lives. It gave us such joy and hope in the middle of our enormous loss."[8] This kind of math is common to both donation campaigns and donor families; Web sites and posters commonly trade on the notion that the sum of the parts can be greater than the whole. In this formulation, grief and caring on the part of the family and the deceased donor become a multiplying force of life. Note, too, that medical vocabulary is commonly stripped from the process and transplant surgeries are often located in passive voice constructions—"were able to be donated" and "he was able to save six lives." The dead donor is the giver of life, not the medical personnel. Medical sociologists Reneé Fox and Judith Swazey concur that such formulations are common among donor families: "it is not uncommon for family members to depict the young donor as an outstandingly humane and generous person and to associate the gift of his or her organs with the admirable things that she or he would have done for others if permitted to live out a normal life span" (34). Recipients are, especially in public, likely to talk of their donors in similarly hyperbolic terms. Connor, the recipient of Kellen's heart, says of his donor: "I was now forever connected with this young man who sacrificed his life and chose to save mine. … He is my hero, my guardian angel and I will be forever grateful for his decision to donate his organs."[9]

The charged, emotional nature of these descriptions—hero, guardian angel, saver of lives—is one reason why medical teams have become reticent to share information between donor families and recipients. Scholars of transplantation describe a standard practice of anonymity that has emerged over the decades. Fox and Swazey describe how, after an early period in which background information was commonly exchanged, "the transplanters were discomfited by the way in which recipients, their kin, and donor families personified cadaver organs, and about how many of them not only arranged to meet but tried to become involved in each other's lives as if they were indebted and related to one another" (37). These new forms of affiliation, founded on emotional connection perceived in the wake of transplantation, demonstrate some of the complexity that emerges in the colliding spheres of medicine and sentiment. According to medical professionals, anonymity protects both donor families and recipients; it prevents recipients' sense of identification with their donors and protects them from the reminder that their continued life was made possible by someone else's death.

Despite the practice of anonymity, the experience of organ exchange on all sides is wrapped up in imaginative acts that seek to make sense of this uniquely twentieth-century experience. These beliefs typically fall under two categories: first, a new valence of "blood relation" emerges as donor families and recipients imagine themselves as a new kind of family; second, individuals commonly describe some form of continuation of life in which something of the donor lives on in the recipient. These imaginative bonds are crucially rooted in the theory of sentiment. From its foundational expression in Adam Smith's *Theory of Moral Sentiments*, we have understood sympathy as an act necessarily rooted in imagination. In the most often-quoted line from that volume, Smith writes, "Though our brother is upon the rack, as long as we ourselves are at our ease, our senses will never inform us of what he suffers. … It is by the imagination only that we can form any conceptions of what are his sensations."[10] Although transplant clinicians have assessed these imaginative ties as pathological, by placing this fantasy of affiliation within the moral philosophy of sympathy, we can understand the binding force between donor families and recipients. In fact, scholars of sentimental literature argue for these forms of imaginative identification as the root of American democracy. For Elizabeth Barnes, Americans do not simply experience "fellow feeling," but are directed by sentimental literature to rely "particularly on familial models. Readers are taught to identify with others in such a way that they come to think of others—even fictional 'others'—as somehow related to themselves."[11] Instead of rejecting these new forms of imaginative attachment between donor family and recipient, we might see them, instead, as an extension of a democratic model, grounded in sympathy, that connects individuals. Of course, American democracy also reminds us of the violence involved in creating an imaginative chain of essentially similar individuals. The cultural figure of the family in the eighteenth century and nineteenth century did much to repress the rights of slaves, women, and the poor.[12] I would argue, nonetheless, that sentimentalism provides a rich and instructive, if complicated, frame by which to understand these imaginative responses.

Lesley Sharp's work on what she calls "biosentimentality" among donor kin and recipients offers an instructive path forward. In her work of medical anthropology, *Strange Harvest*, Sharp argues, "organ recipients and donor kin readily incorporate one another as mothers and fathers, sisters, brothers, and children" (171). Enabled by the sharing of donor flesh and blood, this new "idiom of fictive kinship" forms a powerful way to manage the strange forms of intimacy and hybridity that organ exchange produces (162). Perhaps not surprisingly, given their cultish place in sentimental culture, mothers serve as a special case in these familial fantasies. Sharp includes examples where a donor mother calls the recipient by her dead son's name or where an adult recipient calls his donor's mother "mom" and his sister "sis," despite the fact that the mother is 12 years younger than her new "son" (184, 187). For Sharp, these new sentimental ties are both playful and sacred ways to redefine a new social landscape after the profound disruption of organ exchange. In their own work on transplantation, Fox and Swazey cite similar dynamics; one recipient tells them, "there was another patient, a woman who received a kidney at the same time that I did from the same little girl. We have become brother and sister. That is because our kidneys came from the same donor. … The transplants have created something between us: brotherly love, or what have you" (36). This recipient's use of the term "brotherly love" to describe an imagined affiliation produced through shared blood returns to the democratic roots of family more broadly. While the hedging phrase "or what have you" recalls the strangeness of the new relation, it's important to remember that as an animating principle of national allegiance, such "families" are not so strange in American history.

The second imaginative strategy for managing organ exchange rests in the belief of a continuation of life, a belief commonly held by both donor families and recipients. Both popular coverage and anthropological coverage of transplantation include examples of these sensationalist stories in which a new organ brings with it changes in the recipient. Much of the sentimental literature examined in this chapter begins from some belief in continuation of life after donation. Perhaps unsurprising, given her ruling position among novelists of popular bioethics, Jodi Picoult offers a typical catalog of this mythology in her 2008 novel, *Change of Heart*. In one scene, the mother of a potential recipient worries over "the idea of cellular memory":

> There were dozens of cases. The baby with a clubfoot who drowned and gave his heart to another infant, who began to drag her left leg. The rapper who started playing classical music, and then learned his donor had died clutching a violin case. The cattle rancher who received the heart of a sixteen-year-old vegetarian, and could not eat meat again without getting violently ill.
>
> Then there was the twenty-year-old organ donor who wrote music in his spare time. A year after he died, his parents found a CD of a love song he'd recorded, about losing his heart to a girl named Andi. His recipient, a twenty-year-old girl, was named Andrea. When the boy's parents played the song for her, she could complete the chorus, without ever having heard it.[13]

Picoult's examples seem particularly novelistic in their deployment of seeming opposites—rapper/classical musician, rancher/vegetarian—and objects of special sympathy, infants and tragic lovers. These choices, though, demonstrate through exaggeration a central anxiety of transplantation: Namely, is there an inviolable self and where is it located? If the self is located in the flesh, what happens in a hybrid form? Real-life examples are no less melodramatic. Patients often describe new food preferences, renewed sexual appetites, or changes in personality. In the above-cited case of Kellen and Connor, Connor says, "I feel like I talk to him every day, I feel like I hear his voice all the time."[14] Taken together, these stories in which something of the donor persists beyond death form a central plank in the transplant imaginary. Given the radical nature of the medical procedure, it is neither surprising nor laughable to discover patients and families looking for ways to make sense of an unprecedented embodied condition.

Donor families, in particular, turn to belief in a continuation of life as a pathway through which to channel their grief. The handbook *Caring for Donor Families* even includes a script for a "Continuation of Life Ritual" to be read at the donor's deathbed. The ritual reads, in part, "Although you will no longer be physically present to us, a part of you will remain with us forever. You will continue to be with us through the stories we share and the memories we hold close. Others will continue to experience you through your gift—a gift of life, love, and another tomorrow."[15] Here and elsewhere, a few key terms emerge consistently in non-medical discussions of organ donation, notably "part," "continue," "share," "gift," "love," and "life." This constellation of terms expresses a sentimentalist argument privileging relation, emotion, and an imagined reconciliation after loss (often imagined in heaven in the sentimental novel). In posters for donation campaigns, a similar visual rhetoric emerges; images consistently include hands passing realistic or symbolic illustrations of hearts. Often, these hearts will be wrapped in bows as a gift.

While these recurring tropes of continuation are powerful scripts by which families come to understand donation, they also contain a paradox of the grieving process. In order to come to terms with the donation, families must believe simultaneously that their loved one is, in fact, dead, and also that they will live on through the gift of their organs. In a second best-selling novel on organ exchange called *My Sister's Keeper* (2003), Jodi Picoult captures a common speech found in cases of brain death: "Sweetheart, she's not here. It's the machine keeping her body alive. What makes Anna Anna is already gone."[16] In a true-life case of brain death, a donor family describes feeling similar confusion: "We wanted proof that he was 'dead.' After all, he did not look dead. His chest rose and fell with each breath. His heart was beating. His hands were soft and warm to hold. He looked asleep."[17] The ambiguous circumstances of brain death and the seeming-life of the cadaver can both complicate and animate the "gift of life" rhetoric of most procurement conversations.

Sentimental literary tropes can provide scripts for families to find their way through these uncertain circumstances. In its emphasis on a material reminder, the donated organ can be understood as a contemporary example of the keepsake tradition found in sentimental novels. Locks of hair, memorial photographs, and treasured pieces of clothing all serve as common examples of physical objects that take on the stature of a sacred relic. As Joanne Dobson argues, "Not merely a self-indulgent token or silly relic (although in its more reductive usages it may become such), the sentimental keepsake embodies the memory of love, the anguish of separation, the hope of eventual reunion" (280). Each of these dynamics structures the experience of donor families, and the emphasis on materiality in the keepsake tradition is one way to understand how the organ itself comes to carry the sentimental weight of both loss and hope. Returning to the imagery of donation posters, the translation of the anatomical heart illustration to the symbolic heart demonstrates the conceptual weight attached to the physical object.

The transplanted organ is no less symbolic in the subjective experience of the recipient, who will often believe in a similar continuation of life located in flesh and blood. While donor families are likely to cast the "gift" as heroic or miraculous, a belief in continuation can take on a more ambivalent cast for the recipient. The organ recipient in Picoult's *A Change Heart* imagines her new hybrid identity:

> I have been someone different now for three weeks. It's not something you can tell by looking at me; it's not even something I can tell by looking at myself in the mirror. The only way I can describe it, and it's weird, so get ready, is like waves: they just crash over me and suddenly, even if I'm surrounded by a dozen people, I start to cry.
>
> My mother says that emotion doesn't get transplanted along with the heart, that I have to stop referring to it as *his* heart and start calling it *mine*. But that's pretty hard to do, especially when you add up all the stuff I have to take just to keep my cells from recognizing this intruder in my chest. (445)

In this fictional formulation, anti-rejection drugs are necessary to fool the recipient's own cells from recognizing "this intruder." In this hybrid sense of being "someone else," Picoult follows a sentimental tradition of locating personal identity in emotions, specifically tears as a physical manifestation of feeling. This play of pronouns between what is "his" and what is "mine" shows up in patient testimonials as well. Lesley Sharp quotes one organ recipient who complains of her donor's widow, "She thinks that her husband lives on in me; but I feel uncomfortable about that—I feel they are *my* lungs now" (169). As described below, both of these ambivalent takes on the continuation of life demonstrate the complicated nature of the gift relationship.

These quotes share an emphasis on personal pronouns, signaling identity as a recurring theme in transplant fictions. Shifting and contested pronouns capture an enduring attempt to grapple with the new hybrid physical body and the resulting changes to one's subjectivity. Consider a handful of titles from popular stories of organ exchange: *My Sister's Keeper*, *The Best of Me*, *Return to Me*, *Never Let Me Go*. The repetition of "me" and "my" here suggests a preoccupation with the self: Where does it lie? Can it be changed? Where does it go upon death? Embedded within this preoccupation with the self, however, comes an understanding of the self-in-relation, especially through the intertwined modes of family and romance.

A Gift of Love

Hearts have long occupied a special place in the transplant imaginary. Since the advent of heart transplantation in 1967, stories of love lost and found through transplantation have dominated both fictional and news stories. For Connor and Kellen, the recipient and donor mentioned above, their story of organ exchange is also a love story. Newspapers trumpeted this modern fairy tale under headlines like "How One Heart Healed Two Families: A Valentine's Tale" and "Finding Love After a Heart Transplant." According to news reports, when Connor Rabinowitz approached the mother and sister of his donor, "his new heart began to pound."[18] Connor and Erin, Kellen's sister, fell in love over time, but as Connor reports, "It was a connection at first sight." Connor, Erin, and Kellen's mother all credit the romantic relationship to a connection sparked by the transplanted heart.

This blending of brotherly and romantic love is not surprising in the tradition of the sentimental novel. Such stories offer a big tent conception of love, including affiliation among blood relations, romantic partners, and fellow citizens. As Elizabeth Barnes argues, "sentimental rhetoric conflates the boundaries between familial and social ties. The result is a confusion of familial and erotic attachment: one learns to love those to whom one already feels related" (3). Such happy confusion is a defining feature of Connor and Erin's story, above, but it also serves as plot fodder for a host of films and novels about love after transplantation. In Nicholas Sparks's *The Best of Me*, a mother's affair with a lost love from her youth ends with his sudden death and anonymous organ donation to her ill son. The film version of the novel (2014) closes with a phone call to the now-thriving son who ends the talk by telling his mom, "I gotta go meet a girl."[19] This transfer of erotic love from the mother to the son is never represented as odd or disturbing in the context of the novel; instead, the transfer of the organ is understood as the ultimate romantic gesture, the gift of "the best of me" referenced in the title. Even in sentimental transplant films and novels that don't center on a romance narrative, there is typically a romantic subplot to forward this thematic suffusion of love in the world of the characters. In both *My Sister's Keeper* and *Change of Heart*, Picoult includes plotlines where characters find love in partners who are perfectly "matched" to them but for whom they have had to wait. While such correspondences between the central and subsidiary action might be too on the nose for some readers, they clearly articulate a sentimentalist vision of the world. In 1957, Ian Watt identified "formal realism" as the central characteristic of the eighteenth-century novel, a claim that has remained influential through the last half-century.[20] More recent criticism, however, has been careful to note that while "realistic" is a broadly true appellation, it can also obscure similarly characteristic features of sentimental fiction, notably "the degree to which it relies on palpable artifice, trades in wish fulfillment, and depends on plotting that is too neat to correspond to the course of actual lives."[21] The sentimental fictions under consideration here all trade in these aesthetic strategies, typically to underscore the themes of family, connection, and suffering.

In this sentimentalist worldview, destiny, structure, and design serve as dominant themes. *My Sister's Keeper* includes a recurring motif of amateur astronomy as a way for the family to find meaning in the seemingly punitive or random experience of chronic, debilitating illness to one of its members. In *The Best of Me*, Stephen Hawking and physics textbooks emerge as a metaphor for a design principle that exists but is too complicated to be easily understood. Again, such metaphors, which might feel overwrought in an aesthetic evaluation of the work, serve much the same purpose that belief in continuation of life does among donor families and recipients. In all of these cases, people are seeking ways to understand loss (a familiar search in cultural history), but also to understand the special demands of transplantation: new horizons for prolonging life, the union of flesh between strangers, and the new relationships produced through organ exchange.

The heartbeat, in particular, emerges as a recurring motif that symbolizes both the physical and emotional valences of organ exchange. From Connor Rabinowitz's fast-beating new heart upon meeting his donor's sister (and future girlfriend) to the recipient who told Lesley Sharp, "I can *hear* his heart beating inside my chest whenever I lie down to sleep at night,"[22] the heartbeat serves as an important manifestation of the transplanted organ, one which can be felt and heard by both the recipient and others without specialized medical equipment. The sentimental film *Return to Me* (2000) makes extensive use of the sound of a heart beating to further its romantic vision.[23] In this remarkable story, a man (played by David Duchovny) falls in love with a stranger (played by Minnie Driver) only to discover that she is the recipient of his dead wife's heart. Romantic love, family, and transplantation are inextricably woven together in this story, emblematized for example when the recipient's devoted grandfather tells Duchovny's character, "When Grace met you, her heart beat truly for the first time." The film wholly embraces belief in the continuation of life from donor to recipient; in one key scene, our heroes pass each other without knowing it, but first a ting and then a beating heart sound effect signal their connection for the audience. Later, when they do meet, they experience instant familiarity, asking "do we know each other?" The film expresses no skepticism about the supernatural elements of the couple's affiliation, but in fact underscores them with extradiegetic strategies of sound effects and dramatic irony.

Couples being supernaturally connected or destined for each other is, of course, familiar in romantic fantasies more broadly, but it takes on a specialized meaning in transplant narratives, especially through the weighty concept of "matching." The long-term success of transplants in medical history requires two elements that serve as alternate sides of a single anti-rejection coin: The first was the improvement in immunosuppressant drugs, and the second was the discovery of tissue typing to produce matches for patients.[24] In the seemingly interminable period for families waiting for an organ, a tremendous amount of psychic energy is expended on hoping for a "good match." It is not surprising, then, that this notion of "matching" would become wrapped up in more familiar romantic stories of destined connection. For organ donor Joseph Jacobs, the opportunity to give a kidney to his husband Larry was an expression of love prefigured as the couple's biological destiny. He reports, "I asked a nurse on the evaluation team to do a cross match on our blood while we were there for Larry's evaluation. She said this was not normal protocol but since our relationship seemed so loving she went ahead. At the end of the day she told me we were an *exact* match."[25] For Jacobs, the outward sign of their exceptional love—exceptional for being both "so loving" and for being gay—is matched by the inward fact of their being an "*exact* match" (italics in original). Jodi Picoult deploys a similar metaphor. In a love subplot between potential organ recipients, the couple see their illnesses as the foundation for their connection; Kate says, "He had scars on his hands, from graft-versus-host. … I could feel them when we were holding hands." Her sister asks, "Was it gross?" Kate replies, "No … it was like we matched."[26] In a novel that turns entirely around who is and is not a tissue match for Kate, this word choice significantly draws the medical story into the romance plot, understanding both in a sentimental network of meaning and relation.

Medical professionals, too, have adopted non-medical understandings of matching and compatibility in some circumstances. In addition to screening tests for physical compatibility, medical teams include psychological testing of live donors to ensure that their motives are sound and they can withstand the challenges that follow donation and surgery. In cases where donors have been excluded on the basis of these tests, doctors will commonly tell patients and families that they are "not compatible" with the recipient. According to Fox and Swazey, "medical professionals have stretched the language of immunology, extending it to cover nonbiological factors in an effort to protect the potential live donor, the recipient, and their family" (34). This extension of compatibility beyond strict biology operates according to the same logic of romantic matching above. In both cases, "matching" is understood as a compound property, encompassing both physical and emotional ties.

The conceptual power of donation as a gift of life and love, especially as a mode of establishing affiliation, functions among strangers in the case of donor families and unknown recipients, but can be an even more powerful script in encouraging live donation. Currently most commonly used in kidney, but also increasingly in partial liver and lung transplants, living donation reseats the sentimental narrative of organ exchange within the family itself. Listen to the familiar terms used by this daughter who donated a kidney to her ill father: "I knew the minute that I heard living donation was an option that it was going to be me. I can't explain it but it was a gut feeling. I felt like a hero, excited at the thought of being able to give the gift of life."[27] Although I discuss living donation in more detail below, it is important to understand here how these new filial practices find their expression in the sentimental terms used to understand donation more broadly. Historically, medical professionals have found themselves in a complicated position, since performing surgery on an otherwise healthy patient violates their first precept to do no harm. On the other hand, organs transplanted from living, related donors are likely to have a better success rate than cadaveric transplants (Fox and Swazey, 33). The ethical and legal terms by which the transplant community has resolved these tensions are explored below. At this moment, it is important first to recognize the case Sharon Kaufman makes, that the success of kidney transplantation, especially among living, related donors, "performs radical cultural work … [allowing a family member] to 'see' one's own body as the vehicle for the health and life of a loved one."[28] These are the heroic terms by which the donor daughter above understands her new relationship to her father.

Initially skeptical medical professionals came to justify living donation in exactly these terms as well. According to Fox and Swazey, many were moved by the "understandable and admirable 'altruism,' 'self-sacrifice and love' that motivated many 'close blood relatives' to give of themselves in this fashion" (47). The success of liver transplants, however—and the constant drumbeat of organ shortage—brings back the specter of imagined family affiliations described among donor families and recipients. In this instance, the transplant community began to expand the pool of donors to those "emotionally related" to the recipient, including spouses and family friends. Investing meaning in such relationships echoes arguments quoted from Elizabeth Barnes, in which familial and social connections are necessarily linked in American culture: "America's preoccupation with familial feeling [serves] as the foundation of sympathy, and sympathy as the basis of a democratic republic ultimately confounds the differences between familial and social bonds" (xi). Within the framework of citizenship, the limits of "emotionally related" are tested and expanded, almost to their breaking point in the case of living donation among strangers.

Transplant Surgery as Not-so-Happily-Ever-After

Sentimental stories of love found through transplantation carry the expectation of a "happily ever after," a trope that similarly dominates human-interest stories and public awareness campaigns about organ exchange. Although it's rarely featured on the posters, for most organ recipients, transplantation may lead to a radical improvement in quality of life, but they are still living with a chronic condition. Anti-rejection drugs carry their own side effects; in some cases, the underlying disease will continue to cause debilitating symptoms; and since many transplanted organs have a kind of shelf life in the new body, the first surgery is not always the last. Donors, too, can experience unexpected medical complications from surgery. In both cases, though, the emotional weight attached to the magnitude of giving and receiving an organ can condition patients to deny the negative aspects of their experience. Lesley Sharp argues, "many recipients feel, too, that they are not entitled to speak of ongoing forms of suffering because their surgeries have saved (or, certainly, extended) their lives" (108). As even Jodi Picoult's narrator understands, getting the organ "wasn't the happy ending everyone thought it was."[29]

In the sphere of romance itself, recipients and donors can find themselves surprised by deviations from the fairy-tale script. In the summer of 2015, hopes across the UK were dashed when so-called Transplant Bride Kate Jakes died waiting for her fourth transplantation. Another, more sensational 2014 headline reads "I Gave Him a Kidney and He Dumped Me," capturing the intense sense of betrayal felt in this case of divorce after living exchange. Lesley Sharp chronicles more mundane examples of transplant recipients struggling with romance and intimacy: Many face "failed marriages and relationships, their partners ultimately fatigued after caring long term for a chronically ill person. Some never find love at all because potential partners are wary of a mate with such an extraordinary, chronic condition as an organ transplant" (119). These day-to-day complications have little place in the Technicolor terms that constitute the "gift of life." The radical nature of transplant surgery requires an equally powerful ideology to overcome our reservations to the procedure; the sentimental terms by which we have conducted this conceptual shift operate on an overwhelming principle of universality attached to love, care, and family. It can be hard to find ground for discomforts, failed expectations, and quotidian struggles in the face of such overwhelming ideals.

Renée Fox and Judith Swazey use the striking phrase "tyranny of the gift" to describe the complex interpersonal dynamics that structure organ exchange. They argue:

> This psychological and moral burden is especially onerous because the gift the recipient has received from the donor is so extraordinary that it is inherently unreciprocal. It has no physical or symbolic equivalent. As a consequence, the giver, the receiver, and their families may find themselves locked in a creditor-debtor vise that binds them one to another in a mutually fettering way. We have called these aspects of the gift-exchange dimensions of transplantation, "the tyranny of the gift." (40)

Despite the idealized conceptions of family that populate sentimental fiction, familial ties can be felt as thriving interdependence or as "mutually fettering" burdens (and, often, as both). When the stakes of exchange are so high—understood as life or death—the terms of the relationship will be unavoidably altered or exaggerated through the acts of giving and receiving. Fox and Swazey's work has been influential in encouraging the transplant community to understand the complicated psychological dynamics that condition these choices.

Where donors or recipients do express their struggles post-surgery, they are likely to understand their experiences in the same terms of family that prompted the initial exchange. In the journal *Narrative Inquiry in Bioethics*, Laurie Post describes her "Liver Donor Nightmare" in the following terms:

> [My cousin] wanted to boast of her newfound health, strength and steady improvement in daily life activities, but instead was awash in remorse as I languished. The truth is that it was difficult for me to see her thrive with my liver as I suffered for it. It definitely affected our relationship for about a year. Then, family being family, it was all okay again. We could laugh and moan about it because we had both endured it.[30]

In this essay, Post relies on familiar scripts of affiliation to make sense of her experience, an experience shared with few others in the broader population. The phrase "family being family" covers all manner of unhappiness and failed expectations; ultimately, the cousins use the umbrella of family relationship, emotion ("we would laugh and moan"), and imagined shared struggles (a sense of what they "both endured") to reconcile. The same tropes that prompt the desire to donate in the first place become redeployed in the aftermath of the surgery, reimagining difficulty as an obstacle to be overcome in the highest interests of family connection.

The power of social scripts to make meaning in our lives emerges in ways that are both positive and negative. An important additional consideration falling under the rubric of "not-so-happily-ever-after" is the gender disparity that exists between living kidney donors. According to a series of published studies,[31] gendered differences have been observed among both donors (with two-thirds being women and one-third being men) and recipients (with two-thirds being men and one-third being women). The profound and basic imbalance reflected in these numbers seems tragically unsurprising when understood in the context of the sentimental nature of appeals for organ donors. Read in the context of the history of the sentimental novel—a genre expressly written for and popular among women—the gendered nature of terms like love, feeling, life, sacrifice, and family finds a starkly material manifestation in the far higher numbers of women who are volunteering to give to family and the higher numbers of men who are willing to receive. This disparity reveals the darkest side of sentimentalism as it reminds us that these "universal" values are borne differently among the population.

Giving to Strangers

It was this essential unfairness grounded in personal, sentimental appeals that prompted the National Organ Transplantation Act (1984) in the first place. Lawmakers, led by then-congressman Al Gore, were concerned about both the possible commodification of organs and the unevenness in a private system for organ recipients. Televised public appeals made by families on behalf of specific sick children were compelling, but created clear inefficiencies and inequities. Gore told his congressional colleagues during hearings on the bill, "All of us have been touched by the sight of little children such as those who are here today who suffer from biliary atresia, a fatal liver disease. There is no more compelling plight than that of their parents who must mount nationwide media campaigns to plead for an organ donation or funds to save the lives of their children. … [T]here must be a better way" (7–8). Although Ronald Regan was careful to couch his radio speech on behalf of Ashley Bailey as an appeal for the many infants "like her," his administration did little to support a more systematic approach that could avoid the pitfalls of appeals targeted toward individual patients. In the decades since, the continued practice of directed donation coupled with locals-first allocation policies demonstrates that the creation of UNOS has not solved all of the problems that were rooted in individual, sentimental appeals. The breaking point between the principle of public good and fairness on the one hand and personal autonomy on the other is an enduring problem in organ allocation. At the core of this dilemma are these central questions: who owns donated organs and who can determine how they should be allocated?

In a typical cadaveric organ donation, the organ will be offered first to a patient who is listed at a local transplant center and is a match based on biological factors. If no local match can be found, the organ will be offered to another organ procurement organization in the region, where "local" and "region" are typically defined based on the existence of transplant centers, not an even mapping across US territory or by population. As Rachel Ankeny argues, this "locals first" policy relies on the understanding that, (1) it is morally appropriate to "prefer to donate to members of your local community, and 2) people in fact prefer to donate locally."[32] The latter assumption about donor preferences reaches levels of received wisdom among transplant professionals. This valorization of the local has roots in basic democratic models of affinity, in which people understand their national belonging as lying first in the family, then in the community, then in the nation. In his testimony to a House and Senate joint subcommittee, James Childress laments our narrow definitions of community, advocating instead for a "truly national approach."[33] He argues that timing and distance as it relates to transplantation outcomes should be the only factor in allocation and laments what he calls "accidents of geography" in which patients miss out on needed organs because of where they live. The perceived lack of feasibility of a national transplant list—an idea which would seem to privilege rational models of the broadest extension of fairness—lies in the sense that such an attenuated link between donor and recipient would strain families' sense of affiliation, a sense that we understand as essential to successful donation campaigns. Ankeny also describes cases in which directed donation policies allow recipients to jump the line based on perceived affiliation. In attempting to establish a principle governing what kind of affiliation is morally permissible in cases of directed donation, she argues that "merely coming to care about a potential recipient whom you see night after night on the local news does not count as a morally significant emotional relationship" (392). She cites one case in which a St. Louis family reportedly selected a recipient for their son's heart after reading about his condition in a local newspaper and learning that they were from the same town. Such practices produce a complicated ethical dilemma for bioethicists and transplant professionals, but they are also the direct outgrowth of sentimental media and cultural constructions of affiliation.

Jodi Picoult describes a typical media appeal of this kind in her novel *Change of Heart*: "The camera zeroed in on a girl with fairy-tale blond hair and blue half-moons beneath her eyes. Just the kind of child they'd televise to get you to open up your wallet. 'Claire Nealon,' the reporter's voice-over said, 'is waiting for a heart'" (25). Just as gendered notions of who gives and who receives will shape living donations, so do social constructions of value attach to media appeals for life-saving measures. Children, especially white children from middle-class backgrounds, occupy a special category understood as deserving of extraordinary care and protection in US racial schema. Other examples of extraordinary appeals include a Houston man who received a directed donation in 2004 after advertising on billboards and a Web site named, straightforwardly, toddneedsaliver.com. These forms of public appeal, often amplified by the local news media, continue the tradition of the medical human-interest story that finds its roots in the press of the mid-nineteenth century and which achieved popularity simultaneously with the height of the sentimental novel. As medical historian Susan Lederer argues, thousands of stories on blood transfusion from this time period found an audience because of a few fundamental dynamics: (1) the spectacle of the transfusion procedure, often likened to biblical resurrection, (2) the heroic nature of the donor's act, and (3) the "importance of affiliation" and typical use of family members in transfusion.[34] In these factors, we can see the ground laid for an essential sentimental script that continues in contemporary narratives of organ exchange.

UNOS, in its rejection of a single, national registry, walks a fine ethical line between fairness in allocation policies and the pragmatism of acknowledging local partiality among donor families. Our willingness to accept this bias toward the local in acts of giving and receiving is an expression of the extent to which we have conceived of organ exchange as an extension of basic familial ties. Lesley Sharp describes the remarkable rhetoric of the Donor Memorial found at UNOS headquarters in Richmond, VA. By carving only first names into the stone walls, the agency preserves the practice of anonymity that transplant professionals have come to follow so strongly. In addition to these names, the wall includes relational tags including "friend, wife, son, daughter, mother, sister, husband, brother, father." According to Sharp, "the memorial also standardizes, in a seemingly unproblematic way, the social ties that define who donors are to us. The selective choice of words and first names ultimately obliterates the individual identities and blends them into a larger generic mix. … There is no reference to stepsibling, or ex-wife, or godparent, or lover. Instead, donors fall into highly conventional and unproblematic categories of sociality."[35] Sharp demonstrates effectively the imaginative erasures that take place in a universalizing fiction of family as an umbrella for radically new social connections. Even within the context of the wholly unconventional imagined "family" that exists between recipient and donor kin, this memorial celebration of the donor family is highly normative, inscribed as straight, fertile, and conventional in its mournful relationship to the deceased.

The imaginative power of these social ties lies in their ability to link people and to elide difference; such power is at the heart of the ideological work of sentimentalism. This ideological work gets pursued through a series of metaphors, found in the UNOS Donor Memorial, public awareness campaigns, mourning rituals, and in procurement specialists' conversations with donor families. The notion of blood as a binding force among Americans is an early but enduring idea that finds perhaps surprising valences in organ exchange. As literary theorist Kristin Boudreau argues, in addition to the powerful trope of family to ground the nation, sentimental models of citizenship extended this trope through a metaphor of shared blood. She writes,

> When social bonds are figured as familial bonds, the fiction of shared blood must be managed by imaginary leaps across a space of difference. … [These leaps are enabled by a] cultural fiction of a natural affection alternately called sympathy, charity, and sensibility, a fiction that encouraged a belief in shared feelings even when "consanguinity" remained only a metaphor. (x)

Susan Lederer includes a striking example of this notion of shared blood in an 1880 *Harper's Weekly* cartoon showing the withered and shrouded corpse of democracy receiving a blood transfusion from a hale and hearty military officer (40). In the age of blood transfusion and organ transplantation, the metaphorical belief in consanguinity and the "brotherhood" of American citizens becomes manifest in this literal practice of exchange. The long-standing nature of the metaphor animates public interest in donation, providing a familiar script by which to understand the complicated medical innovation.

The emerging practice of "domino" or "chain" organ exchanges provides another striking example of the ways in which long-standing sentimental models of affiliation offer a path for public understanding of the unconventional practice of stranger donation. A lengthy 2012 *New York Times* article describes one record-breaking chain under the headline, "60 Lives, 30 Kidneys, All Linked."[36] As literary theorist Elizabeth Barnes demonstrates, a culture of sentiment embraces the belief in an essential connection among citizens. Using the very language of "chain," she writes, "The idea of the American people as a single unified body is made possible by imagining diverse individuals connected in a sympathetic chain" (2). "Chain 124" linked 60 individuals in 17 hospitals across 11 states. Descriptions of the effort are likely to blend the language of technical innovation—complex algorithms, business modeling, and sophisticated computer programming—with the sentimental language of love, family, and feeling. The *New York Times* piece emphasizes the family history of Garet Hil, who founded the National Kidney Registry after his daughter became ill. Another section of the article begins, "there were other love stories along the way," and describes the romantic connection that was forged along a hospital corridor between two lost childhood friends who were unrelated and distant links in the chain. Another example valorizes a donor who, despite his divorce from her mother, was motived to donate through his love for their daughter whom he didn't want to grow up without two parents.

In addition to the extraordinary number of patients involved in this chain, the article emphasizes the remarkable nature of the first link required in all such exchanges: a Good Samaritan donor. These donors, also called surgical altruists, are living donors who approach transplant centers to offer their kidneys to strangers. As histories of transplantation demonstrate, such offers have existed since the earliest days of the procedure. Doctors, however, were hesitant to support these donations. As one surgeon argued, these donations would be suspicious from the outset—"such donations would not be an act of love"[37]—and always shadowed by the possibility of financial brokerage. Increasingly, though, as transplant centers began to relax the strict requirement of blood relation between live donor and recipient, thus opening the door to other kinds of affiliation, they also began to understand altruism as a motive in itself. The stronger outcomes attached to live donor organs, long-term studies of live donor health, and improvements in less invasive surgical techniques all extended the perceived permissibility of surgical altruism. By 1999, both Johns Hopkins and the University of Minnesota were prepared to accept kidneys from live donors. By serving as one of the earliest live altruistic donors, Joyce Roush, a nurse from Indiana, hoped to inspire others to donate by publicizing her story. Today, the University of Minnesota Health includes links to donate and videos on their Web site describing the history and process of nondirected kidney donation. They also include a testimonial from "Kris," a donor who was moved to offer her kidney after being unable to donate to an ill family member—"It didn't matter who I gave it to; I just wanted to help someone." Health centers like Minnesota are more likely, now, to credit these donors as heroes and to trust their sentimentally expressed feelings of goodwill and altruism.

Despite this broad evolution from suspicion to support, a 2004 *The New Yorker* article called "The Gift" offers a striking counternarrative to the dominant sentimental tropes that typically structure stories of surgical altruism. In the article, Ian Parker tells the story of real estate millionaire Zell Kravinsky, who, after giving away the vast bulk of his financial fortune decided to give away a kidney to a patient in a Philadelphia hospital serving low-income patients. In contrast to the typically sentimental stories of nondirected donors, Parker casts Kravinsky's gift in terms that are specifically anti-family. His donation is placed rhetorically under the masculine domains of finance and math and against the special ethical demands made by intimate relation. In one moment, Kravinsky assesses, "I had a one-in-four-thousand chance of dying [in the surgery]. … But my recipient had a certain death facing her. … I'd be valuing my life at four thousand times hers if I let consideration of mortality sway me."[38] Kravinsky's math, however, fails to account for his family's interest in his life and health, a factor that plays in nearly all stories of surgical altruism. Family members of the prospective donor often need to be convinced that the risk to their loved one is worth the benefit to a stranger. Kravinsky's lack of family feeling, however, takes on a pathological cast in the article. When asked where he would set the ratio between his love for his own children and that for unknown children, Kravinsky responds: "I don't know where I'd set it, but I would not let many children die so my kids could live. … I don't think that two kids should die so that one of my kids has comfort, and I don't know that two children should die so that one of my kids lives." In the article, M.I.T. philosopher Judith Jarvis Thomson describes this failure to prize the lives of his children as evidence that Kravinsky is "just flatly a defective parent." She argues, "he's deficient in views that parents ought to have, whether it maximizes utility or not." As Parker acknowledges, "arguments about philanthropic extremes tend to be about families," and he draws from a bank of cultural representations by including Dickensian examples of those who would ignore suffering at home to address problems a world away.

Kravinsky's deviation from the determining scripts of sentiment demonstrates how entrenched that script has become. When cast outside of the reassuring mantle of family feeling, even where that "family" is conceived as embodied in a stranger, the motives of surgical altruists can feel radical, excessive, and pathological. In an American context, Zell Kravinsky's choice to give away his kidney is as unthinkable as his choice to give away his millions; where Garet Hil's departure from a lucrative business career to found the National Kidney Register seems emotionally legible because of his daughter's illness, Kravinsky's choices—which are unmoored from family connections and actually in violation of his family's wishes—seem incomprehensible. This response to Kravinsky's donation, a response clearly conditioned by Parker's rhetorical approach in the article, however, can reveal a darker side to the power of sentimental scripts. As Anne Whitehead argues in her reading of Kazuo Ishiguro's *Never Let Me Go* (read at length below), a system of organ donation that is grounded in care and empathy carries with it a key danger; a society based on empathy is often "governed by identity and similarity, and hence is prone to exclusion and ethnocentrism."[39] Although Kravinsky may be a defective parent, he is a hyper-rational citizen, one who rejects inequities conferred to individuals based on special status like relation. That we allow for family status as a privileged category in ethical questions, that we would consider a question like "how much more do you love your children than other children" to be absurd on its face demonstrates the hegemonic status of sentimentalism in some areas.

Heroes and Saviors

Where donations among strangers ask us to imagine the national body as a network that is "like family," increasing success in live donation—especially for bone marrow and kidney transplants—has also resulted in new roles within more traditionally defined families. The "savior sibling" is one new role that has caught the cultural and public imagination in the past three decades. Savior siblings are children who are able to provide stem cells, blood, bone marrow, or organs for their seriously ill siblings. In the most high-profile cases, a child is conceived specifically for this purpose, often with the help of genetic screening of embryos and in vitro fertilization. A *Time* magazine article written in the summer of 1991 characterizes the fraught nature of ethical debates sparked by this practice: The article's tagline reads, "A family's act of lifesaving conception was on the side of the angels, but hovering in the wings is the devilish ghost of Dr. Mengele." Angel or devil, miracle or Nazi—while most public debates seem to land on the side of "miracle," the terms of this article reveal the intensity attached to the ethics of informed consent and medical interventions in conception.

Marissa Ayala is the most famous and among the earliest in a small fraternity of publicly known savior siblings. Marissa was conceived after her parents failed to find a bone marrow match for her 17-years-old sister, Anissa. In his cover story for *Time*, Lance Morrow employs an astonishing mixture of metaphors, citing angels, Dr. Mengele, the Holy Grail, resurrection, spawning salmon, a slippery slope leading to a bottomless abyss, cannibalism, ocean maps, the Donner Party, and Luddites.[40] The diversity of these references suggests that Morrow, like the public spirit he attempts to capture, has trouble reconciling the competing moral principles at play in the Ayala case. His metaphorical exuberance reflects his argument that while transplantation has achieved a level of familiarity, it remains (in 1991) on the outskirts of science, difficult for the public to fully reconcile: "Today the transplant is part of the culture—conceptually dazzling, familiar in a weird way, but morally unassimilated." On the one hand, the parents are "on the side of the angels" for going to such lengths—including a reversed vasectomy and pregnancy at age 43—for a chance to save their dying daughter. On the other hand, as Morrow writes, to some the story "was profoundly, if sometimes obscurely, troubling. It called up brutal images—baby farming, cannibalizing for spare parts." Although many bioethicists argue that children are conceived for all kinds of poor reasons—if for any reason at all—critics of the practice are concerned about what it might mean to the child and the family to be conceived for an instrumentalist purpose. The President's Council on Bioethics, convened by President Bush in 2001, expressed concerns about the practice of therapeutic reproductive engineering, asking, "Is it proper to assign to an unconceived child the burden of being a savior of a sibling, and then give that child life on condition that he or she fulfill that role?"[41]

The linguistic tension expressed by the President's Council—the "burden of being a savior"—is exactly the moral question Jodi Picoult explores in her popular novel *My Sister's Keeper*. In the novel, 13-year-old Anna sues for medical emancipation from her parents to block the donation of her kidney to her ill sister, Kate. Picoult, who was inspired in part by the Ayalas' story, dramatizes many of the terms and dynamics that influence savior siblings. When Kate's mother, Sara, is pregnant with Anna and asked the rote question "what are you having?" she thinks, "I know exactly what I'm having: a miracle" (100). Even before conception, this child is freighted with the hopes and medical demands of the entire family, hopes that find expression in the overdetermining language of "miracle" and "savior." While the rhetorical interplay between science and religion is inescapable in these discussions of conception, medicine's limits, and donation, the locus of these discussions within a single family unit creates a distinctive object of study, making savior siblings a special case by which to understand the new ethical problems created by organ exchange.

These ethical tensions are best understood through registers that are organic to the cases themselves: the language of family, interdependence, and emotion. Traditional ethical concepts—most notably autonomy, neutrality, and rationality—find their limit in these cases of deeply enmeshed interests. Savior siblings extend the ethical principle of interdependence, a value often pressed by feminist philosophers. In *My Sister's Keeper*, Sara advocates for Anna's continued role as a savior sibling in an emotional appeal to her husband, "Would you give blood for Kate? … I would, too. I'd give her half of my heart, for God's sake, if it helped. You do whatever you have to, when it comes to people you love, right? … What makes you think Anna would feel any different?" (169). As we've seen in donor appeals more broadly, Sara makes her case through extended metaphors of love, the heart, and blood. She also describes familial love as a force that produces a fundamental interchangeability among the emotions, affiliations, and desires of the family members.

The sentimental novel, while it may indulge in overdrawn metaphors and constantly escalating plot stakes, is nevertheless a wholly appropriate genre to emphasize the very elements that bioethical debates are prone to ignore. In an article for the journal *Bioethics*, Kimberly Strong, Ian Kerridge, and Miles Little argue that conventional moral theory often rejects contextual issues, including formative experiences of illness or the potential death of a child.[42] Sentimental literature, by contrast, is all about context. The narrative structure of *My Sister's Keeper*, which both jumps among first-person narrators and flashes back to relevant scenes of medical drama in the past, reverses the biases of moral theory and insists upon relational context as a condition for understanding. In their study of families and physicians involved with savior siblings, Strong et al. discovered that the families were easily able to dismiss conventional ethical critiques of their choices. Similarly, concerns of clinicians faded away when asked to consider the choice from the perspective of a parent caring for a sick child. Taken together, these findings suggest a new set of factors rarely considered in bioethical debates, "such as regret, risk perceptions, hope, fear, parental love and the moral obligation to care for sick children."[43]

Because these cases involve minors, savior siblings place special pressure on the legal doctrine of informed consent. In typical cases, informed consent emphasizes autonomy and allows for individuals to weigh complicated factors like risk, hope, and love for themselves. In cases involving legal incompetents, however, the courts use different standards to make decisions in situations that would place persons at risk. Two oft-cited cases of organ exchange within families demonstrate the difficulty of making these kinds of decisions without recourse to an interdependent and emotional understanding of family. In the 1969 case of *Strunk v Strunk*, the Kentucky Court of Appeals upheld a lower court ruling granting a mother the right to consent to a kidney donation on behalf of her developmentally disabled son.[44] According to the decision, Jerry, 27, had an IQ of approximately 53 and a mental age of about 6 years. Her older son, Tommy, 28, had a fatal kidney disease. An extensive search for another qualified donor had been fruitless. Following the legal doctrines of substituted judgment and best interest,[45] the court supported the petition and allowed the donation. Crucial to the court's decision was the testimony of an expert witness who argued that the donation would be beneficial to Jerry himself—not only to Tommy, the recipient—"because Jerry was greatly dependent upon Tommy, emotionally and psychologically, and that his well-being would be jeopardized more severely by the loss of his brother than by the removal of a kidney."[46] Two elements of this expert opinion are striking. First, and explored in more detail below, is the idea that the operation would be not only in the organ recipient's best interest, but also in the best interest of the donor. Second, once again, we see this language of comparison among parts of the body and members of the family. In this case, the removal of a kidney is explicitly weighed against the loss of the brother in a holistic assessment of Jerry's physical and psychological health; Jerry's emotional dependence on Tommy becomes analogous to Tommy's physical dependence on Jerry. In *My Sister's Keeper*, Picoult's fictional psychiatrist makes the case in very similar terms: "If Anna donates a kidney that saves her sister's life, it's a tremendous gift—and not just to Kate. Because Anna herself will continue to be part of the intact family by which she defines herself, rather than a family that's lost one of its members" (365). Granted the license of revision and careful diction in a piece of fiction, Picoult can make the metaphors even more explicit: the loss of a "member," the part and whole of the intact family, and the "gift" that extends beyond the recipient all capture the ideological underpinnings of directed family donation.

A similar case two years later reinforced the Kentucky court's reading of the best interest standard. In *Hart v Brown*, the parents of identical 7-year-old twins sought permission for Margaret to donate a kidney to her dying sister, Katheleen.[47] The much better prognosis of an exchange between the twins and the obviation of the need for immunosuppressant drugs convinced the parents that the risk to Margaret was worth the benefit to Katheleen. This weighing of factors, of benefit to one sibling against harm to the other, however, while it can play a role in cases of informed consent, does not fall under the notion of best interest.[48] That standard is limited to the interest of the individual herself. In this case, the court balanced the physical risk of the surgery with the "grave emotional impact" that would result from the death of her sister and determined that it was, in fact, in Margaret's interest to donate. This ruling, too, rested on the expert testimony of a psychiatrist, who argued that successful transplantation "would be of immense benefit to the donor in that the donor would be better off in a family that was happy than in a family that was distressed and in that it would be a very great loss to the donor if the donee were to die from her illness" (*Hart v Brown*, 375). This early legal precedent involving family organ exchange demonstrates an important ideological Möbius strip connecting family and individual. Live donation is therefore made broadly permissible through terms of sentiment and family. The psychiatrist's explicit call to happiness, distress, and loss among the family demonstrate the success of the sentimental appeal in organ donation; these emotional interests are forces that can overcome even the deep legal prohibition against bodily intrusion.

While these court decisions include language that allows for a complex relation of whole and part constituting membership in a family, the best interest standard relies on a kind of sleight of hand, reframing familial interests as ultimately individual. In their critique of the typical application of "best interest," James Dwyer and Elizabeth Vig argue that the standard approach, in its express appeal to egocentrism, is ultimately a rationalization for conclusions reached through other means. They argue that there is a special moral relationship that exists among families, one that is social and not biological, and that those moral interests should be considered along with physical and psychological interests in determining "best interest." Strong, Kerridge, and Little similarly argue that the best interest standard must be rethought in terms of familial interdependence. Instead of understanding seemingly competing interests within families as "morally problematic" or conflicts, we should recognize that "in reality, parents balance multiple motivations and interests *all the time*. ... The notion that one is making a decision about an individual neutrally or without any consideration of other people in the family is neither ethically coherent nor empirically supportable" (Strong et al., 191). Following from these critics, then, and the foundational work of feminist ethicists before them, emotions, family, and interdependence are not simply the sentimental manipulation of public organ donation campaigns, but important factors in an ethical model that can serve in decision-making about pressing medical problems. A traditional bioethical viewpoint that privileges autonomy but fails to account for the demands of interdependence may be an insufficient tool in medical decision-making.

The necessary tie of emotions and familial interdependence is underscored in the third legal ruling typically cited in discussions of savior siblings. In *Curran v Bosze* (1990), a father petitions to have his 3-year-old twins tested for compatibility with their ill half brother.[49] The case deviates from the earlier precedents, however, because the twins were the offspring of an extramarital affair, had only met their half-siblings on two occasions, and didn't know they were related. The courts decided that since their mother objected to the donation, she would be unable to provide the support necessary for the children during their medical procedure—a key condition in these cases. Furthermore, the court decided that because of the tenuous nature of the relationship, specifically the lack of an emotional bond among the children, to compel the test would not be in the best interest of the twins. *Curran v Bosze* emphasizes feeling as a pillar in medical decisions. Organ procurement personnel and clinicians are used to assessing organ allocation in terms of chance of success, time on the waiting list, and quality of life. As these three interrelated cases demonstrate, however, the sentimental terrain of family and feeling must be taken into account when weighing the risks and benefits involved in live, directed donation.

Some would caution, however, that the courts are too quick to anticipate emotional benefits among organ donors. Jodi Picoult, for one, has certainly explored the complicated facets of family relationships structured around a dying child and her savior sibling. The President's Council on Bioethics's warning about "the burden of being a savior" (96) must also be taken into account in a model of ethical interdependence. In a *Boston College Law Review* article, Cara Cheyette cites studies of the often negative psychological impact of directed donation on both the donor and recipient. Cheyette concludes that while "'organ donor' is an efficient catchall phrase for the process by which human organs are obtained for transplantation, in this context, verbal efficiency masks meaningful differences between the affirmative act of giving and the passive experience of having something taken away" (505–506). As described in the above discussion of the limits of the happily-ever-after rhetoric, the emotional and physical consequences of both donation and transplantation are not always straightforwardly positive, especially when we keep in mind that transplantation is rarely the end of illness. Directed donation within families can produce a kind of symbiotic relationship, where the happiness of the donor is contingent on their sense of the ongoing health of the recipient. This anxious attachment means that while the surgery itself may be a discrete act, the donor's emotional well-being depends on the more long-term success of the transplanted organ (Cheyette, 505).

The continued shortage of cadaver donors as well as the greater success rates attached to live kidney donation have led to a landmark moment in organ donation history: Beginning in 2001, living donors have exceeded cadaver donors for kidney transplantation. For the approximately 5000 individuals who have donated kidneys to loved ones (excluding the exceptional cases of surgical altruists), this decision creates new roles within families. The factors influencing decisions about who will be tested, who will donate, and whether the benefits outweigh the risk are all filtered through a complicated existing and emerging set of emotional and interconnected dynamics within families. Medical anthropologist Sharon Kaufman draws from interviews with recipients and donors to expose the "tyranny of potential" in kidney exchange within families. Extending Renée Fox and Judith Swazey's notion of the "tyranny of the gift," Kaufman argues,

> intergenerational commitment, always complicated, is characterized in [these cases] by the intertwining of medical evidence, love, selflessness, and obligation—all of which are impossible to separate. Tyranny resides in the now routine social fact of offering and giving, accepting and receiving; in the bodily "gift" as a "natural" feature of kin obligation; and in the equation of this kind of gifting with care and love. (61–62)

If national organ campaigns advocate for a "gift of love" among strangers, how much more forceful does this argument become within families where the notions of care and love are already overdetermining forces structuring relations? Where "love" comes to mean accepting an act of bodily intrusion, taking on medical risk—even to extend the life of an aging family member—becomes an appropriate request.

Who among the family, then, will be the one to donate? As Kaufman's interviews illustrate, such decisions are often connected to more long-standing family dynamics, including birth order and the existence of dependent children. Women, in particular, seem to discuss their donation as a way to match the value that other siblings achieved through marriage and children: for example, one donor daughter reports, "We all have different roles in the family. My brother is married and he has two young children. My sister is married and lives across the country. I'm single; I'm here, and I had no one else to consider. So that's just the way it was."[50] Aging parents expressed different degrees of enthusiasm, often casting themselves as needing to be persuaded by children to accept this "hand-me-up."[51] In contrast to this anxiety about violating the traditional direction of care and giving down the generations, one "75-year-old woman guided her children toward living donation when she stated in the clinic, 'I'm thrilled that my four daughters want to donate—that all the sacrifices I've made for them are worth it. I feel wonderful that they want to show their love to me in this way.'"[52] As these examples demonstrate, while directed donation opens up new ways of being, these decisions are often channeled through existing gendered patterns and emotional scripts that have been structuring families for years.

A Novel Case: *Never Let Me Go*

Donor families, savior siblings, and living donors all represent new forms of subjectivity and affiliation. These modes have come into being in the wake of transplantation and have escalated or faded with the changing medical landscape. As I've explored above, families and medical personnel have made sense of these new situations through familiar registers of sentiment: love, loyalty, giving, and feeling. In this final section, I will offer an extended discussion of Kazuo Ishiguro's 2005 novel *Never Let Me Go*.[53] Set in a fictionalized version of "England, late 1990s," the novel deploys many of the central tropes of the sentimental novel—coming-of-age, the discovery of a doomed romance, and illness—but uses these tropes in the service of a story that has more in common with science fiction dystopias. As Ishiguro slowly unspools details of the science fiction plotline, he makes extensive use of oblique reference and euphemism, a strategy we've seen to date in donation campaigns for "the gift of life." From the first paragraph of the novel, seemingly innocuous words seem to take on added weight as we work to understand how they might be used in *this* world, one which feels both familiar and different. Ishiguro opens the novel:

> My name is Kathy H. I'm thirty-one years old, and I've been a carer now for over eleven years. ... Now I know my being a carer so long isn't necessarily because they think I'm fantastic at what I do. ... My donors have always tended to do much better than expected. Their recovery times have been impressive, and hardly any of them have been classified as "agitated," even before fourth donation. (3)

What to make of the word "carer"—repeated 9 times in just 2 pages?[54] How should we understand references to donors and "fourth donation"? Of the ominous ring in the description of donors being "classified" as "agitated"? Nearly every review or critical article on the novel includes a close reading of this opening paragraph and includes descriptions of Ishiguro's intentional use of flat, banal, or muted narrative voice.

From its inaugural moment, euphemism and sentimental tropes in this novel demonstrate how ideology becomes embedded in cultural and social forms, producing new identity categories like "carer" and "donor."

The explicit reveal in the novel comes 81 pages after this opening paragraph. In a series of flashback coming-of-age sections, set in a very British boarding school called Hailsham, one of the teachers finally becomes exhausted by all that is unspoken in this environment; in one of the most direct speeches in the novel, she tells the students: "Your lives are set out for you. You'll become adults, then before you're old, before you're even middle-aged, you'll start to donate your vital organs. That's what each of you was created to do" (81). Even with this striking reference to losing "vital organs," the repeated language of fate or destiny in her speech masks a second layer of complexity in this story. The students were "created" as therapeutic clones. In the repeated phrase of the characters—expressing a dynamic that very much models the way readers are positioned by Ishiguro—we have been "told and not told" (81, 82, 83, 88). Hailsham, then, despite its stated humanist goal of demonstrating to the wider public that these clones "*have souls at all*" (260), is more profoundly a model for the installation of ideology, of raising a class of individuals to accept their limited future and lack of autonomy as natural and to squash resistance.

Another effect of Ishiguro's muted tone in the novel is that the clones become a blank screen for critical projections; readers find in the characters' circumstances an analogy to unstated social identities or conditions. Critics see them as vehicles for socioeconomic class, heteronormativity, the holocaust, and postracialism, among other concepts.[55] My own critical filter is to see organ donation in the novel not as a metaphor, but as an exaggerated yet real expression of a bigger social problem. In my reading, the book works to imagine the social and educational system that would be necessary to inculcate the clones into their roles as carers and donors. Using the tropes of sentiment, Ishiguro depicts a system that expressly values affiliation and exchange. He is concerned, then, with a question similar to the one that I have been asking throughout this book, namely, what ideological and cultural production is necessary to produce a world where practices that should seem repellant are, in fact, normalized and even celebrated?

Ishiguro's world is familiar-yet-strange enough that it can be used as a lens to refocus our understanding of how several of the new subjectivities explored in this chapter have come into being. Ishiguro's setting is most commonly described as dystopic, but, to me, the moral questions of cloning for therapeutic purposes and live donations have been taken seriously, asked and answered by bioethicists. This version of England in the late 1990s represents the very end of the slippery slope, that Mengelian abyss described by *Time* magazine's discussion of savior siblings. The interesting question, then, is not of right and wrong, but of how we use culture to get from here to there. What are the structures by which these new and frightening ways of being are embraced by those embodying them? And how do those structures relate to the terms by which donor families and living donors come to understand their choices in the real world? In *Never Let Me Go*, the answer lies both within the world of the book and in the ways in which Ishiguro positions his reader through narrative structure and genre.

In the value scheme within the novel, three elements are essential to constructing this network of carers and donors: affiliation, exchange, and care. Just as Ishiguro seeds the opening of the novel with charged references to being a "carer," he similarly opens with a naturalized model of affinity. Of her preference for caring for other students from Hailsham, Kathy writes: "when you get a chance to choose, of course, you choose your own kind. That's natural" (4). Tucked away in a kind of no place/every place countryside, the boarding school explicitly functions to create an intense group affiliation among the students. This connection to the social body, to something larger than the self, represents one essential pathway to allow for individual bodily incursion. In addition to its spatial isolation, the school uses a series of related practices to minimize concepts of personal property and elevate the value of others. The students are raised to value creative production highly, but their artistic achievements are not understood as a modernist expression of the imaginative-hero-self.

Instead, through a reified series of practices called Exchanges, Sales, and the Gallery, the students are taught to cast away their own work and embrace material produced by others in an interdependent system. Kathy reflects, "Exchanges had a more subtle effect on us all. If you think about it, being dependent on each other to produce the stuff that might become your private treasures—that's bound to do things to your relationships" (16). This is one of the moments where dramatic irony and re-reading or reflection hits readers with the force of Kathy's words. While the statement can be read as a sinister justification for violation, the value system among these donors is, as Kathy states, subtle, dependent, and deeply felt. The circumstances that have produced this reality are wholly absent from the novel—Ishiguro never fully explains how we have ended up in this alternate near past. These circumstances, however, are materially real, in the same way that the sudden death of a loved one is a tragic reality that becomes the condition for becoming a donor family. Or the fatal illness of one child becomes the catalyst driving parents to conceive a savior sibling. In an interview, Ishiguro describes the insular and inescapable nature of these characters' condition: "the characters do belong to a rather odd community, but they cannot stand outside it. This is why they're so passive about what they're being told to do; they cannot stand outside their situation as individuals."[56] Every grieving parent and spouse would ask to stand outside his or her situation; the role of organ donation campaigns, however, is to articulate a system of value that will lead to donation in the face of stark realities (often with only the most oblique or euphemistic reference to death). The novel does not directly wring its hands about the series of events that have produced these clones; instead it provides an ideology with which to meet this tragic condition.[57]

Where Ishiguro meditates on cloning and subjectivity, he tends to do so through metaphor. In these metaphors, the novel expresses the values of interdependence and personal utility over individualism. In one key scene in the novel, the friends travel to Norfolk on a quest to find Ruth's "possible," their name for the human from which they were copied. Although they fail to confirm Ruth's origin, the scene climaxes with a moment of affinity and burgeoning romance as Tommy and Kathy search out and improbably find a copy of a cassette tape that Kathy had lost years before. Consider, from the perspective of a clone, Tommy's naïve questions: "Do you think it could be the same one? I mean, the *actual* one. The one you lost?" (172). Kathy's caution that there "may be thousands of these knocking about" does not diminish the value of *this* copy, which comes to stand for both her childhood memories of the original and her later memories of the copy's discovery and connection to Tommy. The favorite song on the tape, "Never Let Me Go," is also the title of the novel itself.

Like the treasured cassette copy, two additional symbols argue for the value of emotional connections in place of individualist investment in originals. In the first, Kathy describes a recurring anxious memory of a clown carrying a bunch of balloons through a park. She writes, "I kept worrying that one of the strings would come unraveled and a single balloon would sail off up into that cloudy sky" (213). Rather than a triumphant sign of escape and resistance, Kathy understands the lone balloon as a threatening possibility, one which she connects to continuing to act as a carer while her Hailsham comrades have "completed their fourth donation," leaving her isolated in the world of the living. In a related scene, often read as one of the emotional climaxes of the novel, the three main characters—all friends from Hailsham, but now existing along the spectrum of carer to donor—travel to a wrecked boat, incongruously adrift in a grassy field. This vision of a vessel out of place, severed from its former utility, becomes a powerful motivator in the novel. One character, after seeing it, is both reinvigorated for the trip back to the nursing center and seemingly reconciled to her own fated third and fourth donations.

The final central value within the world of the novel has us circle back to the language of care that names Kathy's subjectivity. Care becomes an expression of extreme selflessness, put to the radical ends of giving up one's vital organs. In an uncharacteristic moment of word play, Kathy writes, "For the most part being a carer's suited me fine. You could even say it's brought the best out of me. But some people aren't cut out for it …" (207). These mild moments of verbal irony—bringing out "the best" in a future organ donor, being "cut out for it"—don't read as bitter in the novel; instead, Kathy looks at her role with good-natured pride. In her philosophical treatise arguing for an ethic of care, Joan Tronto describes the ways in which care work has been traditionally feminized and undervalued as one critical stage in making the case for a positive model of care. She reflects, "care has mainly been the work of slaves, servants, and women in Western history."[58] *Never Let Me Go*'s clones form an extreme example of this caring underclass. Critics, most notably Bruce Robbins, Anne Whitehead, and Josie Gill, argue that while the world Ishiguro describes may be extreme, the idea that societies are segregated among types with different roles and values, especially through the mechanisms of a service economy, should be entirely familiar.[59] Bruce Robbins puts these questions in an especially compelling way:

> How much does it matter that in the novel the split between those who have a future and those who don't results from the biological facts of one's birth, which results in turn from deliberate decisions by the authorities, while in our society it is an effect without originary legislation or identity,

> with no 'they' visibly making the decisions, an outcome that can merely be predicted with high statistical reliability? (292)

Robbins argues that the novel's "official institutionalization of caring reflects on caring generally [and] on failures of caring" (291). These critical perspectives demonstrate the problems with caring as a value limited to a segregated class when the privileged group is conversely taught to pursue autonomy.

The ways in which access and participation fall out along marginalized identity categories in our healthcare system is a stark example of the ways in which a rhetorical deployment of "care" can mask inequities. Joan Tronto describes how both the carer and the recipient of care become objectified in this divided pursuit of autonomy for some and selflessness for others:

> "Otherness" arises out of a failure to recognize care in several ways. In the first instance, because we expect to be autonomous, any form of dependency is treated as a great weakness. The "others" who need care are reduced to an object: "the fracture in bed c" is no longer a person to the care-giver. "Welfare mothers" are perceived as lazy because they are dependent, and the only explanation is their "choice" of this lifestyle. On the other hand, the fear that receiving care makes us dependent requires a pre-emptive strike to make care-givers "other" so that when we receive care, we need not allow it to affect our sense of our own autonomy. (123–124)

The language of organ exchange participates in this kind of objectification, defining individuals by the parts they can either give or receive. By elevating the parts above the whole—or conversely using the reified term "life" as the catchall for discrete organs—organ procurement shares the risks of "care" as a value system that places an inequitable burden with negative consequences for some players involved.

Tronto argues, though, that while care has been devalued in its current context, it represents a powerful ethical possibility, one that could be used to intervene in the false atomization that characterizes the celebration of autonomy. Returning briefly to discussions of savior siblings, we recall how courts have defined "best interest" to include emotions and the interdependent nature of families, not as a violation of a person's interest, but as an essential characteristic of it. Is care as represented in

Never Let Me Go, then, an exposition of the devalued nature of care in our contemporary context? Or a hopeful alternative way of being despite its seemingly dystopic setting? When read as an analogy for the healthcare system and service economy as a whole, the answer seems unquestionably to be the former. If we return, however, to the earlier formulation where we take the tragic circumstance as an unavoidable condition—as in the case of the sudden death or fatal illness of a loved one—the question at hand seems not to be the reader's frustration with the clone's failure to rebel. In this framework, the novel can serve as an interesting thought experiment into the cultural modes that can produce donors and carers, one which acknowledges the sinister elements of the model but not exclusively.

As in real life, of course, organ donation schemes cannot fully overcome a residue of distaste for the process more broadly. For all the work that slogans like "gift of life" and "be a hero" have done to recast the sad and scary physical realities of the process, the repellent elements of donation remain in the public consciousness. Recall here the gap between high rates of public approval for organ donation as a concept compared to lower rates of choosing donation among surviving family members. *Never Let Me Go* dramatizes this residual horror through continued references to the students being viewed as spiders by their more generally sympathetic educators and advocates: "she saw and decided in a second *what we were*, because you could see her stiffen—as if a pair of spiders were set to crawl towards her" (248, also 34, 35). Bioethicist Stuart Youngner argues for an essential act of forgetting as part of organ exchange, where campaigns work to obscure the fact that "some must die" in order for others to live. The walls that exist in exchange, from the anonymous donor rule to the strict segregation of surgical teams, function to maintain a denial of death, especially in the ways we represent recipients. The sentimental fictions explored throughout this chapter seek to offer an alternative mode of intervening in this denial, often embracing an imaginative connection between donor and recipient as an expression of romantic or familial connection. These diverse texts explore how recipients might imagine their donors, asking what tropes they use to reconcile their chance for prolonged life with another's death. Again, we see that these tropes are characteristically sentimental, embracing concepts of destiny, matching, romance, and an inviolable but transferable self.

If care, exchange, and affinity are the values that animate the world within *Never Let Me Go*, similar elements drive the genre and narrative structure of the novel itself. Ishiguro uses a series of familiar devices to place his novel within the sentimental tradition, most notably including direct address to the reader, the conceit of a character writing her memoirs, stories of illness, romantic love, and an emphasis on feeling. Several moments in the novel explicitly place it in the lineage of the Victorian era, including repeated references to Kathy reading and writing about George Eliot's *Daniel Deronda* and physical artifacts like the Victorian furniture in their patron's home. Karl Shaddox explicitly locates the novel in the sentimental traditional, advocating for a connection between Ishiguro's work and the mid-nineteenth-century abolitionist use of sentiment as a universal value that could step outside the terms of purportedly rationalist arguments about slavery.[60] His reminder of the historical and political turn to sentiment, which I have addressed above, offers a means to recast the allegedly apolitical categories of feeling, romance, and family.

For Shaddox, the novel creates what he calls an "affective pact" with its reader. For a novel that emphasizes the importance of affinity and community, it's perhaps no surprise that Ishiguro explores narrative techniques to extend this community to the audience. In one familiar mechanism, Kathy deploys the sentimental tradition of "Dear Reader," using second person direct address to construct a reader whom she imagines as a clone like her. In the repeated phrase, "I don't know how it was where you were" (13, 67, 96), she locates her audience on the side of the carers and donors, allowing for some environmental differences, but requiring an essential affiliation.

For Kathy, the particulars are less important than the feelings. She writes, "I'm sure somewhere in your childhood, you too had an experience like ours that day; similar if not in the actual details, then inside, in the feelings" (36). Affinity, then, extends beyond the previously suggested boundaries of the specific upbringing at Hailsham to the position of being a clone more universally. Her easy assumption, her assurance that the feelings on a particular day will be shared, speak to the fantasy of affect as a tool to overcome difference.[61] The novel acknowledges, however, that emotions can also serve as a coercive force. Ishiguro uses embarrassment and awkwardness as mechanisms that obscure the harsh realities of the situation: "we perhaps even knew that a long way down the line there were donations waiting for us. But we didn't really know what that meant. If we were keen to avoid certain topics, it was probably because it *embarrassed* us. We hated the way our guardians, usually so on top of everything, became so awkward whenever we came near this territory" (69). Among contemporary procurement professionals and grief counselors, the repeated intervention exhorting colleagues to avoid euphemism in discussions with donor families demonstrates how deep the prohibition against naming or discussing difficult topics has become. As lawmakers consider public policies that would increase rates of donation, they have come up against the limits of Required Request. Although it is currently the law in all 50 states to approach donor-eligible families about the possibility of donation upon a diagnosis of brain death, studies reflect unevenness in practice, citing the awkwardness or perceived inappropriateness of the conversation.[62] Feelings, then, function powerfully as both the motivating force for donation through sentimental appeals and a barrier against direct discussions about the realities of death and what happens during donation.

In addition to imagining interpersonal connection through a universal model of feeling, the novel, like many of the more melodramatic fictions explored above, weaves together two subplots: the medical and the romantic. The only chance of resistance entertained by the characters involves a request for a "deferral," rumored to be possible for "a boy and a girl … really, properly in love … [who] could show it" (153). Crucially, Ishiguro repeats the medical language of matching from organ exchange to denote love between donors. The students' collected artwork is imagined as qualifying evidence: "Suppose two people come up and say they're in love. She can find the art they've done over years and years. She can see if they go. If they match. Don't forget, Kath, what she's got reveals our souls. She could decide herself what's a good match and what's just a stupid crush" (176). The end of the novel ultimately dashes this romantic fantasy, but the romantic investment in finding a match dramatizes the terms by which thousands of potential organ recipients wait for an external party to find and confirm their own "match." The feelings of hope, the language of destiny, and the reliance on external validation all hold a strange mirror up to a process that, "if not in the details, then inside, in the feelings" (36), captures some of the emotional valences of transplantation.

This final scene of romantic appeal also functions to pull back the curtain slightly on how they have arrived at this alternative world.

The architects of Hailsham describe their educational experiment and attempt to advocate for the humanity of the clones. Ironically, they cite the very elements of interdependence and concern valued among the students as the same feelings that produced their exploitation in the first place. In one of the longest speeches of the novel, Ishiguro writes:

> After the war, in the early fifties, when the great breakthroughs in science followed one after the other so rapidly, there wasn't time to take stock, to ask the sensible questions. Suddenly there were all these new possibilities laid before us, all these ways to cure so many previously incurable conditions. That was what the world noticed the most, wanted the most. And for a long time, people preferred to believe these organs appeared from nowhere, or at most that they grew in a kind of vacuum. … How can you ask a world that has come to regard cancer as curable, how can you ask such a world to put away that cure, to go back to the dark days? There was no going back. However uncomfortable people were about your existence, their overwhelming concern was that their own children, their spouses, their parents, their friends, did not die from cancer, motor neurone disease, heart disease. (263)

As Anne Whitehead argues, "Here, then, the true horror of Ishiguro's dystopic society is revealed: it is shown to be founded, precisely, on relations of care" (77). Elevated concepts of family—so central to sentimental narratives—have an accompanying dark side; for all their appeal to forms of universalism, they can also pursue an ethics of proximity, which obscures the needs of those perceived as socially or physically distant. The telescoping radius of imagined proximity, ranging from the nuclear family to the nation, is fundamental to the sentimental tradition. Whitehead's word choice, "horror," however, signals an important transition to residual or obscured elements in these tear-jerking cultural scripts of organ exchange. While this chapter has explored a strong tradition of sentiment in news stories, public campaigns, and fictional texts, the following chapter examines its twin genre in our popular imagination: transplantation as horror narrative.

Although *Never Let Me Go* occupies the high literary side of the sentimental tradition, Ishiguro's characters acknowledge that they may, in fact, be players in an entirely different genre:

> You'll have heard the same talk. How maybe, after fourth donation, even if you're technically completed, you're still conscious in some sort of way;

> how then you find there are more donations, plenty of them, on the other side of that line; how there are no more recovery centres, no carers, no friends; how there's nothing to do except watch your remaining donations until they switch you off. It's horror movie stuff, and most of the time people don't want to think about it. Not the whitecoats, not the carers—and usually not the donors. (279)

This speech encapsulates a series of essential elements in the transplantation as horror tradition: references to urban legend, anxiety over lost connections and autonomy, questions about an unnatural end of life, and skepticism about doctors in the dehumanizing term "whitecoats." Where sentiment celebrates destiny, horror recoils from loss of control. Where cellular memory in romantic stories forms the possibility of reconstituted love and redemption, the concept becomes a kind of curse in horror stories in which the transplanted organs of criminals prompt bloodthirsty behavior in recipients. The medical establishment, largely absent or benign in sentimental stories, becomes a sinister force seeking technological progress beyond human limits. In the following chapter, I step across this genre divide, exploring the cultural barriers to transplantation that persist in the popular imagination.

Notes

1. Ronald Reagan, "Radio Address to the Nation on the International Monetary Fund and on Organ Donorship," July 23, 1983, http://www.presidency.ucsb.edu/ws/?pid=41629.
2. The theory of sentiment, especially in literature, falls into three basic categories. First, the foundational work in moral philosophy by Smith, Locke, and Hume. Second, the literary history of the eighteenth-century British novel, see Barbara M. Benedict, *Framing Feeling: Sentiment and Style in English Prose Fiction, 1745–1800* (New York: AMS Press, 1994); Patricia Meyer Spacks, *Novel Beginnings: Experiments in Eighteenth-Century English Fiction* (New Haven: Yale University Press, 2006); Watt, *Rise of the Novel*; and Sydney McMillen Conger, ed., *Sensibility in Transformation: Creative Resistance to Sentiment from the Augustans to the Romantics* (London: Associated University Presses, 1990). And third, the literary history of sentiment in the American tradition, often read through the political context of abolition and woman's suffrage, see Lauren Berlant, *The Female Complaint: The Unfinished Business of Sentiment in American Culture* (Durham: Duke University Press, 2008); Elizabeth Barnes, *States of Sympathy: Seduction and Democracy*

in the American Novel (New York: Columbia University Press, 1997); Kristin Boudreau, *Sympathy in American Literature: American Sentiments from Jefferson to the Jameses* (Gainesville, FL: University Press of Florida, 2002); Joanne Dobson, "Reclaiming Sentimental Literature," *American Literature* 69, no. 2 (1997): 263–288; Ann Douglas, *The Feminization of American Culture* (New York: Alfred A. Knopf, 1977); Markman Ellis, *The Politics of Sensibility: Race, Gender, and Commerce in the Sentimental Novel* (Cambridge: Cambridge University Press, 1996); Julia A. Stern, *The Plight of Feeling: Sympathy and Dissent in the Early American Novel* (Chicago: The University of Chicago, 1997); and Jane Tompkins, *Sensational Designs: The Cultural Work of American Fiction, 1790–1860* (New York: Oxford University Press, 1985).

3. Joanne Dobson, "Reclaiming Sentimental Literature," describes two phases of this reclamation, the first, which brought some sentimental authors into the American canon and demonstrated their expression of American cultural ideals and the second, which she participates in, that seeks to take seriously the literary and aesthetic modes of the genre.
4. Bruce Jennings, "Biopower and the Liberationist Romance," *Hastings Center Report* 40, no. 4 (2010): 16.
5. Although scholarship on organ exchange often uses the term "donor kin," I opt for "donor families" as the term more common in public discourse. While "kin" is likely more anthropologically appropriate, what it makes up for in accuracy it loses in the symbolic weight of cultural signification.
6. Raelynn Maloney and Alan D. Wolfelt, *Caring for Donor Families: Before and After* (Fort Collins, CO: Companion Press, 2001), 43.
7. For more on consent rates among donor-eligible families, factors influencing their decisions, and the potential efficacy of various policies to increase donation see Laura Siminoff et al., "Factors Influencing Families' Consent for Donation of Solid Organs for Transplantation," *JAMA* 286, no. 1 (July 4, 2001): 71–77.
8. Ty Swenson, "How One Heart Healed Two Families, a Valentine's Day Tale," *West Seattle Herald/White Center News*, February 13, 2013, http://www.westseattleherald.com/2013/02/13/features/how-one-heart-healed-two-families-valentine%E2%80%99s.
9. Ibid.
10. Adam Smith, *The Theory of Moral Sentiments*, ed. D. D. Raphael and A. L. Macfie (Oxford: Clarendon Press, 1976), 16.
11. Elizabeth Barnes, *States of Sympathy*, x.
12. For more on the intersections of slavery, sentiment, and the rhetoric of blood, see Shirley Samuels, "The Identity of Slavery," in *The Culture of Sentiment: Race, Gender, and Sentimentality in Nineteenth-Century America*, ed. Shirley Samuels (New York: Oxford University Press, 1992), 157–171.

13. Jodi Picoult, *Change of Heart: A Novel* (New York, NY: Atria Books, 2008), 237.
14. Swenson, "How One Heart."
15. Maloney and Wolfelt, *Caring for Donor Families*, 73.
16. Jodi Picoult, *My Sister's Keeper* (New York: Atria Books, 2004), 417.
17. Maloney and Wolfelt, *Caring for Donor Families*, 5.
18. Jason Gonzales, "Heart Transplant Leads Edina Man to Love," *Star Tribune*, April 10, 2013, http://www.startribune.com/heart-transplant-leads-edina-man-to-love/190399681/.
19. *The Best of Me*, directed by Michael Hoffman (Relativity Media, 2014).
20. Ian Watt, *The Rise of the Novel: Studies in Defoe, Richardson and Fielding* (Berkeley: University of California Press, 1957), 32.
21. Spacks, *Novel Beginnings*, 3.
22. Sharp, *Strange Harvest*, 111.
23. *Return to Me*, directed by Bonnie Hunt (MGM, 2000).
24. For more on the place of tissue typing in the history of transplant medicine, see Hamilton, *A History of Organ Transplantation* and Tilney, *Transplant.*
25. Joseph Jacobs, "Love: The Risk Worth Taking," *Narrative Inquiry in Bioethics* 12, no. 1 (Spring 2012): 17–18.
26. Picoult, *My Sister's Keeper*, 312.
27. Amy K. Lewensten, "A Life for a Life: My Gift to My Dad," *Narrative Inquiry in Bioethics* 2, no. 1 (Spring 2012): 21.
28. Kaufman, "Fairness and the Tyranny of Potential," 56.
29. Picoult, *Change of Heart*, 60.
30. Laurie E. Post, "Liver Donor Nightmare," *Narrative Inquiry in Bioethics* 2, no. 1 (2012): 34.
31. See Nikola Biller-Andorno, "Gender Imbalance in Living Organ Donation," *Medicine, Health Care and Philosophy* 5, no. 2 (May 2002): 199–203; Roger Dobson, "More Women Than Men Become Living Organ Donors," *BMJ: British Medical Journal* 325, no. 7369 (October 19, 2002): 851; and Hanna Hermann et al., "Gender-Specific Differences Associated with Living Donor Liver Transplantation: A Review Study," *Liver Transplantation* 16 (2010): 375–386.
32. Rachel A. Ankeny, "The Moral Status of Preferences for Directed Donation: Who Should Decide Who Gets Transplantable Organs?" *Cambridge Quarterly of Healthcare Ethics* 10, no. 4 (October 2001): 393.
33. James F. Childress, "Putting Patients First in Organ Allocation: An Ethical Analysis of the U.S. Debate," *Cambridge Quarterly of Healthcare Ethics: CQ: The International Journal of Healthcare Ethics Committees* 10, no. 4 (2001): 365–376.
34. Lederer, *Flesh and Blood*, 52.

35. Sharp, *Strange Harvest*, 133.
36. Kevin Sack, "Lives Forever Linked Through Kidney Transplant Chain 124," *The New York Times*, February 18, 2012, http://www.nytimes.com/2012/02/19/health/lives-forever-linked-through-kidney-transplant-chain-124.html.
37. Quoted in Fox and Swazey, *Spare Parts*, 47.
38. Ian Parker, "The Gift," *New Yorker* 80, no. 21 (August 2, 2004): 54–63.
39. Anne Whitehead, "Writing with Care: Kazuo Ishiguro's Never Let Me Go," *Contemporary Literature* 52, no. 1 (2011): 57.
40. Lance Morrow, "When One Body Can Save Another," *Time*, June 17, 1991, http://content.time.com/time/magazine/article/0,9171,973182,00.html.
41. President's Council on Bioethics, *Reproduction and Responsibility: The Regulation of New Biotechnologies* (Washington, DC, 2004), 96, www.bioethics.gov.
42. Kimberly Strong, Ian Kerridge, and Miles Little, "Savior Siblings, Parenting and the Moral Valorization of Children," *Bioethics* 28, no. 4 (May 1, 2014): 189.
43. Ibid.
44. *Strunk v Strunk*, 445 S.W.2d 145 (1969).
45. It is interesting to note that the conventional formulation of the substituted judgment standard—what would this person do if he or she were competent—mirrors the relational nature of Adam Smith's influence formulation of sympathy—how would I feel if I were in the position of the sufferer. In both cases, an act of imagination is required to identify not a universal standard of feeling or correctness, but how another would respond.
46. Quoted in James Dwyer and Elizabeth Vig, "Rethinking Transplantation Between Siblings," *Hastings Center Report* 25, no. 5 (September 10, 1995): 8.
47. *Hart v. Brown*, 289 A.2d (Connecticut Superior Court, 1972).
48. Dwyer and Vig, "Rethinking Transplantation Between Siblings," make a similar point in their critique of the best interest standard.
49. *Curran v Bosze*, 153 Ill. Dec 213 (1990).
50. Quoted in Kaufman, "Fairness and the Tyranny of Potential," 61.
51. Ibid., 60.
52. Ibid.
53. Kazuo Ishiguro, *Never Let Me Go* (New York: Vintage, 2006).
54. This frequency is also noted by Whitehead, "Writing with Care," 59. In his discussion of this paragraph, Bruce Robbins notes usefully that in the UK, where the term "carer" is fairly commonplace, the term would only elicit a "mild chill." Bruce Robbins, "Cruelty Is Bad: Banality and

Proximity in 'Never Let Me Go'," *NOVEL: A Forum on Fiction* 40, no. 3 (2007): 291.

55. Josie Gill offers a similar abbreviated literature review, arguing, "critics have largely concluded that *Never Let Me Go* is not about human cloning," and then offering a list of various interpretation schemes. Josie Gill, "Written on the Face: Race and Expression in Kazuo Ishiguro's *Never Let Me Go*," *MFS: Modern Fiction Studies* 60, no. 4 (2014): 846.
56. Sean Matthews, "'I'm Sorry I Can't Say More': An Interview with Kazuo Ishiguro," in *Kashuo Ishiguro: Contemporary Critical Perspectives*, ed. Sean Matthews and Sebastian Groes (London: Continuum, 2009), 115.
57. Elsewhere in the same interview, Ishiguro seems to support this reading of the novel as an exploration of unavoidable realities of death. He tells Sean Matthews, "I suppose the big thing about Never Let Me Go is that they never rebel, they don't do the thing that you want them to do. They passively accept the program in which they are butchered for their organs. … I suppose, ultimately, I wanted to write a book about how people accept that we are mortal and we can't get away from this, and that after a certain point we are all going to die, we won't live forever. There are various ways to rage against that, but in the end we have to accept it and there are different reactions. So I wanted the characters in Never Let Me Go to react to this horrible program they seem to be subjected to in much the way in which we accept the human condition, accept ageing, and falling to bits, and dying." Matthews, "I'm Sorry I Can't Say More," 124.
58. Joan Tronto, *Moral Boundaries: A Political Argument for an Ethic of Care* (New York: Routledge, 1993), 113.
59. Robbins, "Cruelty Is Bad"; Whitehead, "Writing with Care"; and Gill, "Written on the Face."
60. Karl Shaddox, "Generic Considerations in Ishiguro's *Never Let Me Go*," *Human Rights Quarterly* 35, no. 2 (2013): 448–469. Several critics take up the issue of genre and the novel. Keith McDonald argues for it as a form of "pathography," with its autobiographical elements, meta-fictional references, and positioning of the reader as "witness to trauma and loss" (76). Others focus on the novel's emphasis on emotions, including Myra J. Seaman, "Becoming More (Than) Human: Affective Posthumanisms, Past and Future," *Journal of Narrative Theory* 37, no. 2 (2007): 246–275; Keith McDonald, and Whitehead, "Writing with Care." The other dominant generic consideration of the novel rests in the fact of its being a science fiction novel without science. Gabriele Griffin offers an effective intervention into the idea that "there's no science here," by offering two alternate scientific modes, one called "acute science," which strives for accuracy and attempts to describe scientific knowledge at the time of writing, and "mediated" or "science as effect," that takes up

scientific questions in more oblique ways. As a host of popular fiction—emblematically in the work of Jodi Picoult—demonstrates, the sentimental and science fiction genres can occupy the same place, although Ishiguro's striking push of explicitly scientific elements to the background serves here to elevate the sentimental. It is perhaps interesting to note, however, that the book is often listed commercially as science fiction.

61. In her reading of the novel, Josie Gill, "Written on the Face," agrees that feelings are important, but demonstrates Kathy's inability to articulate these feelings in words. Instead, facial expression becomes an essential object of scrutiny as the face gives meaning to feelings that cannot, for these characters, be named in words.
62. For more on the relationship between proposed policies and their possible efficacy according to measures of public opinion, see Laura Siminoff and Mary Beth Mercer, "Public Policy, Public Opinion." Fox and Swazey similarly argue that studies suggest that early compliance rates under Required Request were as low as 50%, despite their inventor, Arthur Caplan's, continued enthusiasm for the policy.

CHAPTER 6

Murdering Hands and Mad Doctors: The Horrors of Organ Exchange

In the summer of 1978, Robert McFall turned to the Pennsylvania courts in an attempt to save his life. McFall suffered from aplastic anemia and would die without a bone marrow transplant. He had found a match in his first cousin, 39-year-old David Shimp, but Shimp refused to submit to further testing or to the donation. In his ruling, Judge John Flaherty argued that while Shimp's refusal might be "morally repulsive," to compel Shimp's donation would violate the first principle of American society.[1] Flaherty wrote "that society and government exist to protect the individual from being invaded and hurt by another." In its decision, the court—as courts so often do—turned to metaphor to articulate the rationale:

> For a society, which respects the rights of one individual, to sink its teeth into the jugular vein or neck of one of its members and suck from it sustenance for another member, is revolting to our hard-wrought concept of jurisprudence. [Forcible] extraction of living body tissue causes revulsion to the judicial mind. Such would raise the specter of the swastika and the inquisition, reminiscent of the horrors this portends.

At this moment, when McFall's sentimental appeal to family, giving, and mutual responsibility has failed, the principle of individual autonomy trumps alternative arguments. Judge Flaherty's evocation of "horrors" and

E. Russell, *Transplant Fictions*,
Palgrave Studies in Literature, Science and Medicine,
https://doi.org/10.1007/978-3-030-12135-8_6

bloodsucking captures both the content and form of widespread and lingering public fears about organ exchange. Where organ donation pleas tend to be expressed through the generic conventions of sentiment, reservations about the practice take the form of horror narratives. Vampires, mad Dr. Frankensteins, urban legends of kidney heists, and horror movie plotlines in which transplanted organs carry a murderous essence all speak to an underlying force in discussions of organ exchange: the role of popular fears in shaping our attitudes about donation and extraordinary medical experimentation.

Just one year before Judge Flaherty was cautioning against the excesses of a predatory, vampiric society, Robin Cook, M.D., published *Coma*, the first entry in a new genre called the "medical thriller." Cook's best-selling narrative reflects public fears over an unchecked authority of doctors and medical institutions that view individual patients as dehumanized objects of scientific progress. The novel's most enduring image—illustrated on the cover and later memorably staged in the film of the same name (1978)[2]—captures the contours of these anxieties. Late in the novel, the book's protagonist, Susan, makes a startling discovery at an off-site care center for coma patients:

> There were more than a hundred patients in the room, and all of them were completely suspended in midair about four feet from the floor. All of them were naked. Looking closely, Susan could see the wires piercing multiple points on the patients' long bones. The wires were connected to complicated metal frames and pulled taut. The patients' heads were supported by other wires from the ceiling which were attached to screw eyes in the patients' skulls. Susan had an impression of grotesque, horizontal, sleeping marionettes.[3]

Cook's description emphasizes human fears of total vulnerability: bodies naked, displayed, pierced, and suspended. In contrast to the principle of individual autonomy pursued in medical ethics, these patients represent a total loss of control over the body. These "grotesque marionettes" echo a classic horror image: that of the monster laid out on Frankenstein's table, an assemblage of parts stolen from graves and anatomy labs.

But Cook also echoes another powerful image, one less familiar, but nevertheless influential among practitioners and scholars of organ transplantation. In 1974, Willard Gaylin published an article in *Harper's* exploring how technological changes like artificial respiration and transplantation would lead to ideological changes in concepts like life, death, and progress. In part responding to the Harvard criteria for brain death, Gaylin writes:

> To save lives and relieve suffering—traditional motives for violating tradition—we could develop hospitals (an inappropriate word because it suggests the presence of living human beings), banks, or farms of cadavers which require feedings and maintenance, in order to be harvested. To the uninitiated the 'new cadavers' in their rows of respirators would seem indistinguishable from comatose patients now residing in wards of chronic neurological hospitals.[4]

He then outlines a series of imagined uses of "the neomort" (no longer mere "cadaver") housed in a "bioemporium": a training ground for anxious medical students; test dummies for new drugs or surgical techniques; banks for tissues; and manufacturing plants for blood or hormones. Taken together, we see Gaylin, Cook, and *Frankenstein* all turn to a similar image to encapsulate enduring public fears about the outer limits of medical experimentation and the potential for dehumanization, even (or especially) in the quest for medical progress and public good.

This image of the supine body, hovering between life and death, vulnerable to the mastery of the medical scientist, has recurred in horror narratives for nearly two centuries. The image may be familiar, but does it matter for the real work of transplant professionals in the day-to-day? The answer to this question turns out to be both "yes" and "it's complicated." Public surveys and FAQs consistently reveal widespread fears about transplantation, from "is my loved one really dead?" to "will the doctor give up on life-saving measures if I'm a donor?" Throughout this chapter, I will argue that horrific narratives of transplantation dramatize common fears. Rather than criticizing these negative portrayals as a roadblock to greater public acceptance, however, I argue that an outlet for public fears is a necessary part of coming to grips with radically experimental medical practices. Moreover, the hyperbolic nature of the horror genre ultimately serves to not only express but also contain these anxieties. The texts examined in this chapter dramatize these fears, not to limit our acceptance of the practice, but to paradoxically reassure us that such transgressions are located safely at a generic extreme. After all, in the author's letter and press surrounding the publication and reissue editions of *Coma*, Robin Cook tells us that his goal in writing was to increase donations by demonstrating an exaggerated vision of the consequences of organ scarcity.[5]

Anyone who spends time looking at popular media coverage of organ transplantation will find a kind of ritualistic evocation of scarcity in these articles; reports almost always include statistics on the number of individuals currently on transplant lists and how many of these will die waiting for an organ. In scholarly writing about donations, there is a similar refrain, a recurring evocation of the gap between public support for donation and the choices people make when the option of donation is at hand. In 2012, the US Department of Health and Human Services found that survey respondents overwhelmingly expressed positive sentiments toward organ transplantation (94.9%). While rising over time, actual rates of donation among family of eligible donors were only about 50% of those requested in 2002.[6] The gap again emerges between the near-total support expressed on surveys and actual registration (through documents like driver's licenses), which, while still improving, also fall at about 50%.[7] Communication studies scholar Susan Morgan and her research teams have found that negative, sensationalist representations in film and television are an important source of information about organ transplantation for the American public.[8] These portrayals include a series of recurring myths, including: "premature declaration of death, the transference of personality traits from donor to recipient, a US black market for organs, corruption in the medical community, and corruption in the organ allocation system (which allows celebrities to get transplants first)."[9] Morgan and other media studies scholars argue that these myths can influence how a potential donor family might approach the decision to donate. Negative representation, then, does matter for transplant professionals and cannot be dismissed as the silly worries of a superstitious public.

Such myths, cited by families as genuine concerns, are also the barest bones of the hyperbolic horror plotlines that find their expression in tales of murder, monsters, and dystopias. In a process familiar to scholars in cultural studies, popular representation both shapes and reflects public concerns. Negative representation, then, may give shape to common fears, but it cannot be charged with solely inventing them. Understanding the functioning of horror as a genre can offer a path forward in reconciling how representations of negative myths of transplantation can do more than simply confirming public fears about the practice. The bare fact is that transplantation requires a massive ideological shift in which we reset foundational concepts of life, death, self, and other. The move from monstrous violation to medical miracle could never have been seamless. As described in Chapter 5, sentimental narratives offer a script for how to make the positive case for donation, but by contrast, the horror genre can offer a venting mechanism, providing a cultural outlet for lingering concerns about the practice. These anxieties may or may not be resolved to general satisfaction, but we are, at least, given a pathway by which to understand their expression and management.

The Strangely Reassuring Nature of Horror

There's a moment in *Coma* where one character attempts to dismiss the fears of the protagonist by casting her speculation as the stuff of horror movies. He tells her, "Susan, you've been staying up watching old horror movies. ... What do you suspect, some sort of sinister inversion layer spreading evil forces, or is it a crazed killer who hates people with minor ailments?" (Cook 191). The unlikely nature of these suggestions, cast explicitly in the conversation as "absurd" and evidence of a possible "psychotic break," offers a dramatization of the first way in which advocates for organ transplantation manage the concerns of the public—by casting them as exaggerated or superstitious. Of course, in the context of the thriller novel, Susan is more right than crazy. There *is* a syndicate of medical personnel profiting from the sale of organs and justifying their murderous plot as serving the greater good. Readers of *Coma*, however, cannot reasonably cite the novel as evidence for their suspicions about predatory medical institutions. The hyperbolic formal elements of the horror genre deflate such arguments, placing them in a frame that may acknowledge the affective reality of these fears, but that nevertheless denies their material reality. Even the most dystopic visions of transplantation explored below dislocate dramatic possible excesses of organ exchange to a bad (but crucially as yet unrealized) future.

Horror, as a genre, is appropriate to the expression of lingering fears about organ transplant not simply because it is the genre of fear, but because so many shared foundational concerns underpin both horror and transplantation. In theories of horror,[10] critics commonly identify at least two constituent elements of the genre: first, the transgression of boundaries, and second, an emphasis on the physical, both on the page/screen and within the audience. These elements are also central to transplantation and create a productive meeting point to understand how horror narratives play a role in our ideological evolution with regard to organ exchange.

The rehearsal of boundary transgressions prompted by organ exchange should be familiar at this point. Bioethicist Stuart Youngner participates in this chorus, listing as a series of "boundary issues": "the lines between life and death, between human and machine (esp. dialysis), between allowing to die and killing, and between medical progress and hubris."[11] As I have argued throughout this volume, these transgressions are profound and form the ground upon which both material and ideological change is laid. "Transgression" is no less essential in horror narratives. In his work on "body horror," Ian Olney offers a list that reads much like Stephen Youngner's, arguing that the body horror genre "celebrates the breakdown of the normative human body and the emergence of the 'problem' body—a body that resists easy classification because it exists 'in between' established ontological categories like 'alive' and 'dead,' 'self' and 'other, 'human' and 'nonhuman,' 'able-bodied' and 'disabled.'"[12] Stephen Prince echoes this sentiment about horror more broadly, arguing, "The anxiety at the heart of the genre is, indeed, the nature of human being. Within the terrain of horror, the state of being human is fundamentally uncertain."[13] This language of "uncertainty," elsewhere called "anxiety," "indeterminacy," and the "breaking down" of secure categories, achieves a critical consensus among horror theorists. "Transgression" also captures a familiar device in horror stories regarding organ transplantation. I will explore the conceptual and aesthetic meaning of boundary transgression below, in texts ranging from canonical novels like *Frankenstein* to largely forgotten works with outlandish transplant plotlines. I will also draw from accounts of real-life organ exchanges and stories from the frontiers of experimental medicine to explore how these narratives are framed through the tropes of horror.

The second distinguishing feature of the horror genre lies in its striking emphasis on the physical. By definition, horror narratives must be gory, graphic in their portrayals of fear and violence. While this scale has escalated over time, Mary Shelley again provides a template for future practitioners in the genre. She writes of Frankenstein's quest to assemble his creation:

> I collected bones from charnel houses; and disturbed, with profane fingers, the tremendous secrets of the human frame. In a solitary chamber, ... I kept my workshop of filthy creation: my eye-balls were starting from their sockets in attending to the details of my employment. The dissecting room and the slaughterhouse furnished many of my materials; and often did my human nature turn with loathing from my occupation, whilst, still urged on by an eagerness which perpetually increased, I brought my work near to a conclusion.[14]

These dissecting rooms and slaughterhouses not only provide the materials for Frankenstein's "filthy creation," but also alter the scientist's body itself. Here, his "eye-balls were starting from their sockets" and, later, Shelley describes his nervous collapse at this brutal work. This mutually transformative effect on the bodies of both the "patient" and the "doctor" reflects a universal sense of vulnerability in public approaches to organ exchange. Snatching body parts from the anonymous vault of death means that anyone can be subject to violation. Furthermore, the technical and philosophical changes required of cutting-edge science are seen to have costs for the humanity of the practitioner, costs that are borne on the physical frame.

It is not, however, only Frankenstein's eyeballs that are "starting from their sockets." Horror is "sensational" in all valences of the term, especially in the physical nature of its effect on readers and viewers. As Carol Clover argues in her theory of gender and sexuality in the horror film,

> horror and pornography are the only two genres specifically devoted to the arousal of bodily sensation. They exist solely to horrify and stimulate, not always respectively, and their ability to do so is the sole measure of their success: they "prove themselves upon our pulses." Thus, in horror-film circles, "good" means scary, specifically in a bodily way (ads promise shivers, chills, shudders, tingling of the spine ...).[15]

In addition to the pornography and horror that Clover cites, I would include sentimental fiction as a genre proven on the body; the tears and blushes of its readers are often described as the measure of a successful nineteenth-century novel.[16] Horror and sentiment may seem to be strange bedfellows, but their paired exploration across Chapter 5 and this chapter can demonstrate how these narrative modes act concurrently to sweep up and manage public response—both positive and negative—to organ exchange.

In her descriptive catalog of contemporary horror films, Isabel Cristina Pinedo also underscores the centrality of transgression, but emphasizes the body in these disruptions. She uses graphic language to list "physical violence against the body: (typically nonsexual) invasion of bodily cavities or of body surfaces to create cavities, the release of body fluids through stabbing and slashing, the tearing of body parts from each other, the wrenching transformation of bodies."[17] While many contemporary horror films exist in a kind of blood-and-guts arms race to find increasingly novel and extreme ways of violating the sanctity of the body, they also take as their founding premise an often-repressed but inescapable reality of the body as vulnerable. Margrit Shildrick, in her work on theories of embodiment, similarly argues, "To accept ... that the body is intrinsically vulnerable—that embodied vulnerability is indeed the condition of life—is to understand that the well-being associated with medically delivered and maintained health does not offer settled stability."[18] In the sentimental genre, the threat of loss and tragedy binds individuals as ethically and emotionally interdependent. In horror, the constantly imperiled characters showcase a truth of existence so often silenced in stories of medical triumph: to live is to die, to hurt, to become ill.

Of course, patients and medical professionals are closer to these realities than the healthy population at large. A recurring question in horror theory—how can it be that audiences find pleasure in these dramatizations of violence and terror?—offers a useful reminder that individuals will experience horrifying transplant narratives differently depending on their standpoint within the practice. Mary Beth Oliver and Meghan Sanders, for example, cite studies of audience psychology that suggest that people who experience or witness a great deal of violence in their everyday lives are more likely to view horror films and that "witnessing such violence in the safety and comfort of a movie theater or a living room helps viewers cope with their fears of aggression."[19] These studies can help explain the common phenomenon of gallows humor among patients awaiting transplant, who have been known to ask if doctors "had the opportunity to run down any pedestrians on the way to work"; fantasizing about going to the hospital rooftop with a rifle; or hoping for bad weather that might cause a fatal car accident.[20] For patients and families living with terminal illness, the imperiled existence of horror protagonists may not feel entirely distant.

The "Gift of Life" campaign seeks to elide the realities of death in its phrasing and imagery, but lurking just beneath these uplift stories lies an inescapable death, either for the terminally ill patient or for the potential donor family. By contrast, in horror narratives, violence is unavoidably present in everyday life.[21] In *Coma*, Robin Cook includes the following graphic image: "The person next to her turned and Susan recoiled in ill-concealed horror. The man's—or was it a woman's—eyes were surrounded by dark areas of hemorrhage. The nose was swollen and distorted, with nasal packs partially extruding from the nostrils. Several wires came from within the nose and were taped to either cheek. The visage was that of a monster" (229). As reading the passage in context reveals, this "monster" is not part of the murder plot at the center of the novel, but instead a mundane instance of hospital life: a patient who has received plastic surgery. Cook's language intentionally draws from the register of horror, playing up the indeterminacy of the patient's gender and emphasizing the brutality of healing. Such tactics are characteristic of thrillers more broadly, in which atmosphere and imagery combine to suggest terrifying elements in everyday life. According to Pete Boss, this expression of ambivalence about the horrific physical effects of medicine is a determining element in contemporary approaches to the body and medicine: "Modern medicine, its methods of quantification and treatment, its technology and power, stands, at once, as that which improves or prolongs our (physical) existence, and the constant signifier of its limitations, a condition which allows it to slide rapidly from reassurance to disturbance in its imagery."[22] Recall here the above list of boundary transgressions dramatized by both horror and transplant narratives. The mutual "reassurance [and] disturbance" located within these stories—I might get desperately ill ... but I might be saved ... but at what cost?—captures an important indeterminacy that has dogged transplant technology through centuries from its imagination, to its inception, to its standard practice, and imagined future.

Donald Joralemon and Susan Squier share my interest in the conceptual changes that are necessary to make organ transplantation culturally acceptable.[23] Like Joralemon, Squier uses the metaphor of "ideological cyclosporine," exploring what new cultural formations were necessary to prevent social rejection of a radical medical procedure in the same way that immunosuppressant drugs allow the body to prevent rejection of the grafted tissue.[24] These scholars approach transplantation from different fields—Joralemon from medical anthropology and Squier from literary study, particularly science fiction—but both focus on the importance of cultural work done alongside advances in medical technology. The value of the ideological cyclosporine metaphor lies in its insistence that first, acceptance of this revolutionary medicine is not without backlash, and second, it will be unevenly taken up within society. They understand that continued persuasion will be necessary to address ongoing tendencies toward popular rejection. Like the monstrous hand that will pop out of the grave during the closing credits, public acceptance of experimental medicine is unstable and this instability will need to find expression in culture. I argue that horror narratives serve that end, dramatizing the complex push and pull between recoil and reassurance.

Public health research into attitudes about organ exchange offers a fascinating window into the lingering fears that keep people from donating or imagining themselves accepting organs. As described above, investigators are trying hard to account for the gap between public enthusiasm for transplantation as an idea and reticence to actually donate when the signature is required. While much of this research focuses on surveys to determine public attitudes toward donation, Scandinavian social scientist Margareta Sanner has explored these questions by asking about people's attitudes toward *receiving* transplanted organs. The qualitative results of her research reveal fascinating recurring tropes that demonstrate the stickiness of long-held attitudes about the body and the fantasy of its inviolability. Much of the respondents couched their reticence in terms of disgust, especially centered on images where boundaries are transgressed. Respondents said things like, "To get a transplant would be felt as having another person's dirty underwear on" and "Disgusting to have a dirty rotten thing from a deceased."[25] Both of these quotations express a sense of violation, of the transplanted organ as a "dirty" thing that can taint its host through intimate contact. Some went further, imagining the act of transplantation as being akin to cannibalism: "No, I would never accept an organ from a human. I'm no cannibal" and "You don't eat people, but you eat pigs so it would be better to have an animal organ."[26] The terms by which participants express these fears mirror the most common elements of horror films: rotting or decomposition, intimate violation, contamination, and cannibalism.

In particular, these anxieties reveal the slippery interplay so effectively explored in phenomenology between the body that you have and the body that you are. These theorists remind us that a secure split between mind and body is rarely a lived reality. Margrit Shildrick's work on heart transplantation emphasizes the multiple layers of the embodied self:

> In short, [patients] are implicitly encouraged to see the process as one of a *medically* complex transfer, but without implications for what constitutes their self-identity. The ontology, however, is quite different: the other is both integrated within—and indeed essential to—the life of the self, while remaining irreducible to that self. The embodied self is, then, inevitably transformed, not perhaps in any externally dramatic way, but more clearly in the modes by which recipients reflect on their own being.[27]

In contrast to a persistent fantasy of individual autonomy, Shildrick's phrasing of "the other that is both essential and irreducible to the self" offers a powerful theoretical expression of a problem that recurs in both patient and horror stories. In this way, transplant narratives broadly, but transplant horror narratives most emblematically, demonstrate how practices that dismantle the belief in secure corporeal boundaries cause a crisis in one's sense of self.

Something Persists in the Flesh

The archetypical transplant horror narrative centers on this very question: What happens when cadaver tissue is incorporated into a living patient? Does something of the deceased follow its flesh into the new body? This question animates stories about transplantation from the nineteenth through the twenty-first century. Second to worries about transplanted hearts (explored in Chapter 5) and faces, hands seem to serve as a special limit case in our thinking about this relationship between the self and the transmigrated other. Arthur Train's 1907 story, "Mortmain," plays with a mystery plot centered on the transplanted "dead hands" of its title pun.[28] With a remarkably similar plot, Maurice Renard's *Les Mains d'Orlac* (1920) gets credit as the most influential of this breed, inspiring four feature films throughout the twentieth century: Robert Wiene's *Orlacs Hände* (1924), Karl Freund's *Mad Love* (1935), Edmond T. Gréville's *The Hands of Orlac* (1961), and Karl Arnold's *Hands of a Stranger* (1962). Renard's novel tells the story of Stephen Orlac, a piano virtuoso who is injured in a train accident and comes to believe that his transplanted hands carry the criminal identity of their donor. He confesses to his wife, "It seemed to me their flesh was contaminating my own, and that my blood was drawing from them a taste for murder."[29] Over the course of 300 pages, Renard takes his reader through a series of bizarre plotlines, including spiritualism, a criminal cult, and a multi-million dollar inheritance.

While the details of the conspiracy are too intricate to rehearse here, Renard makes a few surprising narrative choices that further our examination of the relationship between self and transplanted other. For example, both Train's short story "Mortmain" and Renard's *Orlac* rely importantly on the emerging science of fingerprinting to move forward their mysteries. In both stories, the protagonists are made vulnerable to prosecution because their newly acquired fingerprints are found at the scene of a crime. With its roots in eugenic theories of reading the "truth" of character upon the surface of the body, fingerprinting touches on questions of both individuality and criminality. In *Orlac*, the detectives on the case express complete confidence in fingerprints as incontrovertible evidence of individual identity. The chief inspector goes so far as to have memorized the prints of an executed criminal and insists, "I'd stake my life on" the recognition of those prints upon the murder weapon. While the signifier of the fingerprints themselves is unchanged, the signified of a unique, personal identity is multiply detached. We learn ultimately that Orlac's transplanted hands are not even those of the criminal named Vasseur, but that Vasseur was also a victim of criminal conspiracy. The exposure of this mistaken identity comes to a head in the final line of the novel, in which the detective reassures Orlac, "Your hands are undefiled" (301). In this concluding moment, Renard preserves the novel's belief in the transmigration of self through the transplanted flesh; after all, if the post-transplant hands were simply "your hands," it would not matter if the donor were criminal or upstanding.

By calling into question the security of fingerprints as a mark of identity, these stories challenge the inalienable tie between body and self. We might imagine a safe retreat to mind/body dualism as a solution to this problem, a fantasy in which the fragmented physical body does not challenge one's mental sense of self. But symbolism of fingerprinting in the stories argues that these marks of unique identity are themselves transferable. For these characters, the psychic transformation is not simply coming to grips with a body that carries multiple signifiers of identity, but with the influence of the body upon the mind. We cannot, then, simply believe that the disrupted body is safely distinct from the mind and therefore the self.

Renard makes interesting stylistic choices to dramatize this interior crisis. In his narrative structure, Renard places Mrs. Rosine Orlac as the center of consciousness in the novel, making it possible to withhold for over 250 pages the crucial fact that Stephen's hands are not simply injured and uncooperative, but secretly transplanted from an executed criminal. While Stephen's wife Rosine (and therefore the reader) attributes the robberies and murders surrounding the couple to the acts of a supernatural cult, Stephen has imagined himself as the culprit, contaminated "as two drops of ink, thrown into a glass of water, stain the whole glass!" (256).

This form of narrative withholding and exposition deviates importantly from film adaptations of the novel, which tend to dramatize the protagonist's sense of alienation from his new hands through camerawork that suggests detachment. The novel, in contrast, withholds this moment of self-discovery; Orlac only later gives voice to a creeping sense of the alienation he has experienced for months of narrative time. In his article-length study of the book and the films it inspired, Ian Olney describes the iconic moment of self-discovery in the films: "Many of the later films inspired by Renard's novel emphasize the fragmentary nature of the pianist's post-operative existence and the newfound autonomy of his hands by showing the renegade limbs almost exclusively in close-up, divorced from the rest of his body through an act of selective framing" (299). In this way, the filmmakers turn to visual metaphors that externalize the changes that Renard describes in the novel through internal metaphors of contamination—"my blood was drawing from [the hands] a taste for murder!" (264). Both of these figurative strategies illustrate the complexities of representing a complex psychic sense of bodily disintegration.

Postoperative transplant patients evince a similar complexity in describing their experience of a fragmented self. Much like Stephen Orlac, it is typical for postoperative patients to report personality changes and newly acquired traits from their donor organ. Such beliefs are common in the literature surrounding transplantation. In one prototypical example, a middle-aged heart recipient credits his 17-year-old donor for inspiring his new preoccupation with loud music, a good stereo, and a different car. Another patient from the same study said that he was calmer, that the donor's "feelings have been passed on to me now."[30] In an article published in the *Journal of Near-Death Studies*, the authors argue that personality changes among heart transplant recipients—including taste in food, music, art and sexual, recreational, and career preferences—both existed and could not be sufficiently explained by stress, drugs, or coincidence.[31] In the article, Pearsall et al. argue for the possibility of cellular or systemic memory as an explanation for these new facets of personality—a function not wholly unlike what authors like Renard and Train imagined.

These hybrid conceptions of personal identity emerge in patients' attempts to represent their new experience—both before and after operations. Consistently, preoperative patients report worries about the changes they will experience through the transplanted organ. Many take comfort in the "spare parts" analogy proffered by health professionals: "But then I thought that it's not going to change me because it's like a water pump in a car; if your car breaks down and the water pump or fuel pump breaks down you just replace it and that's basically what your heart is doing. So it's pumping the blood and oxygen 'round your system, so, I thought, well, it doesn't change your car so it's not going to change me."[32] This mechanistic view of the body recurs throughout both medical and popular coverage of organ exchange. While it may offer comfort to recipients, this view also expresses an important and persistent anxiety among potential donors—their loss of humanity and vulnerability to exploitation.

Early legal approaches to transplantation centered on alleviating anxieties about an increasingly mechanistic view of the body. Then-Congressman Al Gore, in advocating for legal bans on the selling of organs, told reporters in 1983, "We must not allow technology to dehumanize people so that we erode the distinction between things and people. People should not be regarded as things to be bought and sold like parts of an automobile. If this were allowed, it would seriously undermine the values of our society."[33] Where individuals—both patients and medical professionals—seek comfort in a mechanistic view of the body, one which denies lingering beliefs in the persistence of identity in the flesh, others see in this concept a troubling dehumanization, leading inevitably to commercial exchange.

For individual patients, the "spare parts" metaphor offers a conceptual path by which to reconcile the new organ. But for recipients, lived, postoperative realities challenge this fantasy of total incorporation.

Again, like the undead threat that recurs despite seeming closure in the horror narrative, the need for constant vigilance against rejection belies an uncomplicated "happy ending" through transplantation. As Margrit Shildrick describes the phenomenon, "however much a recipient may wish to assert that the graft is now her own, the reality is that her body now hosts alien DNA that will never lose the specificity of its otherness, and that will be the proximate cause of an unremitting bodily response to reject the transplant organ."[34] For the critically ill patient, this sense of alienation from the embodied self has likely begun before transplant. Catherine Waldby reminds us, "People diagnosed with end-stage disease awaiting organ transplant evince a dramatic change in their relationship with their visceral interior. This space becomes highly invested, sensitized, and fragmented."[35] This break between the body and the self, then, is not wholly the result of transplantation; illness itself can prompt a reconsideration of fantasies of the integrated, inviolable self. Organ rejection, then, becomes a multifaceted phenomenon, as the patient first turns from their own ill body and then the "healing" body constantly rejects the transplanted organ.

"Rejection" takes on another layer of complexity in attempts to tease out the distinction between physiological and psychological rejection. In two paradigmatic cases, one involving hand transplant and the other of the first "successful" penis transplant, doctors credit psychological rejection with the ultimate failure of the procedures. The 2006 case of a penis transplant in Guangzhou, China, is especially interesting because the psychological rejection in question is largely reported to come from the recipient's wife. Although the operation was a surgical success, the donor tissue was removed 14 days later. The surgeon in the case reported: "Because of a severe psychological problem of the recipient and his wife, the transplanted penis regretfully had to be cut off."[36] The involvement of the patient's wife in the outcome of the case demonstrates a complicated sense of interdependence; instead of simply a dyad of self/other (where the other is the organ donor), the figures in this case existed in a triad. In this instance, the intimate relation of the wife to her husband's penis meant that her psychological "rejection" of the organ became medically relevant to the course of action.

In another highly publicized case of rejection, the case of Clint Hallam is particularly interesting when placed in conversation with *The Hands of Orlac* and "Mortmain." Credited as the first successful hand transplant in the fall of 1998, coverage of Hallam's operation—and its eventual reversal—includes intersecting elements of criminality, medical experimentation, and horror tropes of transgression. At the time of the procedure, medical controversy erupted over ethical concerns about an operation that would confer mainly aesthetic benefits while carrying severe side effects from the anti-rejection drugs.[37] The ambitious quest to be "first" among the French medical team struck familiar cords of the mad scientist for some onlookers. The nature of the operation itself exacerbated this perception; according to one reporter, "It sounds like something right out of a campy, late-night horror film: eager doctors working to attach the hand of a cadaver to a living person."[38] Hallam, himself, was sensitive to this perception; in the early days following his surgery, he saw himself performing a public service, dispensing with ethical questions troubling transplantation. In an interview with the *New York Times* in 1999, Hallam says, "I still have people that say to me, How do you feel about having the hand of a dead man? And my immediate answer is, Great, because he's very much alive. I made myself the promise that when I had my new hand, it wouldn't just be for Clint, but for everyone. To show people that the hand is not macabre, the hand is not Frankenstein-ish."[39] In these comments, offered one year post-surgery, Hallam falls into the "continuation of life" camp, seeming to celebrate the idea that his donor lives on, that "he's very much alive." By 2001, however, Hallam's language changes substantially; he tells the BBC that "it was like a dead man's hand with no feeling in it" and that his "body and mind had said 'enough is enough.'"[40] This transition from "very much alive" to "a dead man's hand" captures Hallam's increasing sense of disappointment and self-alienation after his surgery. Hallam ultimately had to campaign for over a year to have his hand amputated. In a bizarre twist celebrated by theoreticians everywhere, the surgeons initially refused his request because under French law the body is "inviolable."[41] The removal of Hallam's transplanted hand was particularly public because it also resurrected a series of twists and turns in the story, including Hallam's misrepresentation of the cause of his injury (actually sustained during a prison stay for fraud) and charges that he had stolen money from an organ donation charity. Surgeons argue that Hallam's admittedly erratic use of his anti-rejection medication and lack of exercise led to increasingly limited function in the hand—in other words, they credit psychological, not physiological failure in Hallam's case.

While the specter of prison and a growing enmity between Hallam and his physicians (as captured in the popular press) creates exceptional elements in this instance, both Hallam's case and the failed first penis transplant suggest that medical progress may be hitting limits that are conceptual rather than technological in nature. As the surgical ground of transplantation moves from the interior to the exterior of the body—faces, hands, and penises—medical professionals will have to more seriously confront the deep-seated ideological barriers people hold. As Jean-Michel Dubernard—the French surgeon who performed the world's first face transplant—cautions, "Psychological consequences of hand and face allografts show that it is not so easy to use and see permanently a dead person's hands, nor is it easy to look in a mirror to see a dead person's face."[42] These images, exactly, have been recurring in horror narratives of transplantation for over a century. In "Mortmain," Arthur Train includes an iconic scene of alienation from self as the protagonist contemplates his transplanted limb:

> The hand itself served his purposes well enough, but unmistakably it was not his own. He never laid the two together—never let his eyes fall upon the vicarious fingers if he could avoid it, for inevitably a sickening sensation of repulsion followed. His own fingers were long and tapering, the nails fine with pronounced 'crowns,' the back of his hand slender and smooth; the new one was broader and hairy, the fingers shorter and square at the ends, the nails thick and dull with no 'crowns,' and the veins blue and prominent. There were too many pores! (44–45)

From fingerprints to nails, veins, and even pores, the external features of the body are often cited as signs of internal truths of character. This belief—which has animated a range of systems including fingerprinting, phrenology, physiognomy, and racism—has deep roots in Western culture. The surgeon Dubernard's notion that it is not so easy to "see" a dead person's hands or "look" at a dead person's face in the mirror emphasizes the visual elements of identification, tying into film theorists' work on the scopic regime in modern life. Our ways of looking, especially in moments that have been shaken out of the norm by an act as radical as transplantation, are conditioned by a set of visual expectations created by technology—film, photography, television, and computers.

The sight of one's transplantation, then, becomes mediated in two ways: first, by a belief that the external body will reveal a truth of the self, and second, by a tradition in horror films in which the first vision of the transplanted part dramatizes an almost supernatural alienation from self (recall the iconic shots of isolated hands from the film versions of *Orlac*).

Mortmain's sense of horror at "the dead-alive thing at his wrist" is rooted not only in a conflict between self and other, but also in the instability resulting from a mingling of social categories.[43] The repeated reference to "crowns" in the above quote—Mortmain's original hand has them, the transplanted one does not—reveals the perceived barriers of social class that threatens the incorporation of the new tissue. In a prescient vision of the ways that social economy will play out in black market organ transplantation, Arthur Train writes, "Surely some one will be found who can be induced for a proper consideration to assist in an operation that will restore to usefulness so distinguished a member of society" (32). In this stark expression—the wealthy have value to society, the poor are useful in their support of the wealthy—Train captures the potential for exploitation in organ exchange. In addition to this literal exploitation, the story describes a conceptual break disallowing the integration of rich and poor. Mortmain cannot assimilate the swarthy hand of the other because he believes in an essential, embodied difference according to class. As Susan Lederer argues in her discussion of the story, "It is wealth that enables Mortmain to purchase the hand, … but class difference makes it impossible for the offending tissue to be incorporated into the aristocratic body" (77). This enactment of literal mingling across classes and the disastrous consequences that arise captures the complicated political messages carried in horror films. As a first step, these stories of transgression suggest that social boundaries are not as secure as we might imagine. Horror authors and filmmakers split between, on the one hand, conservative narratives in which these boundaries are ultimately reinscribed and, on the other, progressive visions in which an anxious period of fluidity creates a path for change at a more profound level. In both "Mortmain" and *Orlac*, the stories conclude with a reassuring return to order—Mortmain's horrifying story has all been a dream and his inherited fortune is restored; Orlac's hands are transplanted, but "undefiled."

Ambiguity and transgression are "the stuff" of horror narratives, according to Stephen Prince, editor of *The Horror Film*. As discussed through this chapter, ambiguity can center in a sense of alienation between self and other, but also dramatizes a troubling of social categories. For Train and Renard, these social categories are centered in class boundaries. Robin Cook's *Coma* and Mary Shelley's *Frankenstein*, by contrast, focus on gender. Both of these works transparently describe troubling excesses in pursuit of medical progress, but they also tie the mingling of body parts to violations of patriarchal norms.

Coma opens with a scene in which Nancy Greenly enters the hospital for a gynecological operation—a routine D&C. Throughout the scene, Cook emphasizes Greenly's vulnerability in specifically gendered terms. In the very first paragraph, Greenly expresses feeling embarrassed and fearful, afraid of both the "cruel detached environment of the hospital" and of the uncontrolled bleeding that prompted her to seek medical attention (1). In several references to her menstrual blood, Cook emphasizes the "continued bleeding [that] made her feel messy, unattractive, out of control" (3). In choosing this highly gendered medical condition as the opening scene of the novel, Cook emphasizes womanhood as a porous, vulnerable, fearful, and uncontrollable state. These characteristics of womanhood are then mapped onto the social and professional context of the novel, in which the very presence of a female physician is challenging. When his medical student heroine, Susan, enters the scene, we have been conditioned to understand her presence within the medical field as a threat to an established social order. As a transgressor of the status quo, Susan is uniquely positioned to see abuses in the system, but she is also uniquely subject to fear, intimidation, and disorder—and not just due to the sinister horror plotline.

Mary Shelley's *Frankenstein* similarly uses patriarchal norms to underscore the violation represented by the doctor's transgression. The sideplot of Elizabeth and Victor Frankenstein's marriage sets up a conflict between procreation (standing for natural, civic order) and scientific creation (seen as violation). In the novel, the dying wish of Frankenstein's mother is to see the young couple married: "My children, ... my firmest hopes of future happiness were placed on the prospect of your union. ... Elizabeth, my love, you must supply my place to your younger cousins" (39). In these lines, marriage, motherhood, and procreation have themselves a kind of excess—Elizabeth is to both marry the older son and serve as surrogate mother to the younger siblings—but it's an excess that the novel understands as capacious and life-affirming, not sepulchral and violent.

James Whale's 1931 film version of *Frankenstein* extends the role of the wedding as a suspenseful driver of plot: Will the ceremony happen or not?[44] The climax of the film involves the monster's interruption of wedding preparations in a demonstration of the incommensurate nature of the dueling models of creation. The final scene of the film offers an unequivocal (if bizarre) win for the side of procreation. We see a collection of maids come giggling down the hallway, approaching the room where Frankenstein lies recuperating in bed with Elizabeth at his side. As the maids give the ancestral wine to Frankenstein's overbearing father, he jovially insists: "My son doesn't need this! ... Here's to a son of the House of Frankenstein!" Roll credits. This closing argument for continuation of life through procreation and heredity celebrates the normative frame of heterosexual marriage in contrast to the monstrous excesses of science.

Experimental Medicine and Mad Doctors

The archetypical figure of the mad doctor embodies long-standing popular ambivalence about attempts to use technology as a means of prolonging or creating life. In examining the question "Why Organ Transplant Programs Do Not Succeed," literary critic Leslie Fiedler turns to tales of terror centered on villainous doctors.[45] Fiedler opens his essay with the familiar problem that people express enthusiastic support of organ donation in surveys, but then fail to donate their own organs or those of their loved ones. For Fiedler, this seeming contradiction lies between our conscious celebration of medical progress and our unconscious anxieties about a "seemingly benign surgery" that violates foundational categories. Citing classic horror stories like *Frankenstein*, *Dr. Jekyll and Mr. Hyde*, *The Island of Dr. Moreau*, and *Dracula*, Fiedler argues that these unconscious anxieties become expressed in cultural myths, most commonly embodied by the mad doctor. He writes:

> At the core, the archetypal doctor is portrayed as an enemy (all the more dangerous because of his good intention) of those traditional beliefs that long enabled us to live at peace with our fragile bodies and our sense of their inescapable mortality. ... That archetypal scenario will, of course, continue to be imagined and reimagined for as long as humanity continues to fear death, calls on science to forestall it, and resents it for doing so. (64)

In this closing sentence, Fiedler offers another formulation of the complex push and pull that is so inevitable in public acceptance of experimental medicine. He correctly points out that while fear of death will drive public desires for progress in medical technology, this "progress" does not come without acknowledged costs. As discussed below, sometimes these costs will come in the form of side effects, limited efficacy, or distasteful practices. More profound, perhaps, is the cost to our collective ability to manage the inescapable reality of mortality.

Horror writers understand the compelling undertow produced by reminders of reality. These writers are often excited to position their outlandish plots as an extension of reality, anchoring their work in existing public anxieties about real medical excesses. Writing at the beginning of the twentieth century, Maurice Renard, for example, includes in his novels explicit references to public figures in experimental medicine. A footnote in *Dr. Lerne* cites Giuseppe Boronio's 1803 experiments with skin grafting in sheep as a predecessor for the fantastical xenografting pursued by the titular villain. In the same volume, Renard references real attempts to prolong life in severed heads, claiming that Dr. Lerne "know[s], thanks to Brown-Séquard, that the head of a dog injected with oxygenated blood had survived severance for a quarter of an hour."[46] It makes sense that fiction writers would be attracted to Charles Édouard Brown Séquard—he's one of the most sensational figures in the history of transplant medicine. His experiments at the boundary of life and death included attempts to prolong life in the heads of guillotined criminals and experiments using transfusions of his own blood. With figures like Brown Séquard splashing into public notice, it's not surprising that horrific representations of the mad doctor persist in Western culture.

As our most enduring story of the mad doctor, *Frankenstein* emblematizes the slippage between fact and fiction in transplant horror stories. Shelley's novel, published in 1818, spoke to decades of public worry over cadaver dissection and developments in surgical education. A century later, the makeup artist for James Whale's film version of the novel looked to these same surgical practices to inform his vision of this iconic monster. Jack Pierce describes creating the look of Frankenstein's monster through study of "every operation that would be necessary to create such a body from 'spare parts.'"[47] He vividly connects conceiving of the distinctive head shape of the monster to his quest for medical realism:

> There are six ways a surgeon can cut the skull in order to take out or put in a brain. I figured that Frankenstein, who was a scientist but no practical surgeon, would take the simplest surgical way. He would cut the top of the skull of straight across like a potlid, hinge it, pop the brain in, then clamp it on tight. That is the reason I decided to make the monster's head square and flat like a shoe box and dig that big scar across his forehead with the clamps holding it together.[48]

This description, consistent with the horror genre more broadly, emphasizes an embodied materiality central to storytelling. In discussing his preparation, Pierce's speech is peppered with active verbs that drive home the physical nature of his work; he cuts, digs, pops, clamps, and hinges. The play between excess and reality forms an animating tension in horror narratives, where the most effective stories are typically grounded in a "reality effect" even when the plotlines are at their most outlandish.

The medical thriller, in particular, pursues a reality effect as a central narrative technique. Mass market editions of *Coma*, including those reissued decades later, feature Robin Cook wearing his doctor's white coat,[49] announcing to readers his medical expertise. As a constituent feature of the subgenre, the medical thriller establishes a kind of realism through its use of technical language and (mostly) correct medical information. Within the novel, Cook goes so far as to include a scene in which his protagonist copies relevant medical charts but has to write "… (illegible phrase)" when she fails to decipher the handwriting. While Cook plays on jokes about doctors and their atrocious handwriting, this scene is important because it re-presents several pages of medical jargon that are as indecipherable to the average reader as the occasional scribbled phrase is to Susan (a medical student). Cook employs a reverse dramatic irony in which his character understands something that his reader will not. The work of the scene, then, lies not in what readers comprehend in the content of the chart (e.g., some clue that will move the plot forward). Instead, its meaning lies in a reality effect achieved by the form of the chart as an insular way in which doctors communicate with each other. This feeling of being outside the specialized circle of medical authority is the root of both dependence upon and alienation from doctors for the lay public. The mad doctor trope represents transgressions beyond the outer limits of this authority, but the same exclusive knowledge and skillset that make doctors trusted and valued can breed a suspicious anxiety, creating fertile imaginative territory for frightening tales of doctors who abuse their power.

In his film, James Whale captures public fears over medical transgressions with Dr. Frankenstein's claim, "That body is not dead. I created it. I made it with my own hands from the bodies I took from graves, from the gallows, from anywhere." These lines feature boundary crossing between life and death, technology and natural procreation, and criminality and morality. They form the template for representations of mad doctors because they capture the centuries-old anxieties that I explore in Chapter 2, anxieties prompted by the shift away from ecclesiastical to medical authority over life, health, and death. As an advanced surgical technique, especially when involving cadaver organs, transplantation is a special case within an already fraught field. How appropriate, then, that transplantation recurs as the ground upon which the thriller unfolds—in films like *Coma*, *Muggers*, *Dirty Pretty Things*, *The Donor*, *The Island*, *The Eye*, *21 Grams*, and *Repo Men*.[50] While the specifics vary in each of these films, they all reflect the twin dynamics of transgression and emphasis on the body that link discussions of horror and transplantation.

One emblematic example, *The Brain That Wouldn't Die* (1962), tells the story of Dr. Bill Cortner and his experimental attempts to preserve and transplant human limbs.[51] After a catastrophic car accident escalates his work, he successfully preserves his injured girlfriend's head in a tray of serum and then spends the remainder of the movie searching for a body for transplantation. In a strikingly explicit fashion, the opening scenes of the movie stage a debate about medical experimentation only slightly exaggerated from what one might find in Medical Ethics 101. Dr. Cortner makes the case for progress, insisting, "Today, nothing's hopeless," and asking, "Is it a crime for science to jump ahead by years?" The conservative side of the debate is represented by Cortner's father, also a surgeon, who shuts down his son's argument by warning: "the line between scientific genius and obsessive fanaticism is thin." As the increasingly insane and violent disembodied head of his girlfriend makes clear, Dr. Cortner has crossed that line into the fanatic territory of the mad doctor.

In the same way that the mingling of parts within a physical body (as in transplantation) can mirror public anxieties about boundary crossing in the social body, narratives that question medical progress can reflect popular backlash against social progress as well. In *The Brain That Wouldn't Die*, the film's essentially cautious message about medical experimentation echoes some of the fears described by Robin Cook in *Coma* about changing roles for women. In a piece of on-the-nose scripting, the movie dramatizes Dr. Cortner's search for a body for transplantation as a tour through the many local spaces that objectify women's bodies. This collection of scenes begins with Dr. Cortner cruising around town in his convertible, smooth jazz playing, checking out women walking along the street. This literal expression of the male gaze escalates as he's asked to judge a "Miss Body Beautiful" contest, then visits a burlesque club, and finally visits a woman who works as a "figure model" and who poses in a bikini for a crowd of male amateur photographers in her apartment. In each of these scenes, the camerawork follows Cortner's perspective, inviting viewers to participate in the assessment of each new possible "donor." By crowding the setting with spaces where women are already objectified for masculine pleasure, the film draws a direct parallel between a dehumanizing clinical approach in medicine and the lax morals evident in the changing society of the early 1960s. On the one hand, the location of this sexually exploitive behavior in the person of the film's villain could suggest a critique of patriarchy. When coupled, however, with the anti-experimental argument of the film in its medical plotline, the abiding concern seems to be with the costs of "progress."

Cortner's fictional experiments with preserving life in severed limbs bring us back to Dr. Brown Séquard and his eccentric study of heads delivered from the guillotine. Horror narratives, especially ones rooted in reality, serve a puncturing effect, exposing the fantasy of uncomplicated medical progress narratives. Cutting-edge science necessarily involves crossing boundaries. Horror narratives, in turn, shine a light on these transgressions, bringing to notice practices that most would find at least distasteful and at worst immoral. The writer and director of *The Brain That Wouldn't Die*, after all, are not the first to imagine the possibilities of head transplantation.[52] The history of successful surgical techniques is peppered with "mad" scientists like Brown Séquard. Paging through histories of organ transplantation,[53] one is likely to find images like those in a horror film—of two-headed dogs or monkeys with transplanted heads. Charles Guthrie and Alexis Carrol's pioneering work in anastomosis (stitching together blood vessels) during the early twentieth century included animal experimentation, most famously when Guthrie successfully grafted one dog's head onto the neck of another on May 21, 1908. Russian surgeon Vladimir Demikhov extended the successes of this operation in the 1950s, developing techniques that could prolong the process enough to preserve cerebral function in the transplanted heads—including a dog that nipped at the ear of its new host. As with all advances in transplantation during this era, immune rejection limited its long-term success, but for a few days, Demikhov proved the technical possibility of this radical surgery.

In the decades since Demikhov's experimentation with dogs, others have made headlines for additional forays into this scientific frontier. In 2015, Italian neurosurgeon Sergio Canavero announced his intention to perform the first human head transplantation, and in 2016, he announced that he had found a volunteer patient: a Russian computer programmer who suffers from Werdnig-Hoffman disease, a disorder that kills muscle and nerve cells. Media coverage of the proposed procedure draws on familiar tropes of horror. A *CBS News* article begins: "While severing someone's head and attaching it to another person's body sounds like something straight out of a science fiction or horror movie...."[54] The *Daily Mail* takes a bolder stance, announcing: "The controversial neurosurgeon who wants to carry out the first human head transplant has outlined plans to conduct 'Frankenstein' experiments to reanimate human corpses to test his technique."[55] In a similar vein, *Time* opted for a combination of horror and puns in their 2015 coverage of Chinese surgeon Xiaoping Ren and his roughly 1000 successful transplantations of mice heads; the headline reads, "This Groundbreaking 'Frankenstein' Surgery Will Literally Make Your Head Spin."[56] These headlines are typical of the media coverage that surrounds experimental transplant surgery. The stories themselves follow a common formula: a lead paragraph that evokes "the stuff of a horror film"; an outline of the science behind the procedure and the fearful/hopeful speculation that "it just might work"; followed by a bucket of cold water thrown by a medical ethicist or colleague in the field, who typically casts the experimental surgeon in the role of the ambitious, headline-grabbing mad scientist. In this coverage, calls to horror narratives serve as footholds for public attempts to understand experimental medicine within the frame of the familiar. These stories make explicit connections to horrifying fictional precedents as a way of acknowledging and perhaps exorcising popular anxieties. Rather than getting mired down in alienating technical descriptions, coding such procedures as "Frankenstein experiments" offers a governing frame within which to marvel, scoff at, or dismiss the proposal.

In the USA, Dr. Robert White, a now-retired Cleveland neurosurgeon, is perhaps most familiar with the demands of balancing technical possibility with conceptual objections. In the 1960s and 1970s, White led a series of experiments with rhesus monkeys, including a successful head transplant from one monkey onto the decapitated body of another. In interviews conducted since his published work in the July 1971 issue of *Surgery*, White tends to linger on the conceptual problems associated with the procedure. As chronicled in *Stiff: The Curious Lives of Human Cadavers*, White and Mary Roach discuss the barriers to human head transplantation. White argues that while his experiments proved such an operation would be technically possible, the obstacles to its execution are largely about attitude and practicality. He tells Roach, "You're dealing with a question that is totally revolutionary. People can't make up their minds whether it's a total body transplant or a head transplant, a brain or even a soul transplant" (215). In this discussion, White focuses on our collective inability to sort out the ideological stakes of the operation. White, for his part, calls the surgery a whole-body transplant, telling *Current Science*, "The organ that represents you and me is the brain. … The body is nothing more than a resource to keep the brain alive—a power pack."[57] Although the surgical techniques are new, questions like the ones White asks are long-standing. We could expand the list to include: Is there a soul and where does it reside? What is the relationship between the self and the body? Would the transplant create a new person? Are the mind and body distinct or inseparably enmeshed? Is there a self beyond the brain? The technical ability to sew vessels together does not empty out the conceptual weight of these questions; in some ways, the technical ability to complete the operation makes them even more important. Horror and science fiction narratives understand that the ethical and conceptual debates surrounding experimental medicine only take on real urgency when conducted in the space of technical possibility. They construct a world in which imagined techniques become realized and ask us to examine what that world could look like in its most exaggerated form. These stories push the limit of technical possibility beyond its current frame to explore the complicated contours of these questions with an added element of crisis.

The barriers to head transplantation, though, are not simply conceptual. Important technical barriers exist, forcing us to remember material as well as abstract objections to a proposed operation. One key obstacle on the path to human head transplantation is the constraints on our ability to restore severed spinal nerves. Any recipient of the operation would be quadriplegic, limiting its applicable reach. On the other hand, a quadriplegic person's organs tend to fail more quickly, suggesting an already paralyzed individual might be the most enthusiastic early candidate for such a radical procedure. As Mary Roach writes, however, since insurance companies are unlikely to cover the operation, it is hard to imagine the path by which such a surgery would be funded. Beyond a headline-grabbing experimental case like the kind proposed by Dr. Canavero, the clinical reach of such surgery seems highly limited. White and Roach speculate about a billionaire quadriplegic who had approached White in the 1970s. But she goes on to ask, "Is it sensible to use medical resources to keep terminally ill and extravagantly wealthy people alive? Shouldn't we, as a culture, encourage a saner, more accepting attitude toward death?" (215–216). Roach's questions raise two essential points: First, she reminds us that medical progress exists in a frame of funding, investment that is often directed according to concerns that are (properly and improperly) unrelated to technical feasibility, and second, she puts pressure on the notion of "progress" itself, especially as it lies in an unquestioned goal of prolonging life.

Many scholars of organ transplantation, especially those in medical anthropology, ultimately find themselves with exactly these questions about public attitudes toward death, especially when examining practices at the expanding frontiers of the field. We find that the outer edges of transplantation are a moving limit, especially in practices including: commercial or black market organ exchange; extending eligibility requirements to include older and sicker recipients; and new surgical techniques (like multi-organ operations or hand, face, or penis transplants). This shifting terrain, in which definitions and possibilities are changing year to year, is the very fertile ground upon which horror narratives take place. Horror narratives, though, push beyond the limits of the moment (or the near future) to enact the negative effects of going too far. By staging the transgression of boundaries, horror narratives can work to reinscribe cultural values. Rather than exclusively preying on public fears about actual medical excess, horror narratives use a series of generic conventions to exaggerate the consequences of these excesses, telling its audience that while limits may be expanding, they still should and do exist. In *The Brain That Wouldn't Die*, for example, the movie dramatizes the horrifying effects of medical experimentation: The screen is populated with the failed and monstrous results of previous experiments, culminating in the severed head in a pan, begging to be put to death. Ultimately, through a supernatural telepathy connecting her to a locked-away monster, the severed head ends up causing her own death and the death of the mad scientist. With these deaths, the film signals the conceptual impossibility of such radical experimentation. Its conservative message prompts us to focus on the negative consequences of so-called progress.

In his book *Transplant: From Myth to Reality*, Nicholas L. Tilney, M.D. offers his firsthand account of a career spent participating in rapid advances in organ transplantation. In one particularly vivid section, Tilney describes the horrors he witnessed in the early days of transplantation. Before the advent of cyclosporine, transplant recipients—now removed from the laboratories of "mad scientists" and into clinical settings—were given steroids as a method of immune suppression. Tilney focuses on the often-gruesome physical effects of this treatment:

> Patients developed moon faces, buffalo humps, and protuberant abdomens. Thin skin bruised and tore easily. I vividly remember firmly shaking the hand of a transplant recipient and inadvertently stripping off a patch of skin with my thumb. Wounds did not heal. Healed incisions broke down. After weeks of unexplained fever, the bland-appearing incisions of some individuals would suddenly open and discharge copious amounts of pus. … Infections, often with unusual and relatively unknown bacteria, fungi, and viruses, were prevalent. Mysterious pneumonias developed, impervious to the most powerful antibiotics. (129)

In each phrase in this description, Tilney's imagery intersects with the tropes of horror narratives. With swollen faces, humps, and "protuberant abdomens," patients transform like horror-film monsters. The security attached to the skin as a protective barrier is punctured as it can now be "inadvertently" stripped away or discharge "sudden" amounts of pus. Patients are radically vulnerable to external threats, often invisible and always around, in the form of bacteria, fungi, and viruses. And these infections do not respond to our most powerful antibiotic arsenal. These are the elements of a horror film. Tilney's description offers a shuddering reflection of this time in transplantation; he describes himself and his colleagues as "increasingly concerned, frightened, and horrified by the effects of the treatment" (128).

While the image of the "mad" scientist tinkering with severed limbs or monkeys dramatizes a shadow side to medical advancement, it is important to remember that the history of treatment protocols, especially for fatal conditions, will often include stories of secondary diseases, negative side effects, and very slight prolongation of life. It is worth recalling from the introduction that Christiaan Barnard's first successful heart transplant patient only lived 18 days after his operation. When success is defined according to very slim margins between prolonging life and death, both medical professionals and the public will recoil against the horrifying elements in these experimental procedures.

The Villainous Hospital

As we have seen throughout this chapter, the horrifying elements of transplantation—as seen in both fictional and real accounts of surgeries—underscore the fact that the limits of medical progress are not just technical, but are conceptual as well. Margrit Shildrick argues in her discussion of face transplantation:

> What is interesting is where we locate the limits of what is currently socially tolerable in terms of reconstructive surgery and what is still beyond the pale. As recent press reports indicate, the reality of facial transplants maintains a high yuk! factor—a potent illustration of the abject rejection of an otherness that is indistinguishable from the self-same—explained in large part because of anxieties about the perceived assault on personal identity.[58]

Shildrick's language here illustrates the almost reflexive and often unexamined impulse to turn away from radical medical experimentation: In this case, the phrase "yuk! factor" stands for complex psychological and ideological concepts of self and other. Horror narratives can help to clarify and express these conceptual limits. Consider, for example, the recurrence of the thriller trope in which the transplantation of external limbs—especially hands, eyes, or faces—results in a dramatic (and often criminal) shift in the personality of the recipient. In this familiar formation, our concept of identity as a property of the visible body rises to the top of popular worries. All forms of transplantation are not understood identically, and resistance—in both popular backlash and fictional narratives—to external transplants points to differential understanding of the importance of specific organs as a property of the soul or personal identity. Hearts, then, matter more than kidneys, faces and hands more than livers.

The fact that we treat these surgeries with different amounts of recoil is simply evidence of the fact that the body and its parts carry ideological significance beyond mere biological function. Body parts are enmeshed in a network of meaning, and medical progress must grapple with these conceptual limits. Horror narratives offer an intervention into the sober conduct of medical ethics debates; they emphasize "the yuk! factor" and probe deeper to expose the often-implicit ideas that inform the terms of these debates.

While the trope of the "mad doctor" has never completely fallen away, another related fear has joined the conversation: public distrust in institutions. While the mad doctor has always been seen as a rogue figure made possible by the dehumanizing excesses of the medical field, an increasingly popular vision of medicine as a faceless and corrupt enterprise has produced a new kind of villain. Instead of the highly individual Dr. Frankenstein, we have the impersonal, profit-driven, and anonymous figure of the medical establishment. As medical research solved many of the technical problems of transplant surgery, even positive media representation of the practice began to shift away from portrayals of iconoclastic, hero surgeons. Instead, newspaper, television, and fictional accounts began to focus on the recipient and donor. Gail Moloney and Iain Walker saw this transformation in their decades-long study of the *West Australian* daily newspaper from 1954 to 1995. They document the turn, in the 1980s, away from transplantation as the exclusive domain of the medical world:

> The transplant was now associated with lay people, in a network of meanings and, significantly, values about families and relationships. … An organ transplant involved both a donor and a recipient, and was now understood as a "gift of life"—a gift from one human being to another. … Now it was the donor who gave "life," not the transplant surgeon. (Moloney and Walker 221)

The sentimental dynamics of the "gift of life" are explored more fully in Chapter 5, but I include this quotation here because it signals a historical shift in the stories told about transplantation. As the figure of the surgeon becomes increasingly invisible, dystopic visions of predatory but impersonal institutions are more and more common.[59] If it is the donor who "gives life," then horror narratives can be less shackled by the life-saving motives of the surgeon. After all, our examples of mad doctors—from fictional Dr. Lerne to Dr. White and his "whole body transplant"—were all driven by a desire to heal and prolong life. Understanding medicine as a depersonalized institution, by contrast, emphasizes the profit-driven motives of the enterprise, supporting public fears about unfairness, corruption, and the exploitation of vulnerable populations.

In his 1986 article "Vile Bodies and Bad Medicine," Pete Boss offers a chilling account of this turn to public understanding of medicine as primarily an institution:

> Through the image of fully institutionalized modern medicine, hospitals, banks of life-support equipment, the inscrutable terminology, the rigid regime and hierarchy, one's own body rendered alien, regulated, labeled, categorized, rearranged, manipulated, scrutinized, and dissected, we experience the powerful and pervasive idea of the subject as defenseless matter becoming integrated into a wider frame of reference in which the institutional and organizational aspects of medicine—denuded of bedside manner—focus their conspiratorial attentions upon it. (20)

I concur with Boss's reading of *Coma*, in which the "dispassionate," technical language and monolithic medical institutions—both in its physical and human architecture—produce a highly impersonal view of medicine. This concept is mirrored in Cook's description of the physical campus of Boston Memorial Hospital—all "obtuse angles," "millions of bricks," and "flat monotonous roofs." The metonymic substitution in which "the hospital" becomes a nexus holding together diverse players, actions, and technologies overwhelms humanizing portraits of surgeons to focus on vulnerable patients.

Exploitive institutions dominate the settings of horror films, most notably within the dystopia subgenre. Consider the 2010 film, *Repo Men*, as an emblematic expression of this form. The movie offers a dark and gritty vision of the future in which artificial organs have become common, but prohibitively expensive, and a violent agency has emerged to repossess the unpaid organs, even at the cost of the lives of the recipients. The movie is brutal and bloody, but its dialogue includes uncanny echoes of contemporary appeals and anxieties about organ donation. In one scene, a sales agent for the artificial organ uses a familiar appeal to sentiment, telling the client, "you owe it to yourself; you owe it to your family." In the same scene, the agent characterizes our current system as horrifying: telling the ill client that before the advent of artificial organs, "nearly 200,000 people on transplant lists waited for someone else to die so that they could live." The warning bell of scarcity rings loudly even in this future setting. Robin Cook echoes this notion that a frightening vision of medical exploitation can emerge from beneficent concern about the consequences of organ shortage. In the prefatory letter to the 25th anniversary edition of *Coma*, Cook writes, "Since I had done some transplant surgery myself, I was particularly concerned about [the lack of organ supply], and it became my dream that an entertaining novel and a subsequent movie could influence public policy to nip the developing problem in the bud." One might, of course, question whether a chilling account of medical abuses is an effective propaganda tool for increasing voluntary donation. But films and movies like these take legitimate worries and use hyperbole to both express those concerns while also checking their intensity.

Two science fiction stories published in the early days of transplantation offer similar visions of predatory practices that emerge from institutionalized visions of both donors and medicine. In Larry Niven's "The Jigsaw Man" (1967), the protagonist is on death row, awaiting execution and organ retrieval.[60] In the surrounding cells are two "organleggers," participants in a black market ring of organ theft. In a modern manifestation of eighteenth-century body snatching, one neighbor is the surgeon and the other is the "snatch man." Niven begins his narrative with an open declaration of dehumanization: "Vh83uOAGn7 was his telephone number and his driving license number and his social security number and the number of his draft card and his medical record. Two of these had been revoked, and the others had ceased to matter, except for his medical record" (67). This idea that citizens have become serial numbers whose value lies in their potential as objects of exchange emphasizes the logic of supply and demand that overshadows transplantation narratives. The logics of dehumanization and manufacturing extend from the recipient to the doctor, as authorized retrieval surgeries are conducted not by humans, but by machines along with a conveyor belt. In an evolution of the horrifying image of supine bodies from *Frankenstein* and *Coma* that opened this chapter, Niven describes a hospital organ bank as a "whole vast room filled up with glass tanks" (77).

Writing against the backdrop of the Vietnam War, Robert Silverberg's "Caught in the Organ Draft" (1972) describes a similar Near Bad Future in which elderly leaders conscript the organs of young men and women to extend their own, more socially valuable lives. The story opens with a prospective draftee looking at an elderly couple and describing the secret of their youthful appearance: "She's had at least three hearts, he's working on his fourth set of lungs, they apply for new kidneys every five years, their brittle bones are reinforced with hundreds of skeletal snips from the arms and legs of hapless younger folk, their dimming sensory apparatus is aided by countless nerve grafts obtained the same way, their ancient arteries are freshly sheathed with slick Teflon."[61] Such a mechanistic description is the hyperbolic extension of the "spare parts" logic that comforts many actual organ recipients. While Silverberg's escalating scale from three hearts to four lungs to hundreds of snips may seem excessive, it's not entirely removed from the reality that many organ recipients will need additional transplants as their organs fail again. Silverberg explicitly casts these crises as a cycle of supply that cannot meet demand: "Nobody escapes. They always clip you, once you qualify. The need for young organs inexorably expands to match the pool of available organpower" (144). In the neologism "organpower," Silverberg drives home the reaches of a new medical economy in which individual autonomy is subverted to a fantasy of infinite extension of life.

Like Robin Cook, both Larry Niven and Robert Silverberg draw from a projected crisis in organ supply as the premise for their dystopic societies. In Silverberg's words: "The problem was this: not enough healthy people were dying of highway accidents, successful suicide attempts, diving board miscalculations, electrocutions, and football injuries; therefore there was a shortage of transplantable organs" (147). In Silverberg's work, the organ draft becomes the compulsory structure that attempts to redress this problem. Niven, similarly, places his work in the context of 1970s public debates over the death penalty. In his story, judicial reform efforts come to a screeching halt in the face of successful transplantation; after all, he asks, "What voter would vote against eternal life? The death penalty was his immortality, and he would vote the death penalty for any crime at all" (79). The dramatic twist revealed at the conclusion of the story is that the protagonist finds himself on death row for the relatively mundane crimes of drunk driving and running stoplights. While Niven and Silverberg draw from the dystopic conventions of their genre, it is important to remember the very real historical antecedents of their imagined societies. Silverberg, of course, is writing in a time in which a military draft engineered by elderly political and economic leaders—notably Robert McNamara, both Secretary of Defense and former President of Ford Motor Company—used assembly-line thinking to deliver young soldiers to a dangerous war. Centuries earlier in Britain, parliamentary leaders used the mechanism of the death penalty to deliver cadavers to medical schools. In both of these stories, the "problems" are perceived as real and the mechanisms by which they are solved are not entirely unmoored from reality. By dramatizing the most exaggerated vision of institutional exploitation, however, they reassure an anxious public that their concerns are real, but that we haven't tipped into the realm of our darkest imagination.

Those dark reaches of imagination have been tested, however, perhaps most notably in Britain during the early 2000s with the Alder Hey organ retention scandal. The scandal has all the elements of a popular horror film: a heroic, grieving mother; an eccentric pathologist rumored to keep a baby's head in a jar; and a continuous revelation of dead body parts, with the number finally topping 100,000. In January of 2001, The Royal Liverpool Children's Inquiry (commonly called the "Redfern Report") exposed the horrifying results of a public inquiry into the practices of organ retention at UK hospitals (centering on Alder Hey Hospital and Liverpool University).[62] The inquiry was launched at the instigation of Helen Rickard. Four years after the death of her 11-month-old daughter, Rickard requested the medical records and noticed a notation that the heart had been removed and retained for research. In 1996, she obtained a coroner's ruling to return her daughter's heart, which, according to reports in *The Telegraph*, she kept in a wooden casket in her home for years.[63] It was only through her work with other grieving parents in a local support group that she realized such organ retention after postmortem examination might be much more common than anyone suspected.

Newspaper accounts following the Redfern Report tend to focus on the horrifying material elements of the practice: piling on staggering numbers accounting for body parts kept in dusty containers in the hospital basement. In a report titled, "Growth of a Gruesome Stockpile," *The Guardian* peppers its lead paragraphs with figures like "1,564 foetuses," "188 eyes," and "22 heads."[64] News accounts also follow the Report in focusing attention on Dutch pathologist Dick van Velzen. Employed at Alder Hey between 1988 and 1995, van Velzen is described as "systematically order[ing] the illegal and unethical stripping of every organ from every child who had a postmortem."[65] Since van Velzen was in charge of fetal and child pathology and mostly collected parts from these groups, the scandal took on the added dimension of horror stemming from our desire to protect the most vulnerable bodies. Although he did not ultimately face criminal charges, van Velzen clearly disregarded the express wishes of patients' families against postmortem and was found to have lied to both parents and colleagues.

Although it is tempting to focus on Dr. van Velzen as an idiosyncratic individual with poor supervision—as just another example of a mad doctor—he is simply the most dramatic figure in what the UK came to recognize as a crisis in medicine and public trust. Organ retention, after all, is a modern answer to the centuries-old problem of how to acquire specimens for medical education and research first dramatized in the body-snatching era of the 1800s and explored at length in Chapter 2. In his reflections on the case, David Hall (then-president of the Royal College of Paediatrics and Child Health) argues that "Alder Hey represents the culmination and, perhaps, the final demise of what we have thought of as benign medical paternalism, intended to protect patients and relatives from distressing details. Others have diagnosed our paternalism as arrogance, secrecy, dissimulation, and deception."[66] Hall's words capture the split between doctors' defense of their good intentions and the inescapably horrific elements of medical research, elements like cadaver work that prompted secrecy. The deepest level of critique was levied against these large institutions—public hospitals and universities—for their failure to respect an emerging right of patients' families to direct what happens to the body after death. Hall goes on to explain that "it was widely believed by our profession that 'specimens' could be collected and retained, without the relatives being informed or consent being given." Returning to the public good rationale explored in Chapter 2, these physicians understood cadaver parts as wholly under medical authority.

As the inquiry proceeded, two kinds of atypical and heartbreaking funeral practices emerged. Families who thought they had buried their children years before were driven to hold subsequent burials as retained body parts from these children were identified through the investigation. Sometimes these body parts would be discovered and identified over time and families would have to request multiple exhumations and reburials. In the second kind of funeral, at Allerton Cemetery, anonymous services were held every Thursday between May 2009 and January 2010 to memorialize unclaimed tissue and fetal samples uncovered during the inquiry a decade before. This conflict between "medical retention of specimens" on the one hand and highly sentimental rituals of grief among families dramatizes the conflicting registers operating in this case, between medical authority and familial connection.

The scandal dramatically reformed laws around informed consent and prompted the passage of both the Human Tissue Act of 2004 and the creation of the Human Tissue Authority in the UK. The Human Tissue Act threads together a series of reforms, including allowing for anonymous live organ donation, requiring a license for anyone intending to exhibit human remains (as in *Body Worlds*), and establishing precedence for the wishes of the deceased over that of relatives in cases of organ donation. In providing for altruistic donation to strangers and emphasizing the rights of the deceased, these regulations reflect an elevation of the self-determining individual. This emphasis on autonomy captures a backlash of public fears against the encroaching practices of medical institutions, insisting, as transplant historian Ruth Richardson argues, on patients as informed partners in decision-making.[67]

Historical violations of the principle of informed consent—from both this century and the past—are bound up in the uneven conduct of medical experimentation and treatment among vulnerable populations. In the USA, the poor, prisoners, African Americans, and immigrants have all been subject to unethical or illegal medical exploitation. These incidents are not isolated, but have been the stated and deliberate practice of medical institutions throughout history. From Tuskegee to the forced sterilization of Puerto Rican women, such practices loom large in the contemporary imaginations of marginalized groups, prompting resistance and fear. For example, among African Americans, donor rates lag significantly behind white Americans, resulting in African Americans being overrepresented on transplant lists. Although little empirical research has been done to identify why willingness to donate organs is persistently low among African Americans, a study by Susan Morgan et al., published in the *Journal of Applied Psychology* in 2003, reveals that misconceptions about the facts of transplantation, medical mistrust, fear of bodily mutilation, concerns about funerals, and religious objections were all higher among African Americans who participated in the survey.[68] With the exception of altruism scores, "every known predictor of organ donation willingness … is lower for African Americans than for European Americans."[69]

In these studies of low African American donor rates, we see mistrust in medicine and, specifically, a persistent theme of skepticism about allocation systems. Worries about the fairness of the system extend, of course, more broadly. For example, when former Vice President Dick Cheney received at heart transplant at the age of 71, many felt confirmed in their fears that the system can be manipulated in the interests of the rich and powerful.[70] A 1995 episode of *The X-Files* called "Hell Money" offers a horrific dramatization of these fears.[71] In the episode, FBI agents investigate deaths in a San Francisco Chinese immigrant community, uncovering a lottery that supplies organs for a black market organ ring. When the game is disrupted and a ticket holder reveals that all of the tiles are identical, he shouts "the game is fixed!" This passive voice construction reveals a manipulation of the system by depersonalized and nefarious forces, dramatizing through a horror narrative the common belief in a rigged allocation system. In this case, the disenfranchised immigrants serve as a metaphor for the desperately ill, exploited at the hands of medical institutions.

Perhaps the most common fear surrounding organ transplantation comes in the persistent urban legend of the kidney heist. While some details may vary, versions of this urban legend take strikingly similar form. A person, usually a tourist visiting a large city like New York, takes a night on the town, only to awaken in his or her hotel room in a bathtub full of ice. He or she feels intense abdominal pain and finds a new incision, striking in its surgical neatness. Subsequent medical investigation reveals that a kidney has been skillfully removed, likely by an experienced surgeon. This urban legend has been documented in the *New York Times* and served as inspiration for at least two "ripped from the headlines" episodes of *Law and Order* and *Law and Order: SVU*.[72] In an article for *Western Folklore*, Véronique Campion-Vincent testifies that these heist legends are also international in scope.[73] In these instances, the legends tend to express either xenophobia, for example, blaming gangs of North African immigrants, or to reveal populist fears of exploitation by a wealthy elite. In Bulgaria, anxieties about exploitation by foreigners were intense enough to prompt the requirement of a signed pledge by prospective international adoptive parents: "I will not permit my child to be an organ donor nor allow the child to give organs or be part of any medical experiment."[74] As I discuss in the following chapter, a black market international exchange in organs is an important and very real phenomenon that influences how we understand transplantation more broadly. It is also true, however, that the vibrant details of the heist myth are not attached to any actual, documented crime. Tourists to urban centers do not find themselves waking up in hotel bathtubs full of ice.

But while these stories lack foundation in fact, as a myth the "kidney heist" is striking in its persistence, widespread nature, and similarity of form. These elements reveal exactly the dynamics under discussion throughout this chapter. Although transplantation has been largely celebrated as a medical miracle and a sentimental "gift of life," there is a persistent dark side to public acceptance. These lingering anxieties can serve as one explanation for the low rates of actual cadaver donation, especially when compared to high rates of acceptance of organ transplantation in the abstract. As Campion-Vincent argues, organ theft narratives "articulate the anxieties that are felt but which cannot be expressed openly in societies in which science is touted as a positive force improving human lives. They obliquely attack modern medicine which transgresses boundaries that seemed immutable and which modifies our traditional conception of life and individual identity" (32). An important element of this argument lies in the identification of these persistent myths as the "oblique" expression of a fear that "cannot be openly expressed" in societies where medical innovation is king. Horror narratives like the ones described here provide an outlet for resistant attitudes ranging from the abstract—how does my notion of the self change when mingled with alien parts?—to the practical—how can I protect myself from exploitation by mad doctors or exploitive institutions? The metaphor of immunosuppression offers us a way forward. Resistance to such radical change in our bodies and our ideologies is inevitable. While medical authority and sentimental fictions can serve as powerful suppressant mechanisms, lingering anxiety must find expression. Horror narratives, by using the generic convention of exaggeration, both express these fears while also reassuring us that their most frightening limits have not yet been achieved in the real world. The mutually important elements of the kidney heist urban legend, then, are that it is universally told but also that it is unfounded, both frightening and reassuring in its vibrant specifics. The story suggests that as long as we aren't snatched from the street and placed under the scalpel of a mad, profit-driven surgeon, we can feel reassured that the unsettling elements of our actual system of organ exchange are, in comparison, noble in intent and regulated in practice.

Notes

1. *McFall v Shimp*, 10 PA. D. & C. 3d 90 (July 26, 1978).
2. *Coma*, directed by Michael Crichton (MGM, 1978).
3. Robin Cook, *Coma* (Boston: Signet, 2002), 333.
4. Willard Gaylin, "Harvesting the Dead," *Harper's* 249, no. 1492 (September 1974): 26.
5. Of course, an author's intention can get lost once a book is published and begins to take on a life of its own through popular and critical reception. It is interesting to note that despite Cook's interest in public service, at least one 1978 newspaper article connects it to a recent decrease in organ donors, asking in its headline, "Crisis in Organ Transplants: Did *Coma* Cause It?"
6. Howard M. Nathan et al., "Organ Donation in the United States," *American Journal of Transplantation* 3 (2003): 29–40.
7. According to data published by the US Department of Health and Human Services, Health Resources and Services Administration. "2012 National Survey of Organ Donation Attitudes and Behaviors." US Department of Health and Human Services, 2013. https://www.organdonor.gov. Accessed June 2017.
8. Susan E. Morgan et al., "Entertainment (Mis)Education: The Framing of Organ Donation in Entertainment Television," *Health Communication* 22, no. 2 (2007): 143–151. Statistics from the mid-1990s to late 1990s were even more stark. A series of studies from which Morgan and her team drew as a foundation of *their* study suggest that despite near universal support for donation as a concept (80–90%), only 30–50% of families donated a loved one's organs when given the opportunity, and even fewer Americans in the mid-1990s to late 1990s were registered to donate (about 30%). While it has narrowed, the gap persists today and prompts closer attention to the factors influencing consent rates.
9. Susan E. Morgan et al., "Family Discussions About Organ Donation: How the Media Influences Opinions about Donation Decisions," *Clinical Transplantation* 19, no. 5 (October 1, 2005): 674.
10. For more on horror aesthetics, especially in cinema, see Isabel Cristina Pinedo, "Postmodern Elements of the Contemporary Horror Film," in *The Horror Film* (New Brunswick: Rutgers University Press, 2004), 85–117; Stephen Prince, "Introduction," in *The Horror Film* (New Brunswick: Rutgers University Press, 2004), 1–14; Steven Jay Schneider, "Toward an Aesthetics of Cinematic Horror," in *The Horror Film* (New Brunswick: Rutgers University Press, 2004), 131–149; and Mark Viera, *Hollywood Horror from Gothic to Cosmic* (New York: Harry N. Abrams, Inc., 2003).

11. Youngner, "Some Must Die," 33.
12. Ian Olney, "The Problem Body Politic, or 'These Hands Have a Mind All Their Own!': Figuring Disability in the Horror Film Adaptations of Renard's Les Mains d'Orlac," *Literature/Film Quarterly* 34, no. 4 (October 1, 2006): 295.
13. Prince, "Introduction," 2.
14. Mary Shelley, *Frankenstein*, Reissue edition (New York: Penguin Classics, 2003), 53.
15. Carol Clover, "Her Body, Himself: Gender in the Slasher Film," *Representations*, no. 20 (Autumn 1987): 189.
16. Michael Sappol draws even finer distinctions in the bodily effects produced by nineteenth-century literature: "The nineteenth-century readers of sensationalist fiction expected that the reading of such texts would incite palpable bodily sensations: chills, muscular tension, relaxation, laughter. 'Philosophical' fiction, history, and other high genres, in contrast, were understood to be morally and culturally superior because they principally worked on, and 'elevated,' the reader's mind (or spirit or soul). (Sentimental fiction did both; it moved the reader bodily to sympathetic tears, but tears that are morally redemptive.)" Sappol, *A Traffic of Dead Bodies*, 217.
17. Pinedo, "Postmodern Elements," 91–92.
18. Margrit Shildrick, "The Critical Turn in Bioethics: The Case of Heart Transplantation," *International Journal of Feminist Approaches to Bioethics* 1, no. 1 (2008): 34.
19. Mary Beth Oliver and Meghan Sanders, "The Appeal of Horror and Suspense," in *The Horror Film* (New Brunswick: Rutgers University Press, 2004), 249.
20. Youngner, "Some Must Die," 39.
21. For more on the horrifying elements of everyday life, see Pinedo, "Postmodern Elements."
22. Pete Boss, "Vile Bodies and Bad Medicine," *Screen* 27, no. 1 (January 1, 1986): 19.
23. Joralemon, "Organ Wars."
24. Squier, "Transplant Medicine," 89.
25. Margareta Sanner, "Exchanging Spare Parts or Becoming a New Person?: People's Attitudes Toward Receiving and Donating Organs," *Social Science & Medicine* 52, no. 10 (May 2001): 1496.
26. Ibid.
27. Shildrick, "Critical Turn," 40.
28. Arthur Train, "Mortmain," in *Mortmain* (New York: D. Appleton and Company, 1907), 1–63.

29. Maurice Renard, *Hands of Orlac*, trans. I. White (London: Souvenir Press Ltd, 1981), 264.
30. B. Bunzel et al., "Does Changing the Heart Mean Changing Personality? A Retrospective Inquiry on 47 Heart Transplant Patients," *Quality of Life Research: An International Journal of Quality of Life Aspects of Treatment, Care and Rehabilitation* 1, no. 4 (August 1992): 254.
31. Paul Pearsall, Gary E. R. Schwartz, and Linda G. S. Russek, "Changes in Heart Transplant Recipients That Parallel the Personalities of Their Donors," *Journal of Near-Death Studies* 20, no. 3 (2002): 191–206.
32. Evridiki Kaba et al., "Somebody Else's Heart Inside Me: A Descriptive Study of Psychological Problems After a Heart Transplantation," *Issues in Mental Health Nursing* 26, no. 6 (July 2005): 621. This patient's metaphor finds a striking correspondence in the fictional work of Maurice Renard. Published before the more-famous *Les Mains D'Orlac*, his novel *Doctor Lerne, Sub-God* includes a plotline in which a Dr. Moreau-like scientist experiments with xenotransplantation, moving among plants, animals, humans, and ultimately transplanting his own personality into an automobile. This horrifying vision of man living forever through a machine and its replaceable parts is ultimately thwarted when the protagonist has the vehicle drained of all its fluids and renders it non-functioning.
33. "Network Is Proposed for Organ Transplants," *New York Times*, October 6, 1983, sec. A.
34. Shildrick, "Critical Turn." 39.
35. Catherine Waldby, "Biomedicine, Tissue Transfer, and Intercorporeality," *Feminist Theory* 3 (December 2002): 246.
36. Ian Sample, "Man Rejects First Penis Transplant," *The Guardian*, September 16, 2006, https://www.theguardian.com/science/2006/sep/18/medicineandhealth.china.
37. For coverage of the medical controversy surrounding the procedure, see Valerie Lincy, "Questions for Clint Hallam, the Visible Hand," *The New York Times*, December 26, 1999, sec. Magazine, http://www.nytimes.com/1999/12/26/magazine/the-way-we-live-now-12-26-99-questions-for-clint-hallam-the-visible-hand.html; and "Hand Transplant Surgery Prompts Debate," *American Medical News* 41, no. 48 (December 28, 1998): 31.
38. Quoted in Squier, "Transplant Medicine," 97.
39. Valerie Lincy, "Questions for Clint Hallam."
40. Quoted in Squier, "Transplant Medicine," 99.
41. "Surgeons Sever Transplant Hand," *BBC News*, February 3, 2001, http://news.bbc.co.uk/2/hi/europe/1151553.stm.

42. Quoted in Sample, "Man Rejects."
43. Train, "Mortmain," 47.
44. *Frankenstein*, directed by James Whale (Universal Pictures, 1931).
45. Leslie Fiedler, "Why Organ Transplant Programs Do Not Succeed," in *Organ Transplantation: Meanings and Realities*, ed. Stuart J. Youngner, Renée C. Fox, and Laurence J. O'Connell (Madison, WI: University of Wisconsin Press, 1996), 56–65.
46. Maurice Renard, *Doctor Lerne, Sub-God*, trans. Brian Stableford (Encino, CA: Black Coat Press, 2010), 230.
47. Quoted in Mark Viera, *Hollywood Horror*, 38.
48. Ibid.
49. Catherine Belling, "The Living Dead," also argues for Cook's efforts to enhance the realism of the text by trading on his own status as physician.
50. *Muggers*, directed by Dean Murphy (Instinct Entertainment, 2000); *The Donor*, directed by Damian Lee (Warner Home Video, 1995); *The Island*, directed by Michael Bay (DreamWorks, 2005); *The Eye*, directed by David Moreau and Xavier Palud (Lion's Gate, 2008); *Repo Men*, directed by Miguel Sapochnik (Universal Pictures, 2010).
51. *The Brain That Wouldn't Die*, directed by Joseph Green (1962).
52. Although this paragraph explores the role of head transplantation in actual surgical history, it is worth noting that Maurice Renard's *Dr. Lerne* includes a plot point in which it is revealed that two surgical assistants are thriving examples of successful head swapping: "Oh, those brave men! Who would imagine that their entire bodies had been amputated? And yet each of them, to this day, inhabits his friend's carnal housing. Look!" (231).
53. See, for example, Hamilton, *A History of Organ Transplantation*; and Tilney, *Transplant.*
54. Ashley Welsh, "Russian Man Volunteers for First Human Head Transplant," *CBS News*, August 29, 2016, http://www.cbsnews.com/news/russian-man-volunteers-for-first-human-head-transplant/.
55. Richard Gray, "Head Transplant Surgeon Plans 'Frankenstein' Test to Reanimate Corpses," *Daily Mail Online*, September 20, 2016, http://www.dailymail.co.uk/~/article-3798056/index.html.
56. Jen Wieczner, "This Groundbreaking 'Frankenstein' Surgery Will Literally Make Your Head Spin," *Time*, June 5, 2015, http://time.com/3911435/mice-transplant-head-china/.
57. Quoted in Kirsten Weir, "Getting a Head," *Current Science* 90, no. 7 (December 3, 2004): 5.
58. Shildrick, "Corporeal Cuts," 36.

59. Margaret Lock also discusses how the increasing turn to anonymity for donors has led to an odd position in which their "gift" is celebrated in the abstract, but actual individuals receive little publicity: "donors, who had been disquietingly visible during the first year of heart transplants, disappeared from public view to become nameless ghosts who haunt the transplant world." Lock, *Twice Dead*, 99.
60. Larry Niven, "The Jigsaw Man," in *Tales of Known Space: The Universe of Larry Niven* (New York: Ballantine Books, 1975), 67–79.
61. Robert Silverberg, "Caught in the Organ Draft," in *Caught in the Organ Draft: Biology in Science Fiction*, ed. Isaac Asimov, Martin H. Greenberg, and Charles G. Waugh (New York: Farrar, Straus, Giroux, 1983), 142.
62. Michael Redfern, *The Royal Liverpool Children's Report (The Redfern Report)* (The House of Commons, 2001).
63. Sean O'Neill, "How a Grieving Mother Uncovered the Horror," *The Telegraph*, January 31, 2001, http://www.telegraph.co.uk/news/uknews/1320382/How-a-grieving-mother-uncovered-the-horror.html.
64. Helen Carter, "The Growth of a Gruesome Stockpile," *The Guardian*, January 30, 2001, sec. UK News, https://www.theguardian.com/uk/2001/jan/31/alderhey.helencarter.
65. Sarah Boseley and Helen Carter, "He Stripped the Organs from Every Dead Child He Touched," *The Guardian*, January 31, 2001, https://www.theguardian.com/society/2001/jan/31/health.alderhey.
66. David Hall, "Reflecting on Redfern: What Can We Learn from the Alder Hey Story?," *Archives of Disease in Childhood* 84, no. 6 (June 1, 2001): 455–456.
67. Hall, "Reflections on Redfern."
68. Susan E. Morgan, Jenny K. Miller, and Lily A. Arasaratnam, "Similarities and Differences Between African Americans' and European Americans' Attitudes, Knowledge, and Willingness to Communicate About Organ Donation," *Journal of Applied Social Psychology* 33, no. 4 (April 1, 2003): 693–715.
69. Ibid., 708.
70. For typical coverage of the surgery, see Associated Press, "Cheney's Heart Transplant Sparks Debate," *NY Daily News*, accessed July 14, 2016, http://www.nydailynews.com/life-style/health/dick-cheney-heart-transplant-sparks-debate-old-article-1.1050872. For more politicized coverage, see, for example, Joan Walsh, "Dick Cheney: Even Bigger Monster Than You Thought," *Salon*, November 14, 2013, http://www.salon.com/2013/11/14/dick_cheney_even_bigger_monster_than_you_thought/.

71. *The X-Files*, season 3, episode 19, "Hell Money," directed by Tucker Gates, aired March 29, 1996, on Fox.
72. *Law and Order*, season 1, episode 21, "Sonata for a Solo Organ," directed by Fred Gerber, aired April 2, 1991 on NBC; and *Law and Order: SVU*, season 6, episode 22, "Parts," directed by Matt Earl Beesley, aired May 17, 2005, on NBC.
73. Véronique Campion-Vincent, "Organ Theft Narratives," *Western Folklore* 56, no. 1 (Winter 1997): 1–37.
74. Quoted in ibid., 2.

CHAPTER 7

Kidneyville: Organ Exchange at the Margins

There is a small village in South India where reports suggest that nearly every woman in the community has sold a kidney for transplant. This 2500-person refugee village is called Tsunami Nagar, named after the devastating tsunami of 2004 that necessitated its creation. It is also known locally by another name: "Kidneyville." The story of the village is chronicled in Scott Carney's *The Red Market: On the Trail of the World's Organ Brokers, Bone Thieves, Blood Farmers, and Child Traffickers*. Carney's book lives up to the promise of its title in offering diverse accounts of human tissue crossing boundaries of nations, ethics, legality, and propriety. According to his account, which blends methods from anthropology and investigative journalism, "just about every adult woman" in Tsunami Nagar has sold a kidney to local brokers, often for as little as $700.[1] These patients and brokers are the local links in an extensive international chain of illegal organ trade. Carney's work—reviewed by the *New York Times* and *National Public Radio* and previously published in *Wired*—exposes the hidden realities of contemporary organ exchange to an international, largely Western, audience. Carney shifts the typical media focus away from stories of transplant "miracles" and sentimental appeals for organ donation in order to pull back the curtain on a darker practice in the transnational medical landscape. For the women of Tsunami Nagar, and other communities like it across

E. Russell, *Transplant Fictions*,
Palgrave Studies in Literature, Science and Medicine,
https://doi.org/10.1007/978-3-030-12135-8_7

the Global South, the reasons for selling a kidney are both diverse and painfully similar: most boil down to the promise of mobility, a chance to change one's location or economic circumstances.

In the stories of illegal organ sale that I examine in this chapter[2]—fictional, reported, and anthropological—hope and mobility emerge as a consistent theme across all stages of the process: from the seller's hope for movement out of poverty, to the broker's transport of the organ across regional or national lines, to the recipient traveling as a transplant tourist to sites like Brazil, India, Israel, Turkey, or South Africa. As seen when analyzing descriptions of organ sale more closely below, even this vastly simplified account does not capture the many boundaries crossed by people, capital, and tissue in a typical illegal organ exchange. In a fascinating rhetorical alignment of migration and kidney sale, Carney quotes a local source describing the hopeful promise bound up in the chance for mobility: "In other parts of India people say they are going to Malaysia or the United States with a glimmer of hope in their eyes. In Tsunami Nagar people speak that way about selling their kidneys" (65). Among kidney sellers, however, this promise of movement out of poverty is rarely fulfilled. Some fail to account for the physical and financial toll of major surgery, others find themselves cheated by unscrupulous brokers who refuse additional payments once the kidney has been removed. With no legal recourse among an already disenfranchised population, accounts of kidney sales rehearse stories of dashed hopes and little change. Nancy Scheper-Hughes, an anthropologist at UC Berkeley who co-founded Organs Watch, has done multi-site international fieldwork on organ exchange. Her research suggests that the transplant rhetoric of altruism and self-determination obscures a host of abuses, including: illegal violations of cadavers and disenfranchised patients; coercive practices stemming from gender, class, and race inequalities; and a new "form of debt peonage in which the commodified kidney plays a substantial role."[3] While many sellers cite feeling trapped by poverty as a motivating force in participating in an openly abusive system, these individuals are also crucially rootless, in unstable positions and unfixed locations.

Organ sellers around the globe may not find the promise of movement out of poverty ultimately fulfilled, but their status as a population in flux—as refugees, or prisoners, or urban transplants from rural villages—makes them vulnerable to the appeal of organ brokers. Illegal international organ trade requires a secrecy made possible by drawing from patients and locating in sites that are transitional and outside the notice of established state, juridical, and medical oversight. Consistently, tales of illegal organ exchange center on temporary locations (hotels, refugee camps, airports) and people in transit (illegal immigrants, asylum seekers, and the very poor on one side and economically privileged transplant tourists on the other). The fictional and reported accounts of illegal organ traffic examined in this chapter shed light on these marginal spaces and populations, exposing the underbelly where movement occurs up the global social hierarchy from impoverished sellers to the Western need for organs. These marginal populations are driven by ultimately unfulfilled romantic tropes of hope, transit, and change, which form both the necessary appeal and rarely discussed outcomes of organ sale (for both sellers and buyers). If sentiment structures the affirmative motivation for donation and horror captures the residual anxieties about transplantation, romance is a third genre in transplant culture, constructing a meaningful narrative arc for sellers, brokers, and buyers alike.

Somatic and National Borders

The movement over vast distances that characterizes the contemporary black market organ trade is a trailing consequence of decades of advancement in immunology and tissue typing. In the six decades or so since the advent of organ transplant, a seismic shift has occurred in the conceptual possibility of matching across distance. We have moved from an exceptionally tight practical requirement of identity between donor and recipient to a broadly held hope in which a "match" can be found anywhere in the world. In order to understand current trends, it is necessary to look back briefly at the history of the practice. The first successful human organ transplant took place between twins, Ronald and Richard Herrick, in 1954. Because the brothers were genetically identical, the operation escaped the dangers of organ rejection that had blocked success in organ transplant throughout the first half of the twentieth century. Beginning in 1960, anti-rejection drugs opened the field to transplants beyond identical twins and, as immunology and tissue typing procedures improved, across lines of not just family, but gender and ethnicity as well. In contrast to this early predication on "sameness" and biological relation, current transplant practice typically advocates anonymity between an unrelated donor and recipient, making the exchange more ideologically palatable by diminishing the identity of the donor. As Lawrence Cohen, a professor of medical anthropology at UC Berkeley, describes, "with tissue-typing materializing new sites of sameness and difference, one could screen a large number of potential donors to discover bodies suddenly compatible, far from the family tree."[4]

Nancy Scheper-Hughes extends this point, stressing the strangeness that emerges from the combined practices of donor anonymity and transportation over great distances to find a "match." As described in the chapter on sentiment, new forms of imaginative kinship are deployed "to link strangers, even at times political 'enemies,' from distant locations who are described by the operating surgeons as 'a perfect match—like brothers,' while they are prevented from seeing, let alone speaking, to each other."[5] While the "like brothers" simile uses the language of family and social relation to describe the connection between donor and recipient, the realities of the practice, especially in transnational exchange, eliminate almost entirely the social dimensions of the procedure. Scheper-Hughes goes on:

> Who, for example, would imagine that, in the midst of the long-standing religious and ethnic hostilities and an almost genocidal war in the Middle East, one of the first 'sources' of living donors for Israeli kidney transplant patients would be Palestinian guest workers; or that, as recently as March 2002, Israeli patients would be willing to travel to Istanbul to be transplanted in a private clinic by a Muslim surgeon who decorates his waiting room with photos of Ataturk and a plastic glass eye to ward off evil?[6]

Such phenomena—in which international hostilities dissolve in a pragmatism of desperate scarcity—demonstrate the shifting ideological terrain of organ exchange. The dehumanizing rhetoric of "spare parts" coincides with romantic notions of "matching" and "family" to justify the practice.

The "sites of sameness" Lawrence Cohen describes are not just far from the family tree; they often span thousands of miles. Consider, for example, a 2004 *New York Times* article that follows a sold kidney on a "path of poverty and hope" across four continents.[7] Larry Rohter's article captures hope at both ends of this chain, from the seller's hope of escaping the Brazilian slum where he lives in a two-room shack shared by eleven people to the American recipient's hope for prolonged life. In one form of the conceptual wrangling necessary to make organ sale possible, the seller, Alberty José da Silva, connects his sale of a kidney for $6000 to his mother's work as a prostitute who "'sold her flesh' to survive." In these exchanges, gender, intimacy, and commerce merge to imagine the experience of the peddler of flesh.[8] The imaginative recourse to intimacy that lies in connecting international organ sale to sex work creates a fascinating meeting point between the biological "sameness" required for successful transplants and the differences in social station required for two individuals to buy or sell an organ. While the *NY Times* article focuses on men as the sellers of kidneys in this Brazilian slum—and laments their struggle to perform heavy manual labor for months or years post-surgery—accounts of international trafficking provided by Organs Watch and transplant scholars suggest that women are disproportionately targeted by brokers, who are typically male. As Nancy Scheper-Hughes argues, "*In general*, the organs flow from South to North, from poor to rich, from black and brown to white, and from female to male bodies."[9] Returning, then, to the contrast between the rhetoric of identity and sameness that characterizes voluntary organ gifts among family members, the contours of international organ sale are strikingly conducted across every form of difference.

Some of the anxieties over literally incorporating the "other" into the self are assuaged paradoxically by the First World sense that the impoverished Global South has a surfeit of bodies, that the "expendable" flesh of the poor is their most valuable commodity. As a Los Angeles organ broker said to Scheper-Hughes during an interview, "There's no reason for anyone to die in this country while waiting for a heart or a kidney to materialize. There are plenty of organs to be had in other parts of the world."[10] This all-too-common rationale mirrors more general arguments about global capital in which the laboring bodies of the South serve the goods-and-services-hungry populations of the North.

This transnational flow of bodies (and body parts) asserts parallels between national and somatic borders. More commonly articulated as political and economic crises around undocumented immigrants or asylum seekers, these debates connect to organ trade in two ways: first, as language of a secure body politic shapes public rhetoric about borders, and second, as policies surrounding regulation of organ trade take on national biases about "proper" divisions among populations. Several recent critics, including Sarah Gibson, Emily Davis, and Donna McCormack, have identified these cultural links between national and somatic boundaries as articulated through the transplant narrative.[11] In an analysis of the ethics of organ transplant in contemporary film,

McCormack writes, "Organ donation is currently carrying the weight of cultural anxieties not only regarding divisions between self and other, but also concerning national boundaries of belonging and whether 'different others' are to be welcomed or expulsed" (171). These parallels among anxieties over somatic and national integrity are not merely a clever metaphor, but serve as material forces in the transplant fictions under examination here. In both, the film *Dirty Pretty Things* and the Chris Abani novel *GraceLand*, organ sale or brokerage is made possible among migratory populations by offering the promise of passports or legal resident status. In these narratives, individual body parts are offered up in exchange for legitimacy within the body politic.

In *Dirty Pretty Things*, the simplified logic of organ sale is captured in a speech by the film's villainous organ broker, Juan. He tells Owke, "If you were just some African, the deal would be simple. You give me your kidney, I give you a new identity. I sell your kidney for ten grand so I'm happy. The person who needs the kidney gets cured so he's happy. The person who sold the kidney gets to stay in this beautiful country so he's happy. My whole business is based on happiness." The parallelism in his phrasing accomplishes an ideological sleight of hand in which money, kidney, identity, and happiness exist on an easy plane of exchange. Although the "new identity" Juan references is literally found in a passport, the word choice suggests exactly the flexible attachment to personal identity that makes organ exchange possible. Each element is filtered through the all-powerful function of commodity, resulting in new channels for the flow of capital.

Despite this neat speech, narratives of illegal organ sale more typically taint the promise of hope found in the romantic trope of mobility, recasting the desired passport as acquired through a terrible price. As examined below, immigration in *Dirty Pretty Things* and *GraceLand* takes on a decidedly ambiguous cast; in these cases, the story is arrested in the transitory space of the airport, forever deferring arrival. This turn away from stable paths of immigration mirror contemporary patterns in an era of managed migration. As Ashley Dawson describes in her study of stateless people represented in British culture, global population flow is no longer about a single trip from fixed origin to fixed destination, but instead is characterized by "temporary, circular migrations."[12] While celebrated by Homi Bhabha, Kwame Anthony Appiah, and Salman Rushdie as a transformative cosmopolitanism, these forms of movement are also tempered by concerns about security in the post-9/11 nation-state.[13] By deferring the expected arrival in narratives of crossing geographical and somatic borders, the trope of mobility in these transplant fictions does not equal hope, but a rockier, continued journey. Such ambiguity is appropriate to tales of organ transplant. Since sentimental newspaper accounts or television medical dramas fail to capture the lifetime of complications and anti-rejection drugs endured post-surgery, the medical realities for both organ seller and recipient look much more like the circulatory patterns of contemporary migration than the romantic triumph of arrival.

While their aesthetic strategies stray from the strict realism required by news and scholarly accounts, the film *Dirty Pretty Things* and Chris Abani's novel *GraceLand* serve as emblematic fictional accounts that reveal broader dynamics in the ideology of organ sale. Just as Frears and Abani have drawn from life in representing their fictional worlds, so do representational strategies and imagination structure both lived experiences of and our cultural attitudes toward organ sale. Directed by Stephen Frears, *Dirty Pretty Things* (2002), blends generic elements of horror, romance, and gritty realism to link the British political crisis over policing its national boundaries with the economic complexities of service labor and black market exchange of organs for forged passports.[14] Frears's film and Abani's novel explore two ends of illegal migration: Where the film follows Okwe, a Nigerian doctor turned London taxi driver and hotel clerk, the novel *GraceLand* (2004) is set in Nigeria's slums and explores the economic and political conditions that would incite an individual to sell blood or peddle illegal organs. Placed in critical conversation with accounts of organ sale among refugees, slum dwellers, and undocumented migrants, these fictional stories offer rich, imaginative fodder for interpretation that reveals shared tropes between the real and the fictional. By examining these diverse narratives together, people and spaces characterized by transit, hope, and promised change emerge as the condition of possibility for the illegal sale of organs. As these stories also reveal, however, the romantic promise of organ sale characteristically collapses as illusory or deferred; any of the positive connotations of romance—while they serve as a structuring force in the exchange—remain ultimately unsatisfied.

Dirty Pretty Things: Kidneys for Passports

Throughout *Dirty Pretty Things*, black market organ sale consistently is linked to a requirement of mobility. The film's settings are marked by their transitory nature—airport, hotel, and hospital morgue—and the central characters are all nonnative Londoners, working in service industries characterized by the invisibility and fungibility of their laborers. The most concrete expression of mobility in the film comes with the question: "He swapped his insides for a passport?" The line is delivered incredulously by Okwe, a Nigerian doctor who has fled political persecution through illegal immigration to London, roles which make him uniquely qualified to understand the inherent value and danger attached to both organ exchange and pursuing secure documentation. By "swapping their insides for a passport," desperate organ sellers demonstrate the supremacy of state-sanctioned identification and monitoring. The phrasing "insides" captures a traditional conception of an internal self that is more authentic, personal, and, ironically, imagined as safer from incursion than political allegiances. This equivalence between "insides" and passport sets up an important tie between personal and political identities, laying out an economy in which peddling flesh contains the promise of a new national start.

The film proceeds through the dramatic apparatus of exposure, where the audience follows the characters as they gain increased understanding of the dynamics of the black market. Okwe's surprise at the realities of organ exchange extends to his disbelief that such practices happen in developed countries like Britain. His friend Guo Yi, who works in a hospital morgue, responds, "What do you mean 'not here'? In London? You think it doesn't happen because the queen doesn't approve?. … If I had the courage, I'd sell my kidney, just to get out of here, just to save my brain." Screenwriter Steven Knight employs a subtle vagueness in the repetition of the word "here," in which the term can be metonymic for escaping both London and the demeaning labor of the morgue. In exchanging his kidney "to save his brain," Guo Yi returns to the notion of multiple, fractured facets of identity described above: A distinction in value is made between the personal self—the insides, the brain—and the social self of an exportable kidney. Such fracturing, and the belief that parts of one's body could be excised and shipped off to "save" the rest, is essential to the logic of mobility at the heart of black market organ sale.

In the same way that the film locates the motivation for organ sale in the promise of mobility, it also uses setting to dramatize both the circumstances that would prompt such a desperate move and the fluctuating sites and populations that allow the black market to function. As the film's star, Chiwetel Ejiofor, claims in the DVD commentary, "It's a film about the underbelly, basically." For a film about kidney sale, "underbelly" is of course appropriate to denote the world captured by Frears. In an establishing scene for the film and its preoccupations, Okwe's taxi ferries passengers from the airport on a route that avoids the noteworthy, typically cinematic landmarks of London and instead traverses tunnels and back streets. This behind-the-scenes approach continues in capturing individuals and locations at the periphery: the unadorned staff hallways of the hotel, the graveyard shift, a rented couch, a hospital morgue and laundry. The gritty look of the film—created in part through tinting effects to create a sense of atmosphere in different locations—emphasizes the realism suggested by the camera's ability to move into spaces repeatedly described as "invisible." This invisibility is, in part, due to the transitory nature of individuals through the spaces. Whether hotel guest, taxi passenger, or corpse consigned to the morgue, all of these statuses are impermanent.

The transitory nature of these sites extends, crucially, to the people who live and work there. Within the film, service workers are fungible in the face of an impersonal class system, in the same way that organs are represented as fungible. The film bypasses any question of matching donor to recipient and instead imagines a world (in an exaggeration of the existing black market) in which there will always be a wealthy, unseen buyer for any available organ. Exploiting a population of illegal immigrants or asylum seekers who are unable to legally seek paid employment, the jobs represented in the film—maid, doorman, laundress, taxi driver, sweatshop worker—are vulnerable because there is always another person waiting to take one's place. In a scene, where Okwe must assume the identity of a hospital janitor to steal necessary supplies, he looks skeptically at the false ID badge Guo Yi has offered. "Black is black," his friend replies, driving home the point that for vulnerable populations, differentiating factors of personal and national identity are immaterial.

A similar premise bolsters the expectation that the traffic in falsified passports and visas necessary to complete the organ sale will pass official scrutiny. Despite the villainous presence of the Immigration Enforcement Directive and the repeated shots of security cameras monitoring the maids' entrance to the hotel, the film's heroes thwart both methods of tracking service workers. The service community is represented as excessively targeted by surveillance, but while threatening, it's a surveillance that fails to successfully distinguish among them as individuals. In her *Camera Obscura* article on "The Intimacies of Globalization," Emily Davis describes a tension between film representation and the fact that laborers and people of color are invisible within and yet central to the processes of global capitalism. She writes, "these representations foreground the intimacies of globalization at the same time that they use the visual media of film and television—media that frequently present themselves as transparently immediate, intimately present—to problematize the very idea of intimacy in global exchanges" (36–37). Within *Dirty Pretty Things*, repeated shots within the film of video surveillance mark the invisible, underbelly spaces that Frears is representing as already subject to a viewership that fails to truly see what it monitors. Does the filmed narrative, then, exist in a similar web of intimacy and invisibility?

This emphasis on invisibility is repeated explicitly by all of the major characters in the film, beginning with a prostitute's claim, "I don't exist," and ending at the film's climax with Okwe's oft-cited response to the white organ broker's question, "How come I've never seen you people before?" Okwe answers, "Because we are the people you do not see. We drive your cabs. We clean your rooms. And suck your cocks." Okwe's description of their invisibility dwells on the intimate acts and spaces inherent in the service relationship. The line also recalls Brazilian Alberty José da Silva's quote to the *New York Times* connecting his kidney sale to his mother's prostitution. This intimacy reveals the perverse side of the organ buyer/seller relationship, in which individuals are brought together across difference and through similarly hopeful motivations, but the connection exists through a veil of inequality.

A similar formulation structures the connection between organ seller and recipient in which obscuring layers of brokers, middlemen, hospitals, and the surgical environment create an anonymous organ wholly uprooted from its original host. The practice of shrouding organs in secrecy is similar in legal exchanges where US laws typically prohibit both compensation for and identification of the extra-familial source of the donation. In addition to the biomedical hurdles that have limited organ exchange in the half-century since the practice began, doctors and patients must adjust to a conception of the body that allows for a mobile exchange of parts without entirely unmaking one's sense of coherent identity. *Dirty Pretty Things* captures the social formation of service workers as invisible to demonstrate how these obscuring structures work to make an extensive array of practices—both everyday and exceptional—palatable.

Everything from delivering food after hours, to performing sex work, to organ exchange relies on the invisibility of a class of individuals. This masking is bound up in the romantic nature of hopeful fantasy but is also aided by the intermediary and transitory nature of both location and population. In *Dirty Pretty Things*, Frears focuses on pulling back the obscuring curtain to reveal the relentlessly material realities of this world. His workers are caught in removing the realities of existence from public notice, including: blood, corpses, human medical waste to be incinerated, and a housekeeper's lament that she spends her days "cleaning up after whores." In the film's most dramatic visualization of the return of the abject, Okwe responds to a complaint about an overflowing toilet and discovers a human heart clogging the pipe. The scene is shot with the camera lying in the depths of the toilet: first, a bloom of bright red blood curls up through the water. We see Okwe reaching toward the camera, which then flips to his point of view as he draws out the heart. The quick shifting of perspective suggests that despite his shock at finding the organ in the toilet, there's a kind of equivalence between Okwe's position and blood, waste, and organs. In a similar scene, Guo Yi, to whom we have just been introduced as he swipes blood from an autopsy table and incinerates medical waste, tells Okwe: "I'm a certified refugee, you're an illegal, Okwe. You don't have a position here. You have nothing. You are nothing." The visual metaphor created between the acts of burning bags of discarded flesh and blood with the claim "you are nothing" underscores the larger conceit of the film: Frears captures a population whose official state and class status has reduced them to necessary but disposable byproducts of society.

In populating a film with refugees and undocumented immigrants, Frears focuses on a migratory community caught in an intermediary status between flight and secure arrival. For Senay, a Turkish asylum seeker played by Audrey Tautou, this deferred "arrival" is captured by a postcard of New York City, representing her idealized fantasies of immigration to the USA. Her struggles in London, then, can occupy a temporary position in her imagination, an uncomfortable layover in a long journey. More dangerously, the film conceives of immigrants as consistently vulnerable to both literal deportation and the encroachment of the escaped home nation into the resettled situation. Twice, Okwe describes the shoddy practices of black market medicine as being of another country. Upon finding a Somali victim of bad organ retrieval in Juan's office, Okwe demands, "Where did he have this operation? Which country?" In a repeated expression of his initial naiveté, Okwe can't conceive of such a botched medical procedure as being part of the developed world. In a more extensive expression of this concept, when Senay asks Okwe where he has been after treating the Somali patient in his apartment, Okwe replies, "Africa." In this case, the boundaries of Britain become permeable, not only to migrants, but to practices and realities characteristic of the home country. Migration, then, is not simply the act of individuals, but can occur imaginatively in the overlay of an entire continent into a London apartment. The obvious physical mismatch in this metaphorical site of overlap shows the danger and instability of such a move. The conceptual possibility of these sites of overlap—in which a foreign land finds an island of expression within a larger host nation—serves as a parallel to transplant ideologies in which something of the donor self is seen to linger in the new body. The limits of assimilation offer a powerful connection to lingering fears among recipients about their own somatic incoherence.

The film opens and closes with bookended scenes of the airport,[15] underscoring the overriding theme of transit and the permeability of national boundaries. The closing scene offers two forms of resolution, as Senay and Okwe mouth "I love you" to each other across the crowded terminal and Okwe calls his sister in Nigeria to tell her, "At last, I'm coming home." The sentimental pleasure derived from this scene, however, is enabled by the suspenseful and bloody triumph of our heroes' revenge plot against the organ traffickers. Senay and Okwe's mobility is made possible through the exchange of the exploitative Juan's kidney for cash and new identities. As it reaches its climax, the increasingly dramatic score and rising romantic tension between the leads shifts the film away from the gritty realism of its aesthetic and pushes it more firmly into the territory of both horror and romance. In mingling these genres, Frears casts a pall over the film's positive romantic resolution. Although falling solidly in the category of the "happy ending," arresting the action in the space of the airport—another postponed arrival—recalls the realities articulated early in the film in which Senay acknowledges that New York is "not really like" her fantasy. In an even darker definition of "freedom,"

Senay tells Okwe, "One of the laundry girls did it [sold her kidney] and now she is free." To Okwe's caution that "Others have died," Senay responds, "Then they are free, too." Frears draws together the physicality of horror, the psychic seduction of romance, and the attention to material conditions of realism to demonstrate the structuring narrative forces in organ sale. The tension among these three genres emerges most strongly at the film's conclusion, demonstrating each as the condition for the black market exchange, but denying resolution is an uneasy reminder of the costs of seeking mobility.

GraceLand: Brokering the Abject

If *Dirty Pretty Things* is a film about the "underbelly" of the British service economy and immigration practices, Chris Abani's novel *GraceLand* similarly explores the seldom-seen sites of poverty and violence in metropolitan Lagos. The novel offers a fictional window into the experiences and sharply circumscribed choices available in 1980s Nigeria for Elvis, a sixteen-year old who has recently moved with his father to the city from their village, Afikpo. Abani characterizes Lagos as a city sharply divided, "half slum, half paradise."[16] Much like Okwe's contention in *Dirty Pretty Things* that "we are the people you don't see," Abani argues "it was as if people conspired with the city to weave a web of silence around its unsavory parts" (7) and then sets his novel within that unsavoriness. Read together and alongside anthropological accounts in this chapter, the film and novel can demonstrate shared conceptual dynamics across multiple phases and sites in organ sale. They are emblematic of a commonly encountered story, one which lures impoverished, marginalized individuals into the organ trade. As extended, fictionalized meditations on real-life practices, these stories can support cultural analysis that helps to reveal deeper dynamics structuring transplant ideology more broadly.

If the burbling rise of a human heart in a hotel toilet dramatizes the return of the abject in Frears's film, *GraceLand* follows the cast-off poor of the city to dwell with them in "abject" poverty. Much of the novel takes place in Maroko, a tenement community in Lagos housing almost 300,000 individuals, mostly migrants from across Nigeria. Within the novel, the experience of poverty is emphatically embodied, centered on descriptions of stinking, shared outhouses and make-shift showers or baths, finding money for food purchased at street stalls, and in the limited value of one's body and labor. The latter formulation is most strikingly captured in Elvis's father's speech about familial love and the honor that is passed through the generations—"Do you know why we have a lot of deformed children begging? Because their parents know dey have no future. So at birth, before the child knows pain, dey deform it because it increases its earning power as a beggar. Do you see de love? All dey have to give de child is its deformity" (188). In this speech, the abject image of the deformed child beggar is recast as an expression of parental love and hope for the future.

A similar lens reimagines social value among the poor not as contributions made possible through the laboring body, but as a value inherent in the material products of the body itself. After Elvis befriends a local beggar, Okon, by paying for his meal and sharing conversation, he's surprised to see his friend return barely a week later dressed like Superfly. Wondering how Okon has gone from scrabbling in the dirt for discarded rice to new clothes and eating in a restaurant—a change of state that makes him unrecognizable to Elvis initially—Okon replies that he has been selling his blood at local hospitals, often as many as four in a day. In a simple formulation familiar to any ethics debate around compensation for human tissue, Okon shrugs, "It's illegal, of course, but it's my blood, and it's helping to save lives, including mine, right?" (76). Late in the novel, Okon returns on the scene to reveal that he's given up donating blood and briefly turned to "hijak[ing] corpses from roadsides and even homes which we sold for organ transplants" (308). Both practices are represented in the novel with shuddering distaste, but Abani demonstrates the desperate circumstances that fuel an economy of black market organ exchange. He looks behind the veil of abjection to explore how the sanitized return of blood, organs, and corpses is made possible by a population living at the margins. In Kristeva's traditional formulation of the abject, the psychic and social casting off of reminders of mortality—pus, vomit, feces, blood, corpses—is an inherently unstable affair, marked by the continual return of the abject.[17] Blood and organ sale offer a heightened version of this movement in which the return is facilitated through intermediary spaces of poverty and migratory populations of poor, unemployed, and unskilled citizens. The returned tissue, then, is sanitized through the channels of medical distribution and ascends from its position of abjection to valorized "giver of life."

To underscore the permeability of these boundaries between dead and healthy, local and migrant, Abani offers several establishing scenes of Elvis riding the bus, meditating on spatial boundaries. In one conflation of literal movement with the realities of Nigerian medicine at the margins, a traveling pharmaceutical vendor boards Elvis's bus to pitch his wares to the city travelers. Extolling the wonders of "Pracetmol" (Paracetamol, a fever reducer), he claims, "this is a new drug from de white people's labs and plenty research done go into it. It is manufacture in Yugoslavia.... Today you can obtain your copy at cheap rate from me" (9). Elvis and the bus passengers represent the intersection of options for entering the medical marketplace. Throughout the novel, Abani includes examples of local remedies, Western hospitals (often represented as corrupt or inefficient), and black market dealings in drugs, organs, or blood. These spheres are not discrete entities, but as the vendor's pitch makes clear, rely on channels of exchange among each other—from white (British or American) labs to generic manufacture in emerging economies like Yugoslavia to unauthorized sale on Nigerian buses.

As described throughout this chapter, illegal international organ trade relies on these sites of overlap in which transitory individuals with few options come into contact with mobile intermediaries who can offer them money for an alluring source of value: the body itself. Like the Indian women of "Kidneyville" or the impoverished laborers of Brazil, the precarious circumstances of these individuals create a fractured self/body, allowing for the sale of their organs. In *GraceLand*, Abani captures not only cases where beggars are tempted to sell their own blood or to steal corpses for "spare parts," but also the trail of moral compromises and economic desperation that lead Elvis and his friend, significantly named Redemption, to act as organ brokers. As the last in a series of increasingly dangerous and illegal schemes to make money, Redemption convinces Elvis to join him as an escort for an unknown package to be delivered across the border. Troubled by the secrecy of the mission, but unwilling to disturb the strict prohibition to "ask no questions," Elvis and Redemption are caught in the hidden zone of exchange through which organs travel across international lines from poor to rich. To highlight the veil of secrecy in which even brokers can operate, Elvis and Redemption's realization of their mission is dramatized importantly in a climactic scene of horrific exposure. The climactic device of exposure recurs throughout both fictional and true accounts of organ sale, where the overlooked, extra-national communities and populations that are the condition for the black market come suddenly under the scrutiny of concerned others. In its manifestation in Abani's novel, Elvis goes to the three identical coolers at the back of the truck, opens one looking for sandwiches, but finds six severed heads staring up at him. A second cooler carries loose hearts and livers with their "strange rusty smell" (257). Even more troubling than the gruesome spectacle in the coolers, however, is the acknowledgment that the children they have also picked up are simply "fresher" specimens awaiting surgery (at best) or death to supply wealthy Saudi organ markets.

Elvis and Redemption's discovery of their complicity in this international organ brokering scheme triggers a chain of events in the novel that reveal the impossibility of a coherent individualism expressed within 1980s Nigeria. The figurative alignment of food for the travelers with severed heads and floating kidneys—in the grotesquely comic mix-up involving identical coolers—uses the horrifying materiality of the dis-integrated body to expose the characters' illusions about their peripheral role in violent schemes.[18] Organs and blood have the power to unmake seemingly secure notions of integrity, both bodily and moral (in this case, the fantasy that they are apart from the corruption that surrounds them). This scene offers a harsh reminder of the permeability of self, and stands in contrast to fantasies of the self as a discrete individual. Although most starkly represented in the visual confrontation of heads and kidneys in picnic coolers, the vulnerability of the body's borders is thematized consistently throughout the novel: in scenes of child sexual assault; scars from military brutality during the Nigerian Civil War of 1967–1970; and murder and torture by police. This vulnerability is, in turn, specifically located within charged national and historical sites—Elvis's rape in a colonial church; his father's death in the true-life government demolition of the Maroko ghetto; and his mentor "the King of the Beggars's" death in Freedom Square. Vivid sensory descriptions of both place and bodily effects extend Abani's critique beyond the violent state corruption that keeps Nigerians oppressed to the impossibility of experiencing a coherent individualism within the struggling nation. According to critics of Nigerian literature, Abani's bleak portrait of the nation is consistent with a broader generational discontent with the post-Independent state. For scholar Obi Nwakanma, Elvis's flight to America at the end of the novel "marks, once more, the contemporary Nigerian novelists' tendency to question, as a result of disillusionment, the value of nation and national belonging."[19] Abani uses the scene of organ exchange and kidnapping to dramatize the horror of more fundamentally dis-located individuals.

This brutal transport of organs and unwilling donors across national lines provides a crucial counterpoint to the seemingly hopeful migration story that resolves the book. Hope, again, becomes a crucial trope in the fantasy of organ sale and transplant. From the hope of passport or movement away from refugee life that opened this chapter to the hope of successful surgery and improved quality of life, the recurring themes of hope in these stories are not an accident, but a recurring condition of their possibility. The climactic events of the novel—beginning with Elvis's discovery of the black market organs, through the death of his father and the King, his own brutal torture at the hands of the military, and finally his completely impoverished condition as a caretaker for the beggar children—represent the complete disintegration of Elvis's life and community. Elvis has been brought to a state in which existence within Lagos is impossible. If individualism requires, at its core, self-determination over one's own body, Abani's 1980s Nigeria has failed in that basic condition. Finally, Redemption—with all the symbolic freight of both character and concept—arrives in the slum as a kind of deus ex machina, offering Elvis his own passport and visa as a means of escape to the USA. When Elvis asks why Redemption won't use the passport to fulfill the dreams he once expressed of reaching the USA, Redemption replies, "Because dis na my home. I be area boy, alaye. I no go fit for States" (317). In the interplay of body and place, self and nation that Abani has developed throughout the novel, Redemption is too much of-the-city to escape its disintegrating force; his identity is caught up in the label "area boy." Elvis, by contrast, is consistently marked in the novel as exceptional individual (artistic, well-read, ambitious, autodidact). Adélékè Adéèkó, like Nwakanma and other critics of the novel, places Abani within a cohort of novelists born post-Independence for whom resolving a novel with a character's exile to the USA is a common narrative device. He argues, "In the new novels, the activists' ethical obligations to the self and his or her immediate surrounding are not subordinated to them by their nationality.... The conscientious individual can leave the nation's shores untainted by the odium of betrayal."[20] Abani's novel preserves this structure as Elvis's escape is fiercely desired and made possible by his friends' sacrifice. Full expression of individuality, then, is reserved for an exceptional few, not offered as a model of national uplift as one might expect of earlier Nigerian writers. The final, hopeful note of the novel rings loudly as Elvis, hearing the name on his passport called by an airline clerk, approaches the desk and says, "Yes, this is Redemption."

Of course, individual redemption offered through migration to the USA is a vexed concept within the novel. Given Redemption-the-character's role in unseating Elvis's secure moral positions and his symbolic connection with the underbelly of the Lagos economy, any personal redemption offered through assuming his identity and passport seems shaky at best. Similarly, the too-hasty resolution to Elvis's crisis captured by the sudden re-appearance of the fugitive Redemption, his selfless offer of passport, and the purchase of the airline ticket (with money left over from the organ brokering deal), should prompt suspicion at the improbable and fantastic nature of Elvis's escape. Both *Dirty Pretty Things* and *GraceLand*, then, end on similar notes in airport settings, with central characters poised to flee the difficult circumstances of their former lives. In both cases, however, the weight and tone of the previous action carry onto the final page/frame, recasting these moments of individual escape as coming at a terrible cost of complicity in corrupt systems.

Up to and including this point in *GraceLand*, America represents a fantasy, captured in phrases like "Come and see American wonder" (66) called by local street magicians or in Redemption's early claim that "States is de place where dreams come true" (26). In a crucial reinforcement, however, of the notion of bodily vulnerability that makes individualism impossible, Abani represents 1970s–1980s Nigeria with permeable cultural boundaries, already caught in the global flow of film, music, and books. Elvis and his friends hotly debate the merits of John Wayne vs "Actor"; his mother names him for Elvis Presley, and his favorite authors are James Baldwin and Ralph Ellison. The USA is strikingly present already within Nigeria, infusing Elvis's cultural frame. The title of the novel, *GraceLand*, and its conclusion with Elvis's pursuit of redemption in the States underscore a series of playful double meanings that locate hope and promise first within cultural forms that move across permeable boundaries of self and nation. The dangerous undercurrent, however, to this permeability lies in the possibility of unwanted incursions like rape and organ theft. Ultimately, both Frears and Abani suggest, the hopeful possibilities of migration coexist (or in this case, are literally funded by) the violent disintegration of boundaries.

Deferred Arrival

GraceLand and *Dirty Pretty Things* conclude with uncannily similar scenes located in airports—spaces characterized by hope, mobility, and the permeability of borders. Despite our protagonists' assertions that "this is Redemption" and "I'm coming home," the romantic promise of arrival is deferred crucially in both of these works. Like the hotels, refugee villages, and slums in which many black market accounts of organ sale are set, the airport—despite its typically positive encoding—is also fundamentally a space of flux and transit. These scenes, then, serve as an apt metaphor for the requirement of hope and mobility that animate organ sale coupled with the deferral of an uncomplicated resolution. For both organ sellers and recipients, even successful transplants typically do not take the form of an "ending." Sellers find themselves with complications post-surgery and compromised ability to find work. Recipients must continue a regime of expensive anti-rejection drugs for the remainder of their lives and often struggle with the enduring physical, psychological, and material consequences of chronic illness. In contrast to the fantasy of resolution offered even in mainstream "gift of life" campaigns, both sellers and recipients typically find themselves at odds with the dominant story of organ exchange by living in a state of deferred resolution.

The narrative beats in the fictional accounts examined here are strikingly resonant with anthropological studies of organ sale. In their multi-site fieldwork in Brazil, Argentina, South Africa, Mexico, India, and Bangladesh, Nancy Scheper-Hughes and Lawrence Cohen have encountered evidence of exploitative organ brokering. The stories they recount span tales of outright theft of organs during unrelated surgical procedures to financial crises prompting the sale of kidneys for as little as a thousand dollars. In Scheper-Hughes and Cohen's work, the differing circumstances of the organ loss read as simply variations in a common story: Impoverished individuals in unstable circumstances sell or have an organ stolen and are then left adrift with little possibility of redress, whether financial, medical, or legal. In conversations with female organ sellers in South India—women not unlike the residents of "Kidneyville"—Cohen asks them if the sale made a difference in their lives. The women say yes, temporarily, until the original circumstances of their poverty—borrowing money, high-interest rates, borrowing more—return. He then asks if they would do it again: "Yes, the women answered, what other choice did they have, with the money gone and the new debts piling up? If only there were three kidneys, with two to spare, then things might be better."[21] The circularity of these logics—caught in an unstable cycle of borrowing, wishing for another "spare" kidney to give again—is the structuring force of kidney sale and its outcome. None of the stories related by Scheper-Hughes, Cohen, or Scott Carney describe individuals catapulted to new lives of freedom and stability after their decision to sell an organ. Instead, they are stories of limbo and flux, where moneylenders, doctors, and family members consume profits, and little progress is realized. In addition to the original circumstances of poverty, organ sellers are also often caught in a new snare of medical complications and lost wages from longer-than-expected recovery periods.

While brokers and cultural representations—from news accounts to television melodramas—emphasize the operations themselves as the endings, those close to organ exchange know that such accounts mask the medical realities. Triumphant tales of "the gift of life" collapse "life" into the moment of exchange—frozen in the airport departures lounge—and ignore the journey to come. While longitudinal studies of organ sellers are limited, the data we do have suggests that outcomes for these patients are strongly negative.[22] In Pakistan, among a sample cohort of over 200 organ sellers, 93% said they had sold a kidney to repay a debt and 85% reported no economic improvement in their lives (Budiani-Saberi and Delmonico 927). The news on health-related outcomes is no better. Sellers across the world consistently describe pain, weakness, weight loss, and frequent illness following surgery.[23] These consequences should be understood in contrast to studies of living kidney donors in the USA, which suggest that donation in the USA is very safe. Harvard ethicist I. Glenn Cohen cites another survey of sellers in Pakistan where, despite reporting good health before the transplant, only 1.2% said their health was good after it (270). In exploring the ethical dimensions of transnational organ sale, Cohen emphasizes the temporal conditions of the discussion. While studies like those cited above suggest that sellers both experienced negative outcomes and many regret having donated, Cohen points out that such concerns are after the fact. He uses the language of *ex post* and *ex ante* to argue that organ sale appears to be a case of mutually advantageous exploitation since the fact that they agreed to the transaction "is strong evidence that they *ex ante* believed themselves to be all things considered benefitted rather than harmed" by the sale

(275). Rather than rehearse the ethical debate that Cohen conducts, I point out how the emphasis on *ex ante* mindset draws on the notions of hope represented by the sale. By drawing a bright line between the promise of repaid debts, dowries, and money for migration against the experienced realities of illness and renewed financial trouble, the ethical argument reflects the structuring trope of romantic hope.

Following the language of romance—of matching, journeys, hope, and destination—it is interesting to observe that the same condition of arrested arrival can also describe the experience of the organ recipient. While this chapter focuses largely on the roles of the organ seller and broker, popular representations of organ recipients similarly follow the tropes of romantic fulfillment. The successful transplant surgery promises a "happily ever after," but like most fairy tales, fails to publicize what after truly looks like. Stories of surgical triumph ignore the debilitating effects of immunosuppressant drug therapies and the continued lived experience of diseases like diabetes that may have caused the organ failure in the first place. Recipients often describe post-surgical problems including difficulty sustaining work, failed relationships, fatigue among friends and relatives, and depression.[24] Transplant anesthesiologist Richard I. Cook captures the post-surgical realities experienced by many recipients:

> the transplant recipient is committed to a lifetime of intrusive medical interventions and a future filled with new hazards. Post-implantation immunosuppression takes its toll on the patient, clearing the pathway for exotic infections and cancer, and these changes in the patient's lot are more of a burden than any healthy person would willingly undertake. And the transplanted organs fail, sometimes within months of implantation. The eagerness of patients with end-stage kidney disease or heart failure to undergo transplant is as much testimony to the horrors of those illnesses as to the wonders of transplantation.[25]

Cook's description captures the complex interruptions in more conventional stories tracing an arc from illness, to desperate wait on the transplant list, and ending with restoration to health post-surgery. Like the paths of migration described above, which are most appropriately understood as temporary, circular, or arrested, health and illness are extremes of a spectrum along which patients will shuttle back and forth over time. While this nonlinear and bumpy path is the lived reality for many transplant recipients, it's rarely the narrative structure in traditional accounts of transplant success and failure.

Medical analysts working toward a better understanding of surgical success have begun to deviate from the romantic notions of fulfillment that structure both popular and medical accounts. Increasingly, long-term survival and complication rates are deemed insufficient to account for what might constitute "success" in organ transplantation. As strictly defined survival rates have increased along with better technologies and postoperative therapies, medical analysts are looking toward quantitative measures of "quality of life" to rethink policies around allocation and reconstitute the definition of success.[26] Because of high monetary costs, intensive demand on hospital resources, and the scarcity of available organs, organ transplant is a focus in an emerging area of quality of life assessment for surgical procedures more broadly. Among kidney patients—the organs most typically traded on the black market—measures of quality of life post-surgery reflect the least gain among other solid state organ transplant recipients.[27] This finding is likely because dialysis allows for a relatively high ability to perform daily activities pre-surgery and because the frequency of severe diabetes among these patients will have a continued impact on their health post-surgery. What this turn to quality of life measures suggests is that the teleological thinking that structures most transplant narratives, even black market ones, according to the promise of successful arrival is, in fact, a false happy ending. Bare surgical survival is an insufficient measure of success. The recipient's journey does not end in Israel, South Africa, or other sites of transplant tourism, but continues, often for years, in looping back through medical systems as a patient requiring therapy.

"Transplant tourism" has a kind of cheerful ring that belies the realities of the practice. In an article called "The State of International Organ Trade" (2007), Yosuke Shimazono follows the practice of the World Health Organization in defining transplant tourism as an "overseas transplantation when a patient obtains an organ through the organ trade or other means that contravene the regulatory frameworks of their countries of origin."[28] While transplant tourism is part of a broader commodification of organ exchange (especially as a lucrative source of revenue for medical centers), it is important to remember that not all international organ exchange is illegal.[29] Receiving an organ outside of one's country of residence is legal in several countries, including the USA, Britain, Japan, China, Thailand, Colombia, and the Philippines.[30] In the USA, the United Network for Organ Sharing (UNOS) has established policy allowing up to 5% of organs transplanted within the USA to go to nonresidents. Such operations are often more lucrative for the hospitals as tourists are billed for the full amount of their procedures (although for some patients in countries with low rates of donation, these bills will be channeled through their domestic insurance systems). Web sites have emerged to capitalize on the transplant tourism trend; with catchy names like "kidney4you.org," these sites offer "transplant packages" ranging from $70,000 to $160,000 (as documented in 2007).[31]

Israeli patients and brokers have recently been at the center of a series of international controversies surrounding transplant tourism and organ trafficking. In 2012, Rabbi Levy-Izhak Rosenbaum became the first man ever convicted under a US law banning the sale of organs. An Israeli national living in Brooklyn, Rosenbaum was an orthodox rabbi running a side brokerage in organs between American recipients and Israeli donors. While impoverished Israelis have been sellers of organs in international trafficking rings, their more wealthy compatriots have been recipients of organs off the black market. Nancy Scheper-Hughes tells the story of Avraham, an Israeli who traveled to an undisclosed location in Eastern Europe and bought an organ from a "peasant." Although told by his doctors that transplant surgery would be risky at his age and that dialysis was the best option, "Avraham protested that he was not yet ready for the 'medical trash heap,' which is the way he and many other Israeli kidney patients now view hemodialysis. And, like a growing number of kidney patients, he rejected the idea of a cadaver organ (the 'dead man's organ') as 'disgusting' and unacceptable."[32] This notion of cadaver organs as "disgusting" reflects broader ideological forces within Israel, which act in a kind of Möbius strip of cause and effect, cultural construct, and material conditions. Recipients seek live donors in part because of low consent rates among the families of brain-dead individuals. But low consent rates map onto ideological assumptions about the impermissibility of tampering with one's body before and after death in Judaism and long-standing concepts of the dead in Jewish tradition. Shunning cadaver organs as "disgusting," then, mutually reflects both material and cultural conditions.

JESICA SANTILLAN: AN INTERSECTIONAL CASE

The fraught web of factors influencing international organ exchange is nowhere more evident than in the tragic case of Jesica Santillan. In the years after her birth, Jesica's mother noticed that her daughter had trouble breathing. Her condition worsened and by age twelve she was diagnosed with restrictive cardiomyopathy. Understanding that they would be unable to find adequate medical care in their native Mexico, the family immigrated illegally to the USA and settled in North Carolina. Through the support of a sympathetic wealthy patron, her mother's health insurance from work, and the local community, Jesica and her family gained access to the medical support that placed her on the transplant list. Three years later, at age 17, she learned she would receive new organs. On February 7, 2003, surgeons at Duke University Hospital performed her heart-lung transplantation. Almost immediately, they realized something was wrong—they had transplanted organs of an incorrect blood type. Jesica was type O and the donated organs were type A. Her immune system rejected the new organs and she fell into a coma. Duke admitted the mistake, recriminations were made by the family and their patron, and ultimately a second set of organs was found. But it was too late to correct the mistake. Jesica died on February 23, nearly two weeks after her initial operation.

During those two weeks, while Jesica remained unconscious in the hospital, the national media took up her story and exposed an evolving set of questions that resonate with many of the most profound ethical and political issues of the day. Jesica's case became a flashpoint, drawing together a remarkably diverse series of national concerns. In the early days, Jesica was represented as a tragic victim of medical error, a phenomenon of rising concern in the era of elite medicine. At the point of her second transplant operation, public reaction pivoted and widespread fears about fairness in the allocation system came to dominate coverage; how, onlookers wondered, could someone rise to the top of the list again so quickly? Surely strings were pulled as Duke University Hospital attempted to absolve itself of the earlier error. Then, after her death, a lingering trope in the case—Jesica's immigrant status—became dominant. As California's Proposition 187 and Donald Trump's presidential campaign illustrate, the question of access to medical resources for undocumented immigrants is an animating anxiety of American political life. In their edited volume, *A Death Retold: Jesica Santillan, the Bungled*

Transplant, and Paradoxes of Medical Citizenship, Keith Wailoo, Julie Livingston, and Peter Guarnaccia bring together scholars from diverse fields to explore the many enmeshed features of this case.[33] Their volume, which has become an often-read text in medical anthropology, offers a detailed chronicle of the profound ways in which the death of a 17-year-old Mexican immigrant girl holds together so many social concerns. Medical error, tort reform, elite medicine, immigration, nationalism, fairness in organ allocation, futile treatment, and organ shortages: Each of these topics spirals out from Jesica's case into a rich vein of discussion. In the analysis below, I use the framework already constructed throughout this chapter—that of romantic tropes of hope, mobility, and deferred arrival—and return to these questions from the angle of the organ recipient, rather than the seller or broker.

News coverage of Jesica's case immediately adopts the familiar romantic language of a hopeful journey. The *New York Times* coverage captures this sensibility most emblematically in the following line: The family had "been on an odyssey to save their daughter's life that had taken them from the shacks of Guadalajara to the self-proclaimed City of Medicine."[34] As the "City of Medicine," Durham, NC becomes a kind of Oz, metonymic for elite medicine and its exceptional promise. Coverage is peppered with phrases like "promise," "hope," "brighter future," and "lifesaving medicine." In this case, the typical immigrant story of journey and promise is made more dramatic and literal as the Santillans travel not just to improve the life of their child, but to save it. In this way, Jesica and her family are both the embodiment and a threat to conventional and romanticized formulations of the American Dream. As Susan Morgan and her colleagues also argue, stories that represent the Santillans' achieving the hopeful promise of a better life in America are the fulfillment of the founding American myth. But, the darker nationalist impulses in American culture also see this very achievement as unjust theft, "robb[ing] other American transplant patients … of the 'dream at a chance at life.'"[35] The romantic fantasy of successful odyssey is powerfully motivating—driving the family to pay a smuggler and journey through the desert—but its achievement is also contested. Transplantation, as a literal manifestation of more abstract anxieties about the permeability of borders, serves as a striking cultural touchstone for discussions about immigration and the rights of noncitizens.

As Jesica's story began to evolve in the national consciousness, public discussions of her immigrant status began to evolve as well. While her national origin was a continuing feature of coverage from the beginning, she began to be portrayed less as a tragic victim who had risked everything for a chance at a better life and more as a "racialized foreigner sapping America's resources."[36] Leo Chavez places this evolving coverage into the broader context of American anti-immigrant sentiment in recent decades. He cites Samuel Huntington, writing in 2004 for *Foreign Policy*, as an example of resurgent nativist hostility: "In this new era … the single most immediate and most serious challenge to America's traditional identity comes from the immense and continuing immigration from Latin America, especially from Mexico, and the fertility rates of those immigrants compared to black and white American natives."[37] The hyperbole of Huntington's comments—especially when placed in their post-9/11 geopolitical context—is an example of the depth of anti-immigrant sentiment: *the single most immediate and most serious challenge*? Note, too, the way in which these ideas are typically expressed in embodied terms. Anxieties over the fertility rates of immigrants, the "changing face" of America, focus on manual labor, and metaphors of invading hordes all come together to make immigrant bodies highly contested ground. Abstract conversations about national resources become literal in Jesica's case, especially when viewed through the zero-sum game of organ scarcity and allocation. Reports in the Raleigh *News and Observer* characterize at least one local resident as reconsidering her status as an organ donor in the wake of Santillan's case. Preferring that her organs go to a US citizen, this sixty-five-year-old woman told a reporter, "I definitely do not want them to go to an illegal alien.… I don't think they should be able to come in here and take our hospital and our medicine and turn around and sue us."[38]

Spokespersons from UNOS sought to temper this response, understanding the fragility of public confidence in the allocation system. UNOS policy directs no more than 5% of organs donated within the USA to eligible nonresidents. And immigrants, in fact, donate more organs than they receive. These facts, however, are often lost in high profile and anomalous cases such as Jesica's. The conditions of Jesica's migration to the USA would have precluded her from eligibility under these policies, but neither UNOS nor the hospital is in the business of checking immigration status. In describing this form of legal transplant tourism in America, Nancy Scheper-Hughes argues, "The United States is very democratic in at least one sense—anyone with enough cash, regardless of where they come from, can become a 'medical citizen' of the United States and be transplanted, even with a scarce, 'made in the U.S.A.' transplant organ."[39] The language of trade and citizenship here reinforces the tightly woven strands of this debate. As we've seen throughout this volume, decisions about organ exchange are not simply medical, but also profoundly social. As such, they reveal surprising connections among seemingly unrelated spheres. In this instance, the specter of an undocumented immigrant receiving not one but two American organs raises deeply held anxieties about the distribution of national resources—resources that are, in this case, made strikingly literal.

The over-determining framework of scarce resources for transplantation heightens existing nationalist concerns over their "proper" recipients. But as the specter in almost all discussions of organ exchange, scarcity operates across several debates, often taken as an opening premise. In the evolving and multifaceted discussions surrounding Jesica's case, her second surgery—the fact that she had received not just one, but two heart-lung transplants—puts pressure on many of the prevailing public notions of transplantation. In addition to the nationalist-inflected debate over the fairness of an undocumented immigrant receiving elite care in the USA, reactions to Jesica's second transplant challenge medical standards for how scarce organs are allocated. Where the challenges in the first category are largely political, this second conversation was largely focused on medical concerns about futility. As Keith Wailoo and Julie Livingston argue in their essay, "The Politics of Second Chances," debates over medical futility are a rising concern.[40] Along these lines, Jesica's second operation served as a pivot point in public opinion. News sources consistently represented such a second surgery as rare and many questioned the appropriateness of a surgery whose promise seemed dim. This backlash is, in part, rooted in widely held romantic fantasies about transplantation. As Wailoo and Livingston argue, the public faith in transplantation as "miracle cure" is at odds with both the realities of this case—in which a bureaucracy failed to catch an ultimately fatal error and the heroic doctor could not right the wrong—and in transplant medicine more broadly in which failure of a transplanted organ is often a matter of time. They describe a "broader mythic lay understanding of transplanted organs (perpetuated by donation networks and transplant professionals, to be sure)—that they are 'healthy' organs that effectively and completely replace sick ones, thus fundamentally renewing the body."[41] As in UNOS's anxiety to correct public opinion about nonresident access to American organs, this mythos of assured cure is important in securing public commitment to the donation system. Recipients and their families are equally sustained by this romantic vision. Hope becomes a dominant force in the lives of these patients and the painful realities of deferred arrival described above are pushed away from consciousness.

In addition to the public and patients, a third group approaches the problem of medical futility through hope and promise deferred: doctors. For medical professionals, commitment to individual patients and the promise of future breakthroughs in treatment methods often buttress their position in debates about medical futility. In the 1980s, Thomas Starzl was often criticized for pursuing liver transplantation in an era when patient survival was well below 50%. Whole volumes have been written about the complex ethical calculus conducted by doctors like Starzl and his colleagues and the choice to pursue experimental surgery in a clinical setting. Despite this early criticism, however, Starzl is most often lauded as a "pioneer" in his field, demonstrating how profoundly the romantic metaphors of hope, travel, and the technological frontier structure our acceptance of experimental practices. At the level of the individual patient, Starzl has offered a strong defense of seemingly futile second operations like the one Jesica Santillan received, telling reporter Lee Gutkind, "There is no physician who will withdraw care from patients whose brains are alive, and if you force them to do that, they will quit their practice. The Hippocratic Oath and the bond on the individual basis between the doctor and the patient is still the fundamental credo with which medicine is practiced" (242). In Starzl's speech, we see again how romantic tropes structure participation in organ exchange; he emphatically cites his oath and creed, the bond between individuals, and offers a heroic threat of quitting his practice if asked to compromise his commitment. This romanticized sense of self animates the challenging and high stakes work of transplantation.

Taken together with sentiment and horror, we can see how the genre of romance serves as a structuring frame for organ exchange. Academic debates about ethical models of allocation or compensation and human rights interventions into trafficking networks suggest possible new directions in policy or international law. But a study of the intersections between ideological forces and material realities can both tell us the foundations of our beliefs and practices as well as offering a path toward new attitudes.

Notes

1. Scott M. Carney, *The Red Market: On the Trail of the World's Organ Brokers, Bone Thieves, Blood Farmers, and Child Traffickers*, 1st ed. (New York, NY: William Morrow, 2011), 62. Other estimates of kidney sale in Tsunami Nagar, place the number of kidney removals much lower, citing thirty-five women who have documented sales with local authorities, "Tsunami Nagar: Kidney Case Handed over to Crime Branch," *The Indian Express*, January 19, 2007, http://www.indianexpress.com/news/tsunami-nagar-kidney-case-handed-over-to-crime-branch/21242/. The article concedes, however, that investigators were confident that more women had sold kidneys but were afraid to come forward.
2. It is worth noting that with the exception of Iran, it is illegal to sell organs from a living donor in every other country in the world. Both Israel and Holland have begun discussions of a system of compensation, but have not passed such legislation to date.
3. Scheper-Hughes, "Comodity Fetishism," 33–36.
4. Lawrence Cohen, "The Other Kidney," 9.
5. Scheper-Hughes, "Consuming Differences," 213.
6. Ibid., 219.
7. Larry Rohter, "The Organ Trade: A Global Black Market, Tracking the Sale of a Kidney on a Path of Poverty and Hope," *The New York Times*, May 23, 2004, http://www.nytimes.com/2004/05/23/world/organ-trade-global-black-market-tracking-sale-kidney-path-poverty-hope.html?pagewanted=print&src=pm.
8. Such comparisons to prostitution are not uncommon. Scheper-Hughes also cites the Eastern European country of Moldova as a place where organ sale carries with it the stigma of prostitution. Scheper-Hughes, "Consuming Differences," 217.
9. Nancy Scheper-Hughes, "Commodity Fetishism in Organs Trafficking," *Body and Society* 7, no. 2–3 (September 2001): 45.
10. Ibid., 42.
11. Sarah Gibson, "Border Politics and Hospitable Spaces in Stephen Frears's *Dirty Pretty Things*," *Third Text* 20, no. 6 (November 2006): 693–701; Emily Davis, "The Intimacies of Globalization: Bodies and Borders On-Screen," *Camera Obscura: Feminism, Culture, and Media Studies* 21, no. 2, 62 (January 2006): 32–73; and Donna McCormack, "Initmate Borders: The Ethics of Human Organ Transplantation in Contemporary Film," *Review of Education, Pedagogy, and Cultural Studies* 34, no. 3–4 (2012): 170–183.

12. Ashley Dawson, "The People You Don't See: Immigration and Gender in Monica Ali's *Brick Lane*," *Ariel: A Review of International English Literature* 40, no. 1 (2009): 125.
13. See Homi Bhabha et al., "Cosmopolitanisms," *Public Culture* 12, no. 3 (September 1, 2000): 577–589; Kwame Anthony Appiah, *Cosmopolitanism: Ethics in a World of Strangers*, Issues of Our Time (New York: W. W. Norton & Company, 2006); and on cosmopolitanism as a driving force in Rushdie's fiction see Rüdiger Kunow, "Architect of the Cosmopolitan Dream: Salman Rushdie," *Amerikastudien/American Studies* 51, no. 3 (2006): 369–385.
14. *Dirty Pretty Things*, directed by Stephen Frears (Miramax, 2002).
15. Sarah Gibson focuses on these bookending airport scenes as representing the "doors into the British nation." She goes on to focus on the hotel as the pivotal space for analyzing the break between asylum seekers and tourists, especially where each is caught in political rhetorics of hospitality. Gibson, "Border Politics and Hospitable Spaces," 74.
16. Chris Abani, *Graceland* (New York: Picador, 2004), 7.
17. Julia Kristeva, *Powers of Horror: An Essay on Abjection*, trans. Leon S. Roudiez (New York: Columbia University Press, 1982).
18. Veronica Hendrick situates the characters' role in modern human trafficking in the context of Africans' participation in the transatlantic slave trade. Hendrick draws from Joseph Miller's historical account of slavery to highlight the triangulated relationship among powerful slave trader, marginal local leader, and human cargo to find a series of shifting parallels for these triangulated roles throughout the novel. In the context of my argument, the historical role of the marginal local leader as an intermediary parallels the modern role of the broker and the emerging national sites of transplant tourism in places like South Africa, urban India, and Brazil. Veronica Hendrick, "Negotiating Nigeria: Connecting Chris Abani's *GraceLand* to Africa's Past," in *Emerging African Voices: A Study of Contemporary African Literature*, ed. Walter P. Collins (Amherst, NY: Cambria Press, 2010), 84, 93–95.
19. Obi Nwakanma, "Metonymic Eruptions: Igbo Novelists, the Narrative of the Nation, and New Developments in the Contemporary Nigerian Novel," *Research in African Literatures* 39, no. 2 (Summer 2008): 13. Nwakanma situates the cosmopolitanism and migratory impulses that recur throughout these novels with an "Igbo traveling identity," connecting a seemingly contemporary critique with an enduring historical factor that propels the literature.
20. Adélékè Adéèkó, "Power Shift: America in the New Nigerian Imagination," *The Global South* 2, no. 2 (October 1, 2008), 12.

21. Recounted in Nancy Scheper-Hughes, "Commodity Fetishism," 38. While I have chosen to quote from Scheper-Hughes's description here because of the evocative language of a "spare" kidney and the circularity of the logic, this argument is also informed by Lawrence Cohen's own account of his fieldwork in "The Other Kidney."
22. For accounts of post-surgical outcomes among organ sellers, see Lawrence Cohen, "The Other Kidney"; Scheper-Hughes "Commodity Fetishism"; I. Glenn Cohen, "Transplant Tourism: The Ethics and Regulation of International Markets for Organs," *The Journal of Law, Medicine & Ethics* 41, no. 1 (April 1, 2013): 269–285; D. A. Budiani-Saberi and F. L. Delmonico, "Organ Trafficking and Transplant Tourism: A Commentary on the Global Realities," *American Journal of Transplantation* 8, no. 5 (May 1, 2008): 925–929; Carney, *The Red Market*; and Yosuke Shimazono, "The State of the International Organ Trade: A Provisional Picture Based on Integration of Available Information," *Bulletin of the World Health Organization* 85, no. 12 (December 2007): 955–962.
23. I. Glenn Cohen, "Transplant Tourism," 271.
24. Sharp, *Strange Harvest*, 107–123.
25. Richard I. Cook, "Hobson's Choices," 49.
26. For more on how quality of life measures are used to assess organ transplantation, see C. Wright Pinson et al., "Health-Related Quality of Life After Different Types of Solid Organ Transplantation," *Annals of Surgery* 232, no. 4 (October 2000): 597–607; Matthew Eatough, "The Time That Remains: Organ Donation, Temporal Duration, and *Bildung* in Kazuo Ishiguro's *Never Let Me Go*," *Literature and Medicine* 29, no. 1 (2011): 132–160. Eatough places quality of life assessments from medical discourse in conversation with the representation of affective indifference in Kazuo Ishiguro's *Never Let Me Go*, discussed at greater length in my chapter on sentiment.
27. See Pinson, et al., "Health Related Quality of Life."
28. Shimazono, "The State of the International Organ Trade," 956.
29. For more on the overlap between transplant tourism and international definitions of human trafficking (including organs), see Budiani-Saberi and Delmonico, "Organ Trafficking and Transplant Tourism."
30. Rob Verger, "Israel's Campaign to Halt Organ Trafficking Tourism," *The Daily Beast*, March 18, 2012, http://www.thedailybeast.com/articles/2012/03/18/israel-s-campaign-to-halt-organ-trafficking-tourism.html.
31. Shimazono, "The State of the International Organ Trade."
32. Scheper-Hughes, "Consuming Differences," 216.
33. Keith Wailoo, Julie Livingston, and Peter Guarnaccia, eds., *A Death Retold: Jesica Santillan, the Bungled Transplant, and Paradoxes of Medical Citizenship* (Chapel Hill: University of North Carolina Press, 2006).

34. Jeffrey Gettleman and Lawrence K. Altman, "Girl in Donor Mix-Up Undergoes 2nd Transplant," *The New York Times*, February 21, 2003, http://www.nytimes.com/2003/02/21/us/girl-in-donor-mix-up-undergoes-2nd-transplant.html.
35. Susan E. Morgan et al., "America's Angel or Thieving Immigrant?: Media Coverage, the Santillan Story, and Publicized Ambivalence Toward Donation and Transplantation," in *A Death Retold: Jesica Santillan, the Bungled Transplant, and Paradoxes of Medical Citizenship*, ed. Keith Wailoo, Julie Livingston, and Peter Guarnaccia (Chapel Hill: University of North Carolina Press, 2006), 38.
36. Ibid.
37. Leo R. Chavez, "Imagining the Nation, Imagining Donor Recipients: Jesica Santillan and the Public Discourse of Belonging," in *A Death Retold: Jesica Santillan, the Bungled Transplant, and Paradoxes of Medical Citizenship*, ed. Keith Wailoo, Julie Livingston, and Peter Guarnaccia (Chapel Hill: University of North Carolina Press, 2006), 284.
38. Quoted in Leo R. Chavez, "Imagining the Nation," 290.
39. Scheper-Hughes, "Consuming Differences," 213.
40. As emblems of this rising movement in medical ethics, Wailoo and Livingston cite Lawrence J. Schneiderman and Nancy S. Jecker, *Wrong Medicine: Doctors, Patients, and Futile Treatment* (Baltimore, MD: Johns Hopkins University Press, 2000); Marjorie B. Zucker, Howard B. Zucker, and Alexander Morgan Capron, *Medical Futility: And the Evaluation of Life-Sustaining Interventions* (Cambridge: Cambridge University Press, 1997); and Susan Rubin, *When Doctors Say No: The Battleground of Medical Futility* (Bloomington: Indiana University Press, 1998).
41. Keith Wailoo and Julie Livingston, "The Politics of Second Changes: Waste, Futility, and the Debate over Jesica's Second Transplant," in *A Death Retold: Jesica Santillan, the Bungled Transplant, and Paradoxes of Medical Citizenship*, ed. Keith Wailoo, Julie Livingston, and Peter Guarnaccia (Chapel Hill: University of North Carolina Press, 2006), 124.

CHAPTER 8

Conclusion: Speculative Medicine, Speculative Fictions

A casual exchange in a reception buffet line forced me to reconsider this book. Or at least revealed to me its ending. The president of my college had attended a public talk I had given of the work in progress. Over chaffing dishes and napkin rolls of silverware, he told me that I had "better finish up that book quickly" because "before you know it, organ transplant is going to be obsolete." This kind of optimistic proclamation wasn't out of character for him. He was the kind of physicist-turned-administrator who believed that my preschool-age children will live to be 200 and that we will cure cancer within our lifetimes. In his vision, organ transplant will be obsolete either because we will discover the mechanism to arrest cell decay or we will have fully functioning artificial organs soon or we will have a new species of animal-human hybrid from which to farm kidneys, hearts, and livers. It was not the content of any of these suggestions that gave me pause. It was the conviction from which he dispensed his advice, his genuine concern that the pace of my research might not be fast enough to beat to publication a breakthrough in any of these areas, after which a cultural study of organ exchange would be irrelevant. He was operating as if the imagined and hoped-for future of transplant science had already come to pass or was imminent. And while his timeline is compressed and his optimism extreme, this conversation reminded me that this kind of imagination is a driving force in experimental medicine. Every day, scientists in countries all over the

E. Russell, *Transplant Fictions*,
Palgrave Studies in Literature, Science and Medicine,
https://doi.org/10.1007/978-3-030-12135-8_8

world are seeking advances in exactly these areas. As in the early days of transplantation, this work is often characterized by failures and seemingly insurmountable hurdles. It takes a tremendous effort of imagination and a fundamental temporal reframing to continue such experimentation in the face of these setbacks. This imaginative enterprise represents the final phase in this study of the fictions of transplantation, an enterprise I am calling "speculative medicine" as a parallel to the genre of speculative fiction.

Speculative fiction is most typically associated with science fiction, but can also include fantasy, utopias, the supernatural, and horror (or a combination of the above). In his 1947 essay "On Writing Speculative Fiction," Robert Heinlein distills the genre as a story that follows the question "What would happen if—?" It is the umbrella genre of anticipation, extrapolation, and new problems under imagined conditions. This narrative formula also drives the work of experimental medicine. While all scientists use questioning and hypothesis in their work, highly experimental medicine exists in an altered temporal frame, a "possible world" much like the settings of speculative fiction. In their essay on anticipation and technoscience, Vincanne Adams, Michelle Murphy, and Adele Clarke argue, "The present is governed, at almost every scale, as if the future is what matters most. Anticipatory modes enable the production of possible futures that are *lived and felt* as inevitable in the present."[1] They write that "sciences of *the actual* can be abandoned or ignored," replaced by the "speculative forecast" or "prediction" (247). Like "speculative," the term "anticipation" signals a special emphasis on both imagination and altered temporality. By operating as if imagined outcomes are inevitable achievements, highly experimental researchers can operate in an imagined possible future. In this realm of speculative medicine, the failures of today are consumed by an overwhelming priority given to the promise of the future.

Imagined medical triumphs are, of course, a popular and recurring theme in speculative fiction. In *The Island of Dr. Moreau* (1896), H.G. Wells extrapolates from the late nineteenth-century science of vivisection to an imagined reality in which continued experimentation produces a race of animal-human hybrids. Writing over a century later in *The Scar* (2004), China Miéville imagines a new planet populated by animal- and machine-human hybrids achieved through a combination of surgical technique and magic.[2] These works serve as emblematic bookends framing actual laboratory efforts to find non-human sources for transplantation. In her most recent book, *Transplant Imaginary*, Lesley Sharp looks at xenotransplantation and bioengineering as future-facing attempts to solve the problems of organ scarcity that plague transplantation in the present. Xenotransplantation involves any attempt to transplant animal organs, cells, or tissue into the human body; bioengineering in transplantation accounts for mechanical solutions to the same problem, as in an artificial heart. Sharp, too, frames these medical enterprises as caught up in questions of the future and the imagination. She writes, "Experimental science is by definition an *anticipatory* enterprise. Whereas funding proposals and associated research design are framed and driven by clearly articulated goals, outcomes are always hypothetical and, thus, unknown. In short, the black box of science obscures future knowledge, making way for imagination and desire."[3] The territory Sharp describes is also that of speculative fiction. A brief return to one classic in the genre, *The Island of Dr. Moreau*, can complement Sharp's insights from her ethnographic fieldwork. Where Sharp draws her conclusions from interviews with researchers in the field, H.G. Wells's novel offers another pathway into the medical imaginary and reveals some of its central mechanisms.

Animated by the advances and scandals of vivisection in the late nineteenth century, *The Island of Dr. Moreau* serves as a symbol of scientific experimentation and fantasies of hybridity.[4] In addition to several editions of the novel, at least three popular films have been attempted, a testament to the enduring nature of its speculative form. In the story, our narrator Edward Prendick, also a dilettante scientist, has been marooned on an island dedicated to radical surgical experimentation under the direction of the notorious Dr. Moreau. Prendick encounters a bizarre collection of creatures living in the jungle surrounding the makeshift operating laboratory. Although Prendick believes the creatures to have started their lives as human, Moreau corrects him; they "were not men, had never been men. They were animals—humanized animals—triumphs of vivisection!" (70–71). In an example of the extrapolation so important to speculative fiction, Moreau draws from true historical details of plastic surgery and early transplantation in his explanation. He references Hunter's cockspur, tooth transplants, and the corrective surgery in which noses destroyed by syphilis were repaired by sewing a flap of skin from the patient's own forehead or arm to the damaged area. Although Prendick recoils at these "monsters manufactured!," Wells is careful to place Moreau's work in a speculative lineage of actual science, forcing readers to confront both the opportunities and caution represented by stepping beyond the bounds of what is currently possible.

Upon his first encounter with the creatures, Prendick is struck by "two inconsistent and conflicting impressions of utter strangeness and yet of the strangest familiarity" (42). He studies them from a distance and finds in these human-seeming forms "some now irresistible suggestion of a hog, a swinish taint, the unmistakable mark of the beast" (42). The contemporary science of xenotransplantation is predicated precisely on finding and encouraging this "strangest familiarity." Researchers look to different animal species to discover a link of the familiar that will overcome the divide between human and animal. As Lesley Sharp documents, different animals have found favor at different times over the century, with primates and pigs being elevated most recently as "the ideal match for human bodies."[5] This genetic (primates) and physiological (pigs) familiarity, however, also makes hybrid experimentation troubling. In her study of monstrosity and xenotransplantation, Mary Murray draws upon Sigmund Freud's theory of the uncanny to capture the destabilizing conceptual impact of these experiments. By revealing a typically buried association between human and animal, "genetically modified animals and organs carrying human genes allude to the anxiety-provoking double that Freud identified as arousing dread and creeping horror."[6]

Despite this dread and protest, however, the "strangest familiarity" evoked by laboratory hybrids demonstrates a profound mechanism by which the medical imaginary operates. As in speculative fiction, researchers move from the familiar into the terrain of the increasingly distant. The object of the experiment, even when radical, does not exist outside the realm of what is conceivable, what is in some basic sense known and familiar. Even where Prendick has an impression of "utter strangeness," this feeling is managed simultaneously by a conflicting sense of familiarity. The imagination fills in the gaps of the strange, assimilating it to the terms of our understanding. Often, these reaches of the imagination are made familiar by relying on literary tools of metaphor and reference. At xenotransplantation conferences, researchers commonly make references to the creatures of transnational mythology, from centaurs to sphinxes.[7] Media accounts of these scientific endeavors will illustrate their articles with screenshots of movies like *Planet of the Apes*, *Splice*, or *The Island of Dr. Moreau*. Lesley Sharp also insightfully describes the importance of lab animals as the "fact that they serve as proxies for other things."[8] They must "stand in for something radically different,"[9] specifically humans suffering from the same illness or mutation. Although Sharp does not make her argument in these terms, lab animals, then, operate like metaphors, drawing together seemingly unrelated things through the vehicle of genetic modification. In this form of imaginative and biological substitution, we find both possibility and anxiety. Genetically modified pigs may offer hope that we can conquer the problem of scarcity in transplantation, but it also suggests an "irresistible suggestion of the hog, a swinish taint" already present in us all. Like metaphors, these laboratory substitutions are the ground of speculation; they propose connections, but are not quite identical and therefore require imagination and possibility to make up the gap.

The Island of Dr. Moreau is a warning about the dangerous excesses of scientific experimentation, but it is also an analogy used to explore the prevailing theories of its day. In his extravagant plotline, Wells draws explicitly from contemporary understandings of evolution and devolution. Dr. Moreau describes the central problem of his work as the fact that "somehow the things drift back again," but then insists in the same breath, "I mean to do better things still. I mean to conquer that" (77). This speech cuts to the core of social theories of evolution—things can be changed in their essence and we can pursue that progress through manipulation and experiment. But it also sounds the warning knell of devolution—degeneration is always a looming possibility. Prendick expresses this anxiety most openly in the end of the novel. He has returned to Britain and sees in his fellow citizens a new form of the "strangest familiarity." He writes, "I look about me at my fellow men. And I go in fear. I see faces keen and bright, others dull or dangerous, others unsteady, insincere; none that have the calm authority of a reasonable soul. I feel as though the animal was surging up through them; that presently the degradation of the Islanders will be played over again on a larger scale" (130). In these closing moments, Wells articulates the ideological complexities that exist alongside and animate the ethical and technical challenges of medical experimentation. Human-animal hybrids are difficult, not only because they require cutting-edge advances in immunology and genetics, but because they disrupt our notions of personhood and of the social body. Mary Murray draws from qualitative surveys in the UK and Australia to demonstrate ways that the notion of monstrosity has crept into public attitudes about xenotransplantation. One researcher closely echoes Prendick's worries about the degradation of his fellow men into a lurking inner animal: "my informants feel that something uncontrollable had been released, something that can be pumped through the whole blood system to build up, break down, or otherwise change their bodies."[10] As in earlier discussions of the conflicting logics of the spare parts analogy and the belief in transmigration of the donor, respondents alternated between finding pig organs less or more objectionable. Both attitudes, though, reveal something about how people define humanity, the human-animal order, and the lengths to which we should go to extend life.

Acts of imagination are central to both support of and resistance to speculative medicine. Even this brief analysis of *The Island of Dr. Moreau* reveals the way that speculative fiction about human-animal hybrids can serve as an analogy to unpack larger social concerns. Similarly, speculation about the actual medical use of hybrids reveals no less complex attitudes about foundational ideological categories. Alongside mixed opinion surveys, we find legislative efforts to curb advances in xenotransplantation. In one such example, then-Congressman Sam Brownback (R, Kansas) introduced the "Human-Animal Hybrid Protection Act of 2009."[11] The "Findings" section of the bill (which did not leave committee) demonstrates Brownback's anxiety around hybridity as violating a series of key boundary categories: "human-animal hybrids are grossly unethical because they blur the line between human and animal, male and female, parent and child, and one individual and another individual." But imaginative speculation also serves as a space of possibility, hope, and excitement. In an act that she calls "the biotechnical embrace," Mary-Jo DelVecchio Good argues, "Americans invest in the medical imaginary—the many-possibility enterprise—culturally and emotionally, as well as financially. Enthusiasm for medicine's possibilities arises not necessarily from material products with therapeutic efficacy but through the production of ideas, and potential although not yet proven therapeutic efficacy."[12] Many cite this zeal for innovation—"the many-possibility enterprise"—as the extraordinary character of the USA, a key feature of American Exceptionalism. The pervasive nature of this imaginative speculation underscores the importance of cultural studies methods. Close reading of language and representation can help us understand how we came to the conceptual possibility of transplantation in the first place and what medical evolution may look like in the future. As Susan Squier has argued, science fiction, in particular, because it is a transformative narrative, can enable the transformative practice of transplant medicine.[13]

Speculative fiction shows us how to imagine and live in possible worlds, replacing the disappointments of the actual with a new space of what if.

This projection into the future of transplantation prompts a turn into the past. After all, we are currently living in the once-fantasy world where lives are saved every day by the transplantation of organs from one body into another. Obstacles that once seemed immovable—anastomosis, immunosuppression, heart bypass, dialysis—are now all commonplace strategies to extend or improve the lives of the very sick. How did our predecessors tackle the challenges of their present through optimistic speculation about the future? By looking back at one historical dilemma—with the advantage of knowing how their future would unfold—we find echoes of our own optimistic predictions of the medical frontiers that were seen but as yet out of reach.

In November 1962, *Life* magazine described the work of the awkwardly named "Admissions and Policies Committee of the Seattle Artificial Kidney Center at Swedish Hospital." This group of "seven humble laymen" were tasked with a seemingly impossible task: Determining who should receive potentially life-saving treatment for kidney failure.[14] In this early form of dialysis, patients came to the center twice a week for 10–12 hour sessions with "the miraculous machine." At the time, kidney disease killed around one hundred thousand people in the USA alone, and only one in fifty were considered eligible for the treatment. Once medical eligibility had been established by doctors, the hospital determined that patient selection should be conducted by a committee based on factors they would determine. The group included "a lawyer, a minister, a banker, a housewife, an official of state government, a labor leader, and a surgeon.... all high-minded, good-hearted citizens, much like the patients themselves who were selected as a microcosm of society-at-large" (Alexander 106). Explicit in the work of these individuals, colloquially referred to as the "Life or Death Committee" throughout the piece, is that for every one person they select for treatment, another forty-nine will soon die. The ethical standards by which they made their decisions constitute a fascinating conversation. But in the context of this discussion, what is also important is the way that their visions of the future made this difficult work possible. As Shana Alexander puts it in the article, "As medicine advances and invents assorted other mechanical organs, millions of people with 'fatal' diseases may be given a second chance at life.... But the Brave New World in which people may literally have hearts of gold or nerves of steel is not yet at hand. In the interim, agonizing practical decisions must be made" (104). The choice of which life in fifty to save now is made possible by an extrapolation that medicine will inevitably advance and "millions" of people with formerly "fatal" diseases will be saved. The scope of this conviction in medical progress—from one in fifty to millions—encapsulates the profound work accomplished by imaginative speculation.

One member of the committee, a labor leader, sums up this movement from imagination to accomplishment: "The wonderful thing to me about this work is that we are finally past the stage of experiment. We know we can prolong life. These doctors got an idea and they made it work. With the mass production facilities we have in this country, I believe we can eventually take care of everybody" (Alexander 123). The conviction that someday we will be able to "take care of everybody," is, in the end, the driving force of speculative medicine. In combining altruism with the long-standing desire to conquer death, organ exchange shows us that even the most fundamental boundaries can be crossed in the pursuit of medical progress. It shows, further, that this radical surgical intervention is not just tolerated or feared, but widely embraced and celebrated as a miracle. This simple formulation—"They got an idea and they made it work"—reminds us that technical achievements cannot happen without the animating force of ideology, without a driving idea. *Transplant Fictions* studies the "ideas" surrounding organ exchange and offers an intellectual history of how a practice that should have seemed ghoulish and transgressive became the triumph of twentieth-century medicine.

Notes

1. Vincanne Adams, Michelle Murphy, and Adele E. Clarke, "Anticipation: Technoscience, Life, Affect, Temporality," *Subjectivity* 28, no. 1 (September 2009): 248.
2. China Miéville, *The Scar* (New York: Del Rey, 2004).
3. Sharp, *Transplant Imaginary*, 147.
4. H. G. Wells, *The Island of Doctor Moreau* (New York: Penguin Classics, 2005).
5. Ibid., 50.
6. Mary Murray, "Xenotransplantation, Xenozoonosis and Contemporary Imaginings of Monstrosity," *Sites* 8, no. 1 (2011): 122.

7. Sharp, *Transplant Imaginary*, 67.
8. Ibid., 54.
9. Ibid.
10. Ibid., 112.
11. Sam Brownback, "Human-Animal Hybrid Prohibition Act of 2009," Pub. L. No. S. 1435, Title 19 United States Code (2009), https://www.congress.gov/bill/111th-congress/senate-bill/1435/text.
12. Mary-Jo DelVecchio Good, "The Biotechnical Embrace," *Culture, Medicine, and Psychiatry* 25, no. 4 (December 2001): 397.
13. Squier, "Transplant Medicine," 88.
14. Shana Alexander, "They Decide Who Lives, Who Dies," *Life* 53, no. 19 (November 9, 1962): 106.

Works Cited

Abani, Chris. *Graceland*. New York: Picador, 2004.

Adams, Vincanne, Michelle Murphy, and Adele E. Clarke. "Anticipation: Technoscience, Life, Affect, Temporality." *Subjectivity* 28, no. 1 (September 2009): 246–265.

Adéèkó, Adélékè. "Power Shift: America in the New Nigerian Imagination." *The Global South* 2, no. 2 (October 1, 2008): 10–30.

Agamben, Giorgio. *Homo Sacer*. Stanford, CA: Stanford University Press, 1998.

Alexander, Shana. "They Decide Who Lives, Who Dies." *Life* 53, no. 19 (November 9, 1962): 102–127.

Ankeny, Rachel A. "The Moral Status of Preferences for Directed Donation: Who Should Decide Who Gets Transplantable Organs?" *Cambridge Quarterly of Healthcare Ethics* 10, no. 4 (October 2001): 387–398.

Annas, George J. "From Canada with Love: Anencephalic Newborns as Organ Donors?" *The Hastings Center Report* 17, no. 6 (December 1, 1987): 36–38.

Appiah, Kwame Anthony. *Cosmopolitanism: Ethics in a World of Strangers*. New York: W. W. Norton, 2006.

Ariès, Philippe. *The Hour of Our Death: The Classic History of Western Attitudes Toward Death over the Last One Thousand Years*. Translated by Helen Weaver. 2 edition. New York: Vintage Books, 2008.

Bailey, James Blake. *The Diary of a Resurrectionist, 1811–1812: To Which Are Added an Account of the Resurrection Men in London and a Short History of the Passing of the Anatomy Act*. Urbana, IL: Project Gutenberg. Accessed June 23, 2015. http://www.gutenberg.org/ebooks/32614.

E. Russell, *Transplant Fictions*,
Palgrave Studies in Literature, Science and Medicine,
https://doi.org/10.1007/978-3-030-12135-8

Barkan, Leonard. "Cosmas and Damian: Of Medicine, Miracles, and the Economies of the Body." In *Organ Transplantation: Meanings and Realities*, edited by Stuart J. Youngner, Renée C. Fox, and Laurence J. O'Connell, 221–251. Madison, WI: University of Wisconsin Press, 1996.

Barnard, Christiaan. *The Donor*. London: Penguin Books, 1996.

———. "Human Cardiac Transplant: An Interim Report of a Successful Operation Performed at Groote Schuur Hospital, Cape Town." *South African Medical Journal* 41, no. 48 (December 1, 1967): 1271–1274.

Barnes, Elizabeth. *States of Sympathy: Seduction and Democracy in the American Novel*. New York: Columbia University Press, 1997.

Bates, Stephen. "Bodies Impolitic? Reading Cadavers." *International Journal of Communication* 4 (2010): 198–219.

Beecher, Henry K., Raymond Adams, and Clifford Barger. "A Definition of Irreversible Coma: Report of the Ad Hoc Committee of the Harvard Medical School to Examine the Definition of Brain Death." *JAMA* 205, no. 6 (August 5, 1968): 337–340.

Belling, Catherine. "The Living Dead: Fiction, Horror, and Bioethics." *Perspectives in Biology and Medicine* 53, no. 3 (Summer 2010): 439–451.

Benedict, Barbara M. *Framing Feeling: Sentiment and Style in English Prose Fiction, 1745–1800*. New York: AMS Press, 1994.

Berlant, Lauren. *The Female Complaint: The Unfinished Business of Sentiment in American Culture*. Durham: Duke University Press, 2008.

The Best of Me. Directed by Michael Hoffman. Relativity Media, 2014.

Biller-Andorno, Nikola. "Gender Imbalance in Living Organ Donation." *Medicine, Health Care and Philosophy* 5, no. 2 (May 2002): 199–203.

Boss, Pete. "Vile Bodies and Bad Medicine." *Screen* 27, no. 1 (January 1, 1986): 14–25.

Boucher, Joanne. "Ultrasound: A Window to the Womb?: Obstetric Ultrasound and the Abortion Rights Debate." *The Journal of Medical Humanities* 25, no. 1 (2004): 7–19.

Boudreau, Kristin. *Sympathy in American Literature: American Sentiments from Jefferson to the Jameses*. Gainesville, FL: University Press of Florida, 2002.

Bowers, Charles Gardner. "The Black Hand." *Amazing Stories* 5, no. 10 (January 1931): 909–911, 923.

The Brain That Wouldn't Die. Directed by Joseph Green. American International Pictures, 1962.

Brownback, Sam. "Human-Animal Hybrid Prohibition Act of 2009." Pub. L. No. S. 1435, Title 19 United States Code (2009). https://www.congress.gov/bill/111th-congress/senate-bill/1435/text.

Budiani-Saberi, D. A., and F. L. Delmonico. "Organ Trafficking and Transplant Tourism: A Commentary on the Global Realities." *American Journal of Transplantation* 8, no. 5 (May 1, 2008): 925–929.

Bunzel, B., B. Schmidl-Mohl, A. Grundböck, and G. Wollenek. "Does Changing the Heart Mean Changing Personality? A Retrospective Inquiry on 47 Heart Transplant Patients." *Quality of Life Research: An International Journal of Quality of Life Aspects of Treatment, Care and Rehabilitation* 1, no. 4 (August 1992): 251–256.

Butler, Judith. *Bodies That Matter: On the Discursive Limits of 'Sex'*. New York: Routledge, 1993.

Campion-Vincent, Véronique. "Organ Theft Narratives." *Western Folklore* 56, no. 1 (Winter 1997): 1–37.

Carney, Scott M. *The Red Market: On the Trail of the World's Organ Brokers, Bone Thieves, Blood Farmers, and Child Traffickers.* 1st edition. New York, NY: William Morrow, 2011.

Charon, Rita. *Narrative Medicine: Honoring the Stories of Illness.* Oxford: Oxford University Press, 2006.

Chavez, Leo R. "Imagining the Nation, Imagining Donor Recipients: Jesica Santillan and the Public Discourse of Belonging." In *A Death Retold: Jesica Santillan, the Bungled Transplant, and Paradoxes of Medical Citizenship*, edited by Keith Wailoo, Julie Livingston, and Peter Guarnaccia, 276–296. Chapel Hill: University of North Carolina Press, 2006.

Childress, James F. "Putting Patients First in Organ Allocation: An Ethical Analysis of the U.S. Debate." *Cambridge Quarterly of Healthcare Ethics: CQ: The International Journal of Healthcare Ethics Committees* 10, no. 4 (2001): 365–376.

Clover, Carol. "Her Body, Himself: Gender in the Slasher Film." *Representations*, no. 20 (Autumn 1987): 187–228.

Cohen, I. Glenn. "Transplant Tourism: The Ethics and Regulation of International Markets for Organs." *The Journal of Law, Medicine & Ethics* 41, no. 1 (April 1, 2013): 269–285.

Cohen, Lawrence. "The Other Kidney: Biopolitics Beyond Recognition." In *Commodifying Bodies*, edited by Nancy Scheper-Hughes and Loïc J. D. Wacquant, 9–29. London: Sage, 2002.

Conger, Syndey McMillen, ed. *Sensibility in Transformation: Creative Resistance to Sentiment from the Augustans to the Romantics.* London: Associated University Presses, 1990.

Cook, Richard I. "Hobson's Choices: Matching and Mismatching in Transplantation Work Processes." In *A Death Retold: Jesica Santillan, the Bungled Transplant, and Paradoxes of Medical Citizenship*, edited by Keith Wailoo, Julie Livingston, and Peter Guarnaccia, 46–69. Chapel Hill: University of North Carolina Press, 2006.

Cook, Robin. *Coma.* Boston: Signet, 2002.

Coma. Directed by Michael Crichton. MGM, 1978.

Culler, Jonathan. *Literary Theory: A Very Short Introduction.* Oxford: Oxford University Press, 1997.

Davis, Alex, and Lee M. Jenkins, eds. *The Cambridge Companion to Modernist Poetry.* Cambridge: Cambridge University Press, 2007.

Davis, Emily. "The Intimacies of Globalization: Bodies and Borders On-Screen." *Camera Obscura: Feminism, Culture, and Media Studies* 21, no. 2 (62) (January 2006): 32–73.

Dawson, Ashley. "The People You Don't See: Immigration and Gender in Monica Ali's *Brick Lane.*" *Ariel: A Review of International English Literature* 40, no. 1 (2009): 124–141.

DelVecchio Good, Mary-Jo. "The Biotechnical Embrace." *Culture, Medicine, and Psychiatry* 25, no. 4 (December 2001): 395–410.

Desmond, Jane. "Postmortem Exhibitions: Taxidermied Animals and Plastinated Corpses in the Theaters of the Dead." *Configurations* 16, no. 3 (Fall 2008): 347–378.

de Voragine, Jacobus. *The Golden Legend: Readings on the Saints.* Translated by William Granger Ryan. Princeton: Princeton University Press, 1993.

Dirty Pretty Things. Directed by Stephen Frears. Miramax, 2002.

Dobson, Joanne. "Reclaiming Sentimental Literature." *American Literature* 69, no. 2 (1997): 263–288.

Dobson, Roger. "More Women Than Men Become Living Organ Donors." *BMJ: British Medical Journal* 325, no. 7369 (October 19, 2002): 851.

The Donor. Directed by Damian Lee. Warner Home Video, 1995.

Douglas, Ann. *The Feminization of American Culture.* New York: Alfred A. Knopf, 1977.

Dwyer, James, and Elizabeth Vig. "Rethinking Transplantation Between Siblings." *Hastings Center Report* 25, no. 5 (September 10, 1995): 7–12.

Eatough, Matthew. "The Time That Remains: Organ Donation, Temporal Duration, and *Bildung* in Kazuo Ishiguro's *Never Let Me Go.*" *Literature and Medicine* 29, no. 1 (2011): 132–160.

Edwards, Erin E. "Extremities of the Body: The Anoptic Corporeality of *As I Lay Dying.*" *MFS: Modern Fiction Studies* 55, no. 4 (2009): 739–764.

Ellis, Markman. *The Politics of Sensibility: Race, Gender, and Commerce in the Sentimental Novel.* Cambridge: Cambridge University Press, 1996.

Emanuel, Linda. "What Is Wrong with 'Dead'?" In *Brain Death*, 47–56. Proceedings of the Second International Conference on Brain Death. Amsterdam: Elsevier, 1995.

The Eye. Directed by David Moreau and Xavier Palud. Lion's Gate, 2008.

Farrell, James. *Inventing the American Way of Death, 1830–1920.* Philadelphia: Temple University Press, 1980.

Faulkner, William. *As I Lay Dying.* Edited by Michael Gorra. Norton Critical Edition. New York: W. W. Norton, 2010.

Fiedler, Leslie. "Why Organ Transplant Programs Do Not Succeed." In *Organ Transplantation: Meanings and Realities*, edited by Stuart J. Youngner, Renée

C. Fox, and Laurence J. O'Connell, 56–65. Madison, WI: University of Wisconsin Press, 1996.
Foucault, Michel. *The Birth of the Clinic an Archaeology of Medical Perception.* World of Man: World of Man (London, England). New York: Pantheon Books, 1973.
Fox, Renée C., and Judith P. Swazey. *Spare Parts: Organ Replacement in American Society.* New York: Oxford University Press, 1992.
Frankenstein. Directed by James Whale. Universal Pictures, 1931.
Friedman, Alan Warren. *Fictional Death and the Modernist Enterprise.* Cambridge: Cambridge University Press, 1995.
Gawande, Atul. *Being Mortal: Medicine and What Matters in the End.* New York: Metropolitan Books, 2014.
Gaylin, Willard. "Harvesting the Dead." *Harper's* 249, no. 1492 (September 1974): 23–30.
Ghosh, Sanjib Kumar. "Human Cadaveric Dissection: A Historical Account from Ancient Greece to the Modern Era." *Anatomy & Cell Biology* 48, no. 3 (September 2015): 153–169.
Giacomini, Mita. "A Change of Heart and a Change of Mind? Technology and the Reinvention of Death in 1968." *Social Science & Medicine* 44, no. 10 (1997): 1465–1482.
Gibson, Sarah. "Border Politics and Hospitable Spaces in Stephen Frears's *Dirty Pretty Things.*" *Third Text* 20, no. 6 (November 2006): 693–701.
"The Gift of a Heart." *Life*, December 15, 1967.
Gill, Josie. "Written on the Face: Race and Expression in Kazuo Ishiguro's *Never Let Me Go.*" *MFS: Modern Fiction Studies* 60, no. 4 (2014): 844–862.
Gilman, Sander. *Picturing Health and Illness: Images of Identity and Difference.* Baltimore: Johns Hopkins University Press, 1995.
Gorer, Geoffrey. "The Pornography of Death." *Encounter* 5, no. 4 (October 1955): 49–52.
Grosz, Elizabeth. *Volatile Bodies: Towards a Corporeal Feminism.* Bloomington: Indiana University Press, 1994.
Gunning, Tom. "Phantom Images and Modern Manifestations: Spirit Photography, Magic Theater, Trick Films and Photography's Uncanny." In *Fugitive Images: From Photography to Videa*, edited by Patrice Petro, 42–68. Bloomington: Indiana University Press, 1995.
Gutkind, Lee. *Many Sleepless Nights: The World of Organ Transplantation.* Pittsburgh, PA: University of Pittsburgh Press, 1988.
Hadders, Hans. "Enacting Death in the Intensive Care Unit: Medical Technology and the Multiple Ontologies of Death." *Health: An Interdisciplinary Journal for the Social Study of Health, Illness, and Medicine* 13, no. 6 (2009): 571–587.
Halevy, A., and B. Brody. "Brain Death: Reconciling Definitions, Criteria, and Tests." *Annals of Internal Medicine* 119, no. 6 (1993): 519–525.

Hall, David. "Reflecting on Redfern: What Can We Learn from the Alder Hey Story?" *Archives of Disease in Childhood* 84, no. 6 (June 1, 2001): 455–456.

Hamilton, Charles V., Lynn Huntley, Neville Alexander, Antonio Sérgio Alfredo Guimarães, and Wilmot James, eds. *Beyond Racism: Race and Inequality in Brazil, South Africa, and the United States*. Boulder, CO: Lynne Rienner, 2001.

Hamilton, David. *A History of Organ Transplantation: Ancient Legends to Modern Practice*. Pittsburgh, PA: University of Pittsburgh Press, 2012.

Haraway, Donna Jeanne. "A Cyborg Manifesto: Science, Technology, and Socialist-Feminism in the Late Twentieth Century." In *Simians, Cyborgs, and Women: The Reinvention of Nature*. New York: Routledge, 1991.

Harvey, Janet. "The Technological Regulation of Death: With Reference to the Technological Regulation of Birth." *Sociology* 31, no. 4 (November 1997): 719–735.

Hellmann, Ellen, and Henry Lever, eds. *Race Relations in South Africa 1929–1979*. New York: St. Martin's Press, 1979.

Hendrick, Veronica. "Negotiating Nigeria: Connecting Chris Abani's *GraceLand* to Africa's Past." In *Emerging African Voices: A Study of Contemporary African Literature*, edited by Walter P. Collins, 75–99. Amherst, NY: Cambria Press, 2010.

Hermann, Hanna, Burghard F. Klapp, Gerhard Danzer, and Christina Papachristou. "Gender-Specific Differences Associated with Living Donor Liver Transplantation: A Review Study." *Liver Transplantation* 16 (2010): 375–386.

Hochberg, Benjamin. "Bringing Jim Thorpe Home: Inconsistencies in the Native American Graves and Repatriation Act." *Rutgers Race and the Law Review* 13 (2012).

Hoffenberg, Raymond. "Christiaan Barnard: His First Transplants and Their Impact on Concepts of Death." *BMJ: British Medical Journal* 323, no. 7327 (December 22, 2001): 1478–1480.

Homer, Sandra. *Heavensbrook Angels*. Accessed July 12, 2017. http://heavensbookangels.com/.

The Island. Directed by Michael Bay. DreamWorks, 2005.

Ishiguro, Kazuo. *Never Let Me Go*. New York: Vintage, 2006.

Jacobs, Joseph. *The Dying of Death*. Tucker Publishing Company, 1900.

———. "Love: The Risk Worth Taking." *Narrative Inquiry in Bioethics* 12, no. 1 (Spring 2012): 17–19.

Jennings, Bruce. "Biopower and the Liberationist Romance." *Hastings Center Report* 40, no. 4 (2010): 16–20.

Joralemon, Donald. "Organ Wars: The Battle for Body Parts." *Medical Anthropology Quarterly*, New Series, 9, no. 3 (September 1995): 335–356.

Kaba, Evridiki, David R. Thompson, Philip Burnard, Deborah Edwards, and Eleni Theodosopoulou. "Somebody Else's Heart Inside Me: A Descriptive

Study of Psychological Problems After a Heart Transplantation." *Issues in Mental Health Nursing* 26, no. 6 (July 2005): 611–625.
Kantorowicz, Ernst Hartwig. *The King's Two Bodies: A Study in Mediaeval Political Theology*. Princeton: Princeton University Press, 1957.
Kaufman, Sharon R. "Fairness and the Tyranny of Potential in Kidney Transplantation." *Current Anthropology* 54, no. S7 (October 1, 2013): S56–S66.
Kemp, Martin, and Marina Wallace. *Spectacular Bodies: The Art and Science of the Human Body from Leonardo to Now*. Berkeley: University of California Press, 2000.
Kristeva, Julia. *Powers of Horror: An Essay on Abjection*. Translated by Leon S. Roudiez. New York: Columbia University Press, 1982.
Kunow, Rüdiger. "Architect of the Cosmopolitan Dream: Salman Rushdie." *Amerikastudien/American Studies* 51, no 3 (2006): 369–385.
Kuppers, Petra. "Visions of Anatomy: Exhibitions and Dense Bodies." *Differences: A Journal of Feminist Cultural Studies* 15, no. 3 (Fall 2004): 123–156.
Law and Order. Season 1, episode 21, "Sonata for a Solo Organ." Directed by Fred Gerber. Aired April 2, 1991, on NBC.
Law & Order: SVU. Season 6, episode 22, "Parts." Directed by Matt Earl Beesley. Aired May 17, 2005, on NBC.
Lederer, Susan E. *Flesh and Blood: Organ Transplantation and Blood Transfusion in Twentieth Century America*. Oxford: Oxford University Press, 2008.
Lewensten, Amy K. "A Life for a Life: My Gift to My Dad." *Narrative Inquiry in Bioethics* 2, no. 1 (Spring 2012): 21–24.
LifePoint, Inc. "Donation After Cardiac Death." Accessed May 29, 2014. http://www.lifepoint-sc.org/facts_cardiac.htm.
Lock, Margaret. *Twice Dead: Organ Transplants and the Reinvention of Death*. Berkeley: University of California Press, 2001.
Lupton, Deborah. *Medicine as Culture: Illness, Disease, and the Body*. 3rd edition. London: Sage, 2012.
MacDonald, Helen. *Human Remains: Episodes in Human Dissection*. Melbourne, VIC: Melbourne University Press, 2005.
Malan, Marais. *Heart Transplant: The Story of Barnard and the 'Ultimate in Cardiac Sugery'*. Johannesburg: Voortrekkerpers, 1968.
Maloney, Raelynn, and Alan D. Wolfelt. *Caring for Donor Families: Before and After*. Ft. Collins, CO: Companion Press, 2001.
Matthews, Sean. "'I'm Sorry I Can't Say More': An Interview with Kazuo Ishiguro." In *Kashuo Ishiguro: Contemporary Critical Perspectives*, edited by Sean Matthews and Sebastian Groes, 114–125. London: Continuum, 2009.
McCormack, Donna. "Intimate Borders: The Ethics of Human Organ Transplantation in Contemporary Film." *Review of Education, Pedagogy, and Cultural Studies* 34, nos. 3–4 (2012): 170–183.

Menikoff, Jerry. *Law and Bioethics: An Introduction*. Washington, DC: Georgetown University Press, 2001.

Miéville, China. *The Scar*. New York: Del Rey, 2004.

Mitford, Jessica. *The American Way of Death Revisited*. Revised edition. New York: Alfred A. Knopf, 1998.

Moloney, Gail, and Iain Walker. "Messiahs, Pariahs, and Doctors: The Development of Social Representations of Organ Transplants." *Journal for the Theory of Social Behaviour* 30, no. 2 (2000): 203–227.

Moore, Wendy. *The Knife Man: The Extraordinary Life and Times of John Hunter, Father of Modern Surgery*. New York: Broadway Books, 2005.

Morgan, Susan E., Tyler Harrison, Lisa Chewning, LaShara Davis, and Mark DiCorcia. "Entertainment (Mis)Education: The Framing of Organ Donation in Entertainment Television." *Health Communication* 22, no. 2 (2007): 143–151.

Morgan, Susan E., Tyler R. Harrison, Lisa Volk Chewning, and Jacklyn B. Habib. "America's Angel or Thieving Immigrant?: Media Coverage, the Santillan Story, and Publicized Ambivalence Toward Donation and Transplantation." In *A Death Retold: Jesica Santillan, the Bungled Transplant, and Paradoxes of Medical Citizenship*, edited by Keith Wailoo, Julie Livingston, and Peter Guarnaccia, 19–45. Chapel Hill: University of North Carolina Press, 2006.

Morgan, Susan E., Tyler R. Harrison, Shawn D. Long, Walid A. Afifi, Michael S. Stephenson, and Tom Reichert. "Family Discussions About Organ Donation: How the Media Influences Opinions About Donation Decisions." *Clinical Transplantation* 19, no. 5 (October 1, 2005): 674–682.

Morgan, Susan E., Jenny K. Miller, and Lily A. Arasaratnam. "Similarities and Differences Between African Americans' and European Americans' Attitudes, Knowledge, and Willingness to Communicate About Organ Donation." *Journal of Applied Social Psychology* 33, no. 4 (April 1, 2003): 693–715.

Morison, Robert S. "Death: Process or Event?" *Science* 173, no. 3998 (1971): 694–698.

Morrow, Lance. "When One Body Can Save Another." *Time*, June 17, 1991.

Muggers. Directed by Dean Murphy. Instinct Entertainment, 2000.

Murray, Mary. "Xenotransplantation, Xenozoonosis and Contemporary Imaginings of Monstrosity." *Sites* 8, no. 1 (2011): 108–128.

Nathan, Howard M., Suzanne L. Conrad, Philip J. Held, Keith P. McCullough, Richard E. Pietroski, Laura Siminoff, and Akinlolu O. Ojo. "Organ Donation in the United States." *American Journal of Transplantation* 3 (2003): 29–40.

Niven, Larry. "The Jigsaw Man." In *Tales of Known Space: The Universe of Larry Niven*, 67–79. New York: Ballantine Books, 1975.

"The No-Nonsense Heart Man of Houston." *Life*, August 2, 1968.

Nwakanma, Obi. "Metonymic Eruptions: Igbo Novelists, the Narrative of the Nation, and New Developments in the Contemporary Nigerian Novel." *Research in African Literatures* 39, no. 2 (Summer 2008): 1–14.

Oliver, Mary Beth, and Meghan Sanders. "The Appeal of Horror and Suspense." In *The Horror Film*, 242–259. New Brunswick: Rutgers University Press, 2004.

Olney, Ian. "The Problem Body Politic, or 'These Hands Have a Mind All Their Own!': Figuring Disability in the Horror Film Adaptations of Renard's Les Mains d'Orlac." *Literature/Film Quarterly* 34, no. 4 (October 1, 2006): 294–302.

Parker, Ian. "The Gift." *New Yorker* 80, no. 21 (August 2, 2004): 54–63.

Pearsall, Paul, Gary E. R. Schwartz, and Linda G. S. Russek. "Changes in Heart Transplant Recipients That Parallel the Personalities of Their Donors." *Journal of Near-Death Studies* 20, no. 3 (2002): 191–206.

Petchesky, Rosalind Pollack. "Fetal Images: The Power of Visual Culture in the Politics of Reproduction." *Feminist Studies* 13, no. 2 (1987): 263–292.

Picoult, Jodi. *Change of Heart: A Novel.* 1st Atria Books Hardcover edition. New York, NY: Atria Books, 2008.

———. *My Sister's Keeper.* New York: Atria Books, 2004.

Pinedo, Isabel Cristina. "Postmodern Elements of the Contemporary Horror Film." In *The Horror Film*, 85–117. New Brunswick: Rutgers University Press, 2004.

Pinson, C. Wright, Irene D. Feurer, Jerita L. Payne, Paul E. Wise, Shannon Shockley, and Theodore Speroff. "Health-Related Quality of Life After Different Types of Solid Organ Transplantation." *Annals of Surgery* 232, no. 4 (October 2000): 597–607.

Poe, Edgar Allan. "A Premature Burial." In *The Complete Tales and Poems of Edgar Allan Poe*, 258–268. New York: Vintage Books, 1975.

Pollock, Sheldon I., Homi K. Bhabha, Carol Appadurai Breckenridge, and Dipesh Chakrabarty. "Cosmopolitanisms." *Public Culture* 12, no. 3 (September 1, 2000): 577–589.

Porter, Roy. *Bodies Politic: Disease, Death and Doctors in Britain, 1650–1900.* Ithaca: Cornell University Press, 2001.

Post, Laurie E. "Liver Donor Nightmare." *Narrative Inquiry in Bioethics* 2, no. 1 (2012): 31–34.

President's Commission for the Study of Ethical Problems in Medicine and Biomedical and Behavioral Research. *Defining Death: Medical, Legal, and Ethical Issues in the Determination of Death.* Washington, DC, 1981.

President's Council on Bioethics. "Reproduction and Responsibility: The Regulation of New Biotechnologies." Washington, DC, 2004. www.bioethics.gov.

Prince, Stephen. "Introduction." In *The Horror Film*, 1–14. New Brunswick: Rutgers University Press, 2004.

The Princess Bride. Directed by Rob Reiner. Twentieth Century Fox, 1987.

Prior, Lindsay. "Reflections on the 'Mortal' Body in Late Modernity." In *Health, Medicine, and Society: Key Theories, Future Agendas*, edited by Simon Williams, Michael Calnan, and Jonathan Gabe, 186–202. London: Routledge, 2000.

Quigley, Christine. *The Corpse: A History*. Jefferson, NC: McFarland, 1996.

Reagan, Ronald. "Radio Address to the Nation on Organ Donorship and on Reform 88." July 30, 1983. http://www.presidency.ucsb.edu/ws/?pid=41663.

———. "Radio Address to the Nation on the International Monetary Fund and on Organ Donorship." July 23, 1983. http://www.presidency.ucsb.edu/ws/?pid=41629.

Redfern, Michael. *The Royal Liverpool Children's Report (The Redfern Report)*. The House of Commons, 2001.

Reifler, Douglas R. "'I Actually Don't Mind the Bone Saw': Narratives of Gross Anatomy." *Literature and Medicine* 15, no. 2 (1996): 183–199.

Renard, Maurice. *Doctor Lerne, Sub-God*. Translated by Brian Stableford. Encino, CA: Black Coat Press, 2010.

———. *Hands of Orlac*. Translated by I. White. 1st edition. London: Souvenir Press Ltd, 1981.

Repo Men. Directed by Miguel Sapochnik. Universal Pictures, 2010.

Return to Me. Directed by Bonnie Hunt. MGM, 2000.

Richardson, Ruth. "Human Dissection and Organ Donation: A Historical and Social Background." *Mortality* 11, no. 2 (May 2006): 151–165.

Roach, Mary. *Stiff: The Curious Lives of Human Cadavers*. New York: W. W. Norton, 2003.

Robbins, Bruce. "Cruelty Is Bad: Banality and Proximity in *Never Let Me Go*." *NOVEL: A Forum on Fiction* 40, no. 3 (2007): 289–302.

Rubin, Susan. *When Doctors Say No: The Battleground of Medical Futility*. Bloomington: Indiana University Press, 1998.

Ruby, Jay. *Secure the Shadow: Death and Photography in America*. Cambridge, MA: MIT Press, 1995.

Rufus, Anneli. *Magnificent Corpses: Searching Through Europe for St. Peter's Head, St. Chiara's Heart, St. Stephen's Hand, and Other Saints' Relics*. Cambridge, MA: Da Capo Press, 1999.

Samuels, Shirley. "The Identity of Slavery." In *The Culture of Sentiment: Race, Gender, and Sentimentality in Nineteenth-Century America*, edited by Shirley Samuels, 157–171. New York: Oxford University Press, 1992.

Sanner, Margareta. "Exchanging Spare Parts or Becoming a New Person?: People's Attitudes Toward Receiving and Donating Organs." *Social Science & Medicine* 52, no. 10 (May 2001): 1491–1499.

Sappol, Michael. *A Traffic of Dead Bodies: Anatomy and Embodied Social Identity in Nineteenth-Century America*. Princeton, NJ: Princeton University Press, 2002.

Scheper-Hughes, Nancy. "Commodity Fetishism in Organs Trafficking." *Body and Society* 7, nos. 2–3 (September 2001): 31–62.

———. "Consuming Differences: Post-Human Ethics, Global (In)Justice and the Transplant Trade in Organs." In *A Death Retold: Jesica Santillan, the Bungled Transplant, and Paradoxes of Medical Citizenship*, edited by Keith Wailoo, Julie Livingston, and Peter Guarnaccia, 205–234. Chapel Hill: University of North Carolina Press, 2006.

Schneider, Steven Jay. "Toward an Aesthetics of Cinematic Horror." In *The Horror Film*, 131–149. New Brunswick: Rutgers University Press, 2004.

Schneiderman, Lawrence J., and Nancy S. Jecker. *Wrong Medicine: Doctors, Patients, and Futile Treatment*. Baltimore, MD: Johns Hopkins University Press, 2000.

Schwartz, Margaret. *Dead Matter: The Meaning of Iconic Corpses*. Minneapolis: University of Minnesota Press, 2015.

Seaman, Myra J. "Becoming More (Than) Human: Affective Posthumanisms, Past and Future." *Journal of Narrative Theory* 37, no. 2 (2007): 246–275.

Seymour, Jane Elizabeth. "Negotiating Natural Death in Intensive Care." *Social Science & Medicine* 51, no. 8 (2000): 1241–1252.

Shaddox, Karl. "Generic Considerations in Ishiguro's *Never Let Me Go*." *Human Rights Quarterly* 35, no. 2 (2013): 448–469.

Sharp, Lesley A. *Strange Harvest: Organ Transplants, Denatured Bodies, and the Transformed Self*. Berkeley: University of California Press, 2006.

———. *Transplant Imaginary: Mechanical Hearts, Animal Parts, and Moral Thinking in Highly Experimental Science*. Berkeley: University of California Press, 2014.

Shelley, Mary. *Frankenstein*. Reissue edition. New York: Penguin Classics, 2003.

Shildrick, Margrit. "Corporeal Cuts: Surgery and the Psycho-Social." *Body and Society* 14, no. 1 (March 2008): 31–46.

———. "The Critical Turn in Bioethics: The Case of Heart Transplantation." *International Journal of Feminist Approaches to Bioethics* 1, no. 1 (2008): 28–47.

Shimazono, Yosuke. "The State of the International Organ Trade: A Provisional Picture Based on Integration of Available Information." *Bulletin of the World Health Organization* 85, no. 12 (December 2007): 955–962.

Silverberg, Robert. "Caught in the Organ Draft." In *Caught in the Organ Draft: Biology in Science Fiction*, edited by Isaac Asimov, Martin H. Greenberg, and Charles G. Waugh, 141–156. New York: Farrar, Straus, Giroux, 1983.

Siminoff, Laura, Nahida Gordon, Joan Hewlett, and Robert Arnold. "Factors Influencing Families' Consent for Donation of Solid Organs for Transplantation." *JAMA* 286, no. 1 (July 4, 2001): 71–77.

Siminoff, Laura, and Mary Beth Mercer. "Public Policy, Public Opinion, and Consent for Organ Donation." *Cambridge Quarterly of Healthcare Ethics* 10, no. 4 (October 2001): 377–386.

Simon, John K. "The Scene and Imagery of Metamorphosis in *As I Lay Dying*." *Criticism* 7 (1965): 1–22.

Slankard, Tanya. "'No Such Thing as Was': The Fetishized Corpse, Modernism, and as I Lay Dying." *The Faulkner Journal* 24, no. 2 (Spring 2009): 7–28.

Smith, Adam. *The Theory of Moral Sentiments*. Edited by D. D. Raphael and A. L. Macfie. Oxford: Clarendon Press, 1976.

Southwest Transplant Alliance. "Saving More Lives: Organ Donation After Cardiac Death." Accessed May 29, 2014. http://www.organ.org/v2/assets/documents/brochures/Brochure_DonationAfterCardiacDeath.pdf.

Spacks, Patricia Meyer. *Novel Beginnings: Experiments in Eighteenth-Century English Fiction*. New Haven: Yale University Press, 2006.

Squier, Susan. "Transplant Medicine and Transformative Narrative, or Is Science Fiction 'Rubbish'?" In *Biotechnological and Medical Themes in Science Fiction*, edited by Domna Pastourmatzi, 87–110. Thessaloniki: University Studio Press, 2002.

Stafford, Barbara Maria. *Body Criticism: Imaging the Unseen in Enlightenment Art and Medicine*. Cambridge, MA: MIT Press, 1993.

Steinbrook, Robert. "Public Solicitation of Organ Donors." *New England Journal of Medicine* 353, no. 5 (August 4, 2005): 441–444.

Stephens, Elizabeth. *Anatomy as Spectacle: Public Exhibitions of the Body from 1700 to the Present*. Representations: Health, Disability, Culture. Liverpool: Liverpool University Press, 2011.

Stern, Julia A. *The Plight of Feeling: Sympathy and Dissent in the Early American Novel*. Chicago: University of Chicago Press, 1997.

Stern, Megan. "Dystopian Anxieties Versus Utopian Ideals: Medicine from Frankenstein to the Visible Human Project and Body Worlds." *Science as Culture* 15, no. 2 (2006): 1–24.

Stevens, Wallace. "The Emperor of Ice-Cream." In *The Collected Poems of Wallace Stevens*, Reissue edition. New York: Vintage, 1990.

Stevenson, Robert Louis. "The Body Snatcher." In *The Body Snatcher and Other Stories*, 1–19. New York: Signet Classics, 1988.

Strong, Kimberly, Ian Kerridge, and Miles Little. "Savior Siblings, Parenting and the Moral Valorization of Children." *Bioethics* 28, no. 4 (May 1, 2014): 187–193.

"The Telltale Heart." *Ebony*, March 1968.

Tilney, Nicholas L. *Transplant: From Myth to Reality*. New Haven: Yale University Press, 2003.

Timmermans, Stefan. "Resuscitation Technology in the Emergency Department: Towards a Dignified Death." *Sociology of Health & Illness* 20, no. 2 (1998): 144–167.

Tompkins, Jane. *Sensational Designs: The Cultural Work of American Fiction, 1790–1860*. New York: Oxford University Press, 1985.

Train, Arthur. "Mortmain." In *Mortmain*, 1–63. New York: D. Appleton and Company, 1907.

Tronto, Joan. *Moral Boundaries: A Political Argument for an Ethic of Care*. New York: Routledge, 1993.

Troyer, John. "Embalmed Vision." *Mortality* 12, no. 1 (2007): 22–47.

UNOS. Accessed July 11, 2017. https://www.unos.org/.

US Congress. National Organ Transplant Act: Hearing Before the Subcommittee on Heath of the Committee of Ways and Means, House of Representatives, Ninety-Eighth Congress, First Session, on H.R. 4080, July 29, October 17 and 30, 1983 (1984).

US Department of Health and Human Services, Health Resources and Services Administration. "2012 National Survey of Organ Donation Attitudes and Behaviors." US Department of Health and Human Services, 2013. https://www.organdonor.gov.

van Dijck, Jose. "Bodyworlds: The Art of Plastinated Cadavers." *Configurations* 9, no. 1 (Winter 2001): 99–126.

Viera, Mark. *Hollywood Horror from Gothic to Cosmic*. New York: Harry N. Abrams, Inc., 2003.

von Hagens, Gunter. *Bodyworlds*. Heidelberg: Institute for Plastination, 2001.

———. "Bodyworlds." *Bodyworlds*. Accessed June 29, 2015. http://www.bodyworlds.com/en.html.

———. "On Gruesome Corpses, Gestalt Plastinates and Mandatory Interment." *Brave New Body Worlds: The Question of the Exhibition*. Accessed May 11, 2016. http://www.koerperwelten.com/Downloads/OnGruesomeCorpses.pdf.

Wagner, Corinna. *Pathological Bodies: Medicine and Political Culture*. Berkeley: University of California Press, 2013.

Wailoo, Keith, and Julie Livingston. "The Politics of Second Changes: Waste, Futility, and the Debate over Jesica's Second Transplant." In *A Death Retold: Jesica Santillan, the Bungled Transplant, and Paradoxes of Medical Citizenship*, edited by Keith Wailoo, Julie Livingston, and Peter Guarnaccia, 119–141. Chapel Hill: University of North Carolina Press, 2006.

Wailoo, Keith, Julie Livingston, and Peter Guarnaccia, eds. *A Death Retold: Jesica Santillan, the Bungled Transplant, and Paradoxes of Medical Citizenship*. Chapel Hill: University of North Carolina Press, 2006.

Waldby, Catherine. "Biomedicine, Tissue Transfer, and Intercorporeality." *Feminist Theory* 3 (December 2002): 239–254.

———. *The Visible Human Project: Informatic Bodies and Posthuman Medicine*. London: Routledge, 2003.

Walter, Tony. "Body Worlds: Clinical Detachment and Anatomical Awe." *Sociology of Health & Illness* 26, no. 4 (May 2004): 464–488.

Watt, Ian. *The Rise of the Novel: Studies in Defoe, Richardson and Fielding*. Berkeley: University of California Press, 1957.

Weir, Kirsten. "Getting a Head." *Current Science* 90, no. 7 (December 3, 2004): 4–5.

Wells, H. G. *The Island of Doctor Moreau*. New York: Penguin Classics, 2005.

Werbel, Amy. *Thomas Eakins: Art, Medicine, and Sexuality in Nineteenth-Century Philadelphia*. New Haven: Yale University Press, 2007.

"What and When Is Death?" *JAMA* 204 (1968): 219–220.

Whitehead, Anne. "Writing with Care: Kazuo Ishiguro's *Never Let Me Go*." *Contemporary Literature* 52, no. 1 (2011): 54–83.

Wieczner, Jen. "This Groundbreaking 'Frankenstein' Surgery Will Literally Make Your Head Spin." *Time*, June 5, 2015.

The X-Files. Season 3, episode 19, "Hell Money." Directed by Tucker Gates. Aired March 29, 1996, on Fox.

Youngner, Stephen, C. Landefeld, C. J. Coulton, B. W. Juknialis, and M. Leary. "'Brain Death' and Organ Retrieval: A Cross-Sectional Survey of Knowledge and Concepts Among Health Professionals." *JAMA* 261, no. 15 (April 21, 1989): 2205–2210.

Youngner, Stuart J. "Some Must Die." In *Organ Transplantation: Meanings and Realities*, edited by Stuart J. Youngner, Renée C. Fox, and Laurence J. O'Connell, 32–55. Madison, WI: University of Wisconsin Press, 1996.

Youngner, Stuart J., and Robert Arnold. "Philosophical Debates About the Definition of Death: Who Cares?" *Journal of Medicine and Philosophy* 26, no. 5 (2001): 527–537.

Youngner, Stuart J., Robert Arnold, and Renée C. Fox. *The Definition of Death: Contemporary Controversies*. Baltimore: Johns Hopkins University Press, 1999.

Yurchak, Alexei. "Bodies of Lenin: The Hidden Science of Communist Sovereignty." *Representations*, no. 129 (Winter 2015): 116–167.

Zucker, Marjorie B., Howard B. Zucker, and Alexander Morgan Capron. *Medical Futility: And the Evaluation of Life-Sustaining Interventions*. Cambridge: Cambridge University Press, 1997.

Index

E. Russell, *Transplant Fictions*,
Palgrave Studies in Literature, Science and Medicine,
https://doi.org/10.1007/978-3-030-12135-8

S

Kolibri 360 GmbH
Ferdinand-Jühlke-Straße 7
99095 Erfurt, Deutschland
produktsicherheit@kolibri360.de